Investigative Techniques and Ocular Examination

Dedications

To my wife Bhavna and my sons Jai and Kiran. I hope that one day the boys will understand why daddy was so often unable to play.

Sandip Doshi

Thanks to Heidi, Tallulah, Kitty, Spike and Black Sabbath for all their inspiration.

William Harvey

For Butterworth–Heinemann:
Publishing Director: Caroline Makepeace
Development Editor: Kim Benson
Production Manager: Yolanta Motylinska
Copy Editing/Project Manager: John Ormiston
Design and Layout: Judith Campbell

Investigative Techniques and Ocular Examination

Sandip Doshi PhD, MCOptom
Optometrist in private practice, Hove, East Sussex, UK
Examiner, College of Optometrists, London, UK
Formerly Clinical Editor, *Optician*

William Harvey MCOptom
Visiting Clinician and Boots Opticians' Tutor Practitioner,
Fight For Sight Optometry Clinic, City University
London, UK
Clinical Editor, *Optician*
Reed Business Information
Sutton, UK
Examiner, College of Optometrists, London, UK

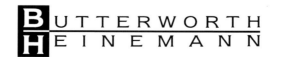 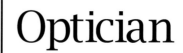

EDINBURGH LONDON NEW YORK OXFORD PHILADELPHIA ST LOUIS SYDNEY TORONTO

Butterworth–Heinemann
An imprint of Elsevier Science Limited

First published 2003
ISBN 0 7506 5404 X

British Library Cataloguing in Publication Data
A catalogue record for this book is available from the British Library

Library of Congress Cataloging in Publication Data
A catalogue record for this book is available from the Library of Congress

Note
Medical knowledge is constantly changing. As new information becomes available, changes in treatment, procedures, equipment and the use of drugs become necessary. The author/contributors and the publishers have taken great care to ensure that the information given in this text is accurate and up to date. However, readers are strongly advised to confirm that the information, especially with regard to drug usage, complies with the latest legislation and standards of practice.

Cover illustration, fundus view (right): copyright and courtesy of Andrew Field; also published in *Optometry Today*.

The
Publisher's
policy is to use
**paper manufactured
from sustainable forests**

Printed in Spain by Grafos SA., Arte sobel papel, Spain

Contents

Foreword

This is a timely publication that focuses on the rapidly developing areas of clinical investigation and ocular examination. I particularly welcome this book during the current period of rapid evolution of the scope of optometry as a profession – the contents are directly relevant to the much greater emphasis now placed on the key role optometrists play in the detection, diagnosis and management of ocular disease.

The book comprises seventeen chapters arranged in three sections. Section 1 deals with the assessment of vision and colour vision. In keeping with the remainder of the book, modern technology is placed firmly in the foreground, notably in the chapter on the use and development of computer-based test charts, which have gained recent and deserved popularity. A striking feature of the book is the superb figures, and this exceptional quality is very much in evidence in the schematic diagrams found in this section.

Section 2 is devoted to the assessment of the eye, and begins with two comprehensive chapters, again beautifully illustrated, on the principles and clinical use of the slit-lamp biomicroscope, which lead to the examination of the anterior chamber and assessment of its depth. In Chapter 7 the measurement of intraocular pressure is thoroughly covered, from the early Schiotz instrument through to the most sophisticated of modern tonometers. It is a natural progression, and a fascinating topic for future optometric practice, to then consider the measurement of ocular blood flow. A major chapter is devoted to the assessment of the fundus, concentrating on indirect methods. Laser imaging techniques to assess the ocular fundus is the subject of the final chapter in this section, and features recent advances such as the Scanning Laser Ophthalmoscope.

As a long-term visual fields enthusiast I am delighted to see the high profile given to this topic in Section 3. This excellent section opens with a helpful glossary of terms used in perimetry. Frequency doubling and short-wave perimetry are relatively recent additions to the range of techniques available to optometrists, and are given a chapter to themselves. Other chapters are devoted to visual field defects caused by neurological disease and glaucoma, the analysis of visual field data, and common errors in visual field analysis. The section closes with two contrasting chapters: the first on the often neglected but important topics of catch trial responses, fixation errors and test intensities, and the second on the more qualitative assessment of visual fields using Amsler charts.

The text is thoroughly referenced throughout. Each section closes with a series of multiple-choice questions, which will prove popular with all those who wish to test their knowledge, especially students at both undergraduate and pre-registration level. The answers to all the MCQs, plus the rationale for the choice of each correct answer, are given at the end of the book.

The editors are to be congratulated on assembling such a distinguished panel of authors to contribute to this text. Each chapter is written by an acknowledged expert in the field, all of whom are at the cutting edge of knowledge in this rapidly expanding area. They have combined to produce an up-to-date and readable text that will be an indispensable part of any student's or practice's library. This book provides ideal support to clinical skills training on undergraduate optometry courses, both in the UK and beyond. Pre-registration students and those registered optometrists from overseas who seek registration in the UK will regard this book as invaluable. Furthermore, such is the pace of expansion of clinical knowledge in our specialism that registered practitioners will undoubtedly benefit from the wealth of clinical experience and expertise contained herein.

Dave Edgar
Head of Department
Department of Optometry and Visual Science
Institute of Health Sciences
City University
London

Preface

The role of the optometrist is an evolving one. Developments in technology and education have complemented the ever-increasing eyecare requirements of the public. For this reason, a series of articles was commissioned for the *Optician* between 1998 and 2002 in an attempt to describe and explain the many techniques used by the practitioner to assess the ocular health and optical state of a patient's eyes. It is these articles that form the basis of this book.

To make this book as useful as possible we have combined descriptions of the latest techniques with established methods and theory. By doing so, it is our aim to provide a useful reference to all in optometric practice.

The book is divided into three sections. The first section deals with the various methods of establishing what a patient can see. It contains an appraisal of the Snellen chart, the mainstay of optometry over many decades, and descriptions of colour vision assessment. Alongside this, newer ideas of vision assessment are described.

The second section is concerned with the many ways to evaluate and visualise ocular health. We include established techniques, such as the use of the slit-lamp biomicroscope, and where these techniques have been adapted and developed we reflect this. Many techniques, such as binocular indirect ophthalmoscopy and gonioscopy, that are now standard procedures in optometry were once mainly the responsibility of the ophthalmologist, so these are described in detail. We have also included newer techniques used by our research colleagues that are of interest and may have potentially significant clinical application.

The final section deals with the evaluation of visual fields. Using specified stimuli to evaluate the health of the visual system has been essential to the successful screening of eye health, and advances in technology have led to great improvements in the methods used. We reflect these developments by including chapters on both the established methods of field evaluation, such as the Amsler grids, and newer techniques, such as frequency doubling.

Throughout the book, we have encouraged authors to present practical information. It is hoped that this makes the book useful for optometrists who wish to develop their practical skills. As well as the qualified practitioner, this book will appeal to those who are training and developing their skills, such as the undergraduate and pre-registration optometrist.

Each author has considerable experience in his or her chosen topic; we are grateful for their individual contributions and hope that collectively their work will prove useful and enjoyable to the reader.

Sandip Doshi
William Harvey

Contributors

Jennifer Birch
BSc MPhil FCOptom FAAO

Kamlesh Chauhan
BSc PhD MCOptom

Robert Cubbidge
BSc PhD MCOptom

Frank Eperjesi
BSc PhD MCOptom FAAO

Andrew Franklin
BSc DipCLP DipOrth FCOptom

William Harvey
BSc MCOptom

David Henson
BSc MSc PhD FCOptom

Sarah Hosking
BSc PhD DBO MCOptom FAAO

Anita Lightstone
BSc FCOptom FAAO

Andrew Morgan
BSc FCOptom

Geoff Roberson
BSc FCOptom

David Ruston
BSc DipCLP FCOptom FAAO

Chris Steele
BSc DipCLP DipOC FCOptom

David Thomson
BSc PhD MCOptom

Section 1
ASSESSMENT OF VISION AND COLOUR VISION

1
The assessment of vision

David Thomson

The Snellen chart (*Figure 1.1*) is currently the most widely used test of visual capability. The chart is familiar, quick and easy to use, and for most patients the results seem to correlate well with the subjective description of their vision – but not in all cases. The following extract from a letter received from an elderly relative describes succinctly an exception to the rule:

My vision has definitely got hazier over the past year. The funny thing is that under some conditions, I can still see quite well, and yet at other times I feel that I am practically blind. I very seldom go out nowadays because I feel that I cannot see well enough to cross the road safely, especially when it is sunny. Yet at home I seem to see the television quite well and I can still read even quite small print. The frustrating thing is that every time I go to the hospital I seem to be able to read quite small letters on the chart and they tell me that my cataracts are not yet ready to be operated on.'

Such accounts, which are not uncommon in clinical practice, suggest that Snellen acuity does not always provide an adequate description of visual capability in the 'real world'.

Background

It is likely that letters of different sizes have been used to grade vision for more than 200 years. However, Snellen is generally credited with producing the first standardised test based on letters of decreas-

ing size in 1862.[1] This chart has survived the test of time and the vast majority of clinicians still use it, based on his original scheme.

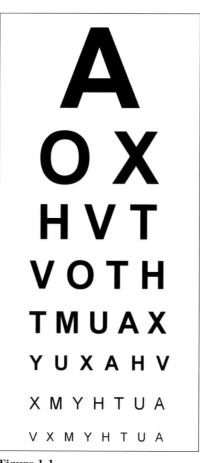

Figure 1.1
The standard Snellen chart

Although there are several ways to specify the size of letters on the chart, the most widely used system is the Snellen notation. Snellen assumed that an 'average' eye could just read a letter if the thickness of the limbs (and the spaces between them) subtended one minute of arc at the eye. Consider the letter E – such a letter would subtend five minutes of arc vertically and between four and six minutes of arc horizontally, depending on the letter and the style.

In simple terms, Snellen notation can be described as 'The testing distance over the distance at which the letter would subtend five minutes of arc (vertically).' Thus, at 6 metres a 6/6 letter subtends five minutes of arc vertically, a 6/12 letter subtends 10 minutes, and a 6/60 letter 50 minutes. The Snellen fraction may also be expressed as a decimal, for example 6/6 = 1, 6/12 = 0.5.

An alternative method is to record the minimum angle of resolution (MAR). The MAR relates to the resolution required to resolve the elements of a letter. Thus 6/6 equates to a MAR of one minute of arc, 6/12 equates to two minutes of arc, and so on. LogMAR is simply the $\log_{10}$ of the MAR (see *Table 1.1*).

Table 1.1 The relationship between different acuity scales			
Snellen	*Decimal*	*MAR*	*logMAR*
6/60	0.10	10	1.000
6/24	0.25	4	0.602
6/12	0.50	2	0.301
6/6	1.00	1	0.000
6/4	1.50	0.667	−0.176

Design flaws of the Snellen chart

While letters provide a convenient series of test stimuli, some letters are easier to recognise than others, and some combinations of letters are easily confused. Furthermore, the relative legibility of letters depends to some extent on the magnitude and the axis of any uncorrected astigmatism. For these reasons, most charts use a limited subset of the alphabet. However, many charts fail to adhere to the recommendations and standards that relate to the selection of letters.

Most Snellen charts have one 6/60 letter and an increasing number of letters on their descending lines. Although this means that the chart can be accommodated in a small rectangular frame, there are a number of problems with this aspect of the design:

- First, patients with poor acuity are required to read fewer letters than those with good acuity.
- Second, the letters on the lower lines are more crowded than those towards the top of the chart. It is well known that crowding increases the difficulty of the task, particularly for children and some amblyopes.
- Additionally, the spacing between each letter and each row of letters bears no systematic relationship to the width or height of the letters. Thus, the task required of the patient changes as they read down the chart. For this reason, visual acuity measured at a distance of less than 6 metres cannot be equated easily to a 6m equivalent, as the patient will inevitably read further down the chart and will have therefore carried out a different task.
- The small number of larger letters also limits the chart's usefulness when assessing vision and/or acuity of low-vision patients.

Most charts contain a 6/60 line and a 6/6 line with an assortment of other lines. The letter sizes follow an approximate geometrical progression, with letter size doubling every other line. However, the progression is irregular, with extra lines at the bottom of the chart and lines omitted at the top. This characteristic of the Snellen chart precludes the use of parametric statistics for the analysis of results, which greatly reduces the value of the test for research purposes.

The Snellen chart is scored by noting the lowest line of letters that can be read. However, in practice, patients seldom read all of one line and no letters on the line below, and the endpoint may even spread over three lines, in which case the clinician is left to try and convey the result in the format: $6/6^{-3}$. As there are no agreed standards for the exact notation in these situations, there is ample scope for confusion.

Design improvements to the Snellen chart

There have been many attempts to improve the design of the Snellen chart. However, one chart design, originally proposed by Bailey and Lovie, has emerged as the test of choice in vision research and is beginning to be adopted in clinical practice.[2]

The Bailey–Lovie chart overcomes many of the shortcomings of the Snellen chart (*Figure 1.2*). In this there are five letters on each line, and the spacing between each letter and each row is related to the width and height of the letters, respectively. Thus, each row is simply a scaled-down version of the row above. This means that the task remains the same as the patient reads down the chart and therefore the results obtained at different viewing distances can be equated easily.

The progression of letter sizes is uniform, increasing in a constant ratio of 1.26 (0.1 log unit steps) from the bottom to the top of the chart. The result is usually recorded in terms of a logMAR score. With this notation, 6/6 is equivalent to a logMAR of zero ($\log_{10} 1 = 0$), while smaller letters have a negative logMAR score (as the log10 of any number less than one is negative) and larger letters a positive score. As letter size changes in units of 0.1 logMAR units per row, each letter can be assigned a score of 0.02 (there being five letters on each line). For example, if all five letters on the 6/6 line are read, the logMAR score is zero. If one letter is missed on the zero line (all other letters being read

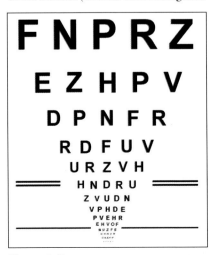

Figure 1.2
The Bailey–Lovie chart

on the lines above), the logMAR score is taken as +0.02, two letters +0.04, and so on. In other words, 0.02 is added for each letter incorrectly read. Thus, the final logMAR score takes account of every letter that has been read correctly, which avoids the confusion that may occur with Snellen notation.

The Bailey–Lovie chart therefore has a number of advantages over a conventional Snellen chart. However, both charts measure just one aspect of visual capability, that is the ability to resolve small high-contrast letters. While this relates well to a patient's ability to read high-contrast text, it relates less well to the ability to drive a car or cross the road. Such tasks involve the detection of objects of various sizes and a range of contrasts.

In the early 1960s, Campbell and colleagues looked to the world of engineering for inspiration.[3] They realised that the key to describing the properties of any complex system was to choose appropriate test stimuli. These stimuli must be simple, but at the same time be able to serve as building blocks to construct more complex stimuli. A sine wave is an example of such a stimulus.

Techniques based on this principle have been used for many years in engineering to assess the characteristics of a wide range of systems, including lenses, amplifiers, loudspeakers, and microphones. In essence, the technique involves measuring the response of the system to sine waves of various frequencies, which gives rise to a function known as the modulation transfer function (MTF). The value of this function arises because more complex waveforms can be constructed by adding together sine waves of different amplitudes, frequencies, and phases (a technique known as Fourier synthesis). Thus, by measuring the response of the system to sine waves of different frequencies, it is possible to predict the response of the system to virtually any input.

Campbell and colleagues were the first to apply this technique to the visual system. Their technique involves measuring the response to sine-wave gratings (*Figure 1.3*). A sine-wave grating can be described in terms of four parameters:

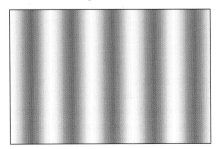

Figure 1.3
A sine-wave grating

- spatial frequency in cycles per degree (cpd);
- contrast, defined as:

$$\frac{L_{max} - L_{min}}{L_{max} + L_{min}}$$

where L_{max} and L_{min} are the maximum and minimum luminances, respectively (the Michelson contrast);

- phase (the position in space); and
- orientation.

The patient is shown a grating of a certain spatial frequency and the contrast is adjusted until the bars can only just be seen (i.e., the contrast threshold). Contrast sensitivity (CS) is defined as 1/contrast threshold. This is normally repeated for at least five different spatial frequencies.

The resultant contrast sensitivity function (CSF; *Figure 1.4*) provides information about how well a patient sees over a range of spatial frequencies and is therefore analogous to an MTF. Within certain constraints, the CSF can be used in the same way as an MTF to predict the perception of more complex images.

Figure 1.5 shows how the CSF may be related to acuity. Visual acuity is a measure of the highest spatial frequency that can be detected at a high contrast (usually >90 per cent) and can be shown to relate, approximately, to the intersection of the CSF with a horizontal line at a corresponding contrast. As such, visual acuity is sensitive to conditions that produce a loss of CS at high spatial frequencies, such as refractive error. However, it is not so good at quantifying the quality of vision when there is a loss of sensitivity at lower spatial frequencies (as may occur in some neurological conditions, cataracts, corneal disturbance, or contact lenses).

Until relatively recently, the measurement of CS required complex computer-based equipment, but now a number of chart-based systems have become available. These are cheaper, less bulky, and allow rapid assessment of CS. The Vistech

chart consists of a matrix of sine-wave gratings of different contrasts and spatial frequencies printed on a wall-mounted chart.[4] This allows CS to be measured for five different spatial frequencies.

The Pelli–Robson chart[5] consists of rows of letters of the same size, but decreasing contrast (*Figure 1.6*). The chart is normally viewed from 1 metre, from where the letters equate approximately to one cycle per degree. Thus, the Pelli–Robson chart gives a measurement of CS at one spatial frequency.

Another approach is to measure visual acuity at a lower contrast, such as 10 per cent. This method provides a second point on the CSF, as shown in *Figure 1.6*.

While the Pelli–Robson and low-contrast acuity charts provide only a single point on the CSF, a second point can be obtained easily by measuring visual acuity with a normal high-contrast letter chart. These two measurements are usually adequate to predict the shape of the entire CSF and therefore provide a powerful description of a patient's visual capability.

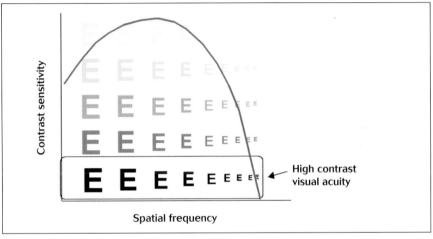

Figure 1.5
Relating visual acuity to the contrast sensitivity function

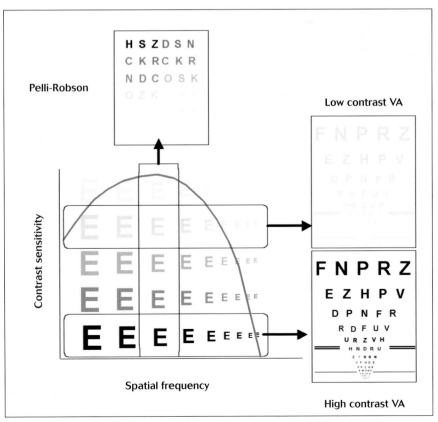

Figure 1.6
Relating high- and low-contrast visual acuity and Pelli–Robson contrast sensitivity to the contrast sensitivity function

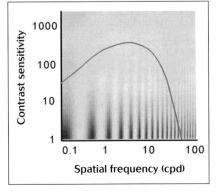

Figure 1.4
Contrast sensitivity function

Light scatter and glare

The limitations of high-contrast visual acuity are perhaps most apparent in patients with media opacities. Such patients often complain of poor vision (especially in bright conditions) and yet achieve surprisingly good visual acuity in the consulting room. To understand how this can occur, it is necessary to consider the nature of the image degradation caused by media disturbances.

The discussion here concentrates on cataracts, but similar principles apply to disturbances in the cornea, aqueous, or vitreous. The effects of cataracts on vision are varied, but can usually be attributed to one or more of the following:
- reduction in retinal illuminance;
- decrease in optical quality; and
- light scatter.

Reduction in retinal illuminance

The normal crystalline lens acts as a filter and plays an important role in protecting the retina from shorter wavelengths, particularly in the UVA region of the spectrum. The absorption of the lens increases with age, particularly towards the blue end of the spectrum (hence the yellow appearance of the ageing lens). Therefore, even in the normal eye, the average retinal illuminance tends to decrease with age.

The eye has a remarkable dynamic range, being capable of operating over about 10 log units (10,000 million:1) and therefore even a 50 per cent drop in retinal illuminance does not significantly affect visual performance under normal daylight conditions. However, when there is less light available or under low-contrast conditions, the reduced retinal illuminance may become an important factor.

All cataracts tend to reduce retinal illuminance to some extent, but (with the probable exception of nuclear sclerosis cataract) it is generally agreed that the reduction in retinal illuminance is not usually the main factor responsible for the degradation of vision.

Decrease in optical quality

Changes in the structure of the lens may result in 'pockets' of material of higher or lower refractive index. This, in effect, makes parts of the lens more powerful than others and causes rays that pass through different parts of the lens to come to a focus at different points. This results in blurring of the retinal image that cannot be corrected fully with a spectacle lens. This tends to reduce sensitivity at high spatial frequencies, and hence visual acuity, but will have less effect on sensitivity to lower spatial frequencies.

Light scatter

There has been a great deal of research on the transparency of the ocular media. The key to transparency seems to lie in the tight spacing and regular arrangement of the elements. Although the normal cornea and lens achieve good transparency, some scatter does occur. Any disruption to the regular structure of the cornea or lens will cause an increase in the proportion of light scattered and a corresponding loss of transparency.

The size and irregularity of distribution of the scattering particles largely determines the type of scattering. For very small particles (less than the wavelength of light), the distribution of the scattered light has little or no relation to the direction of the incident beam (Rayleigh scattering). When the scattering particles are larger, the angular distribution of the scattered beam tends to follow more closely the direction of the incident beam.

Even in a normal eye, diffraction, and other aberrations, cause the image of a point source of light to be spread out on the retina. This is described by the point-spread function. The effect of scattered light is to increase the proportion of light distributed outside the region of the point-spread function. Therefore, the effect of scatter is to spread the light from the brighter parts of the image onto the darker parts, and thus reduce the contrast (*Figure 1.7*).

Although the image is in focus, it is degraded by the loss of luminous and chromatic contrast. While this has a dramatic effect on the quality of vision, it has surprisingly little effect on high-contrast

visual acuity (*Figure 1.8*). Therefore, high-contrast visual acuity tends to overestimate the visual capability of patients with increased scatter.

The effect of scatter on the contrast sensitivity function

Any loss of contrast in the retinal image results in a corresponding reduction in CS. The effect on spatial frequency of the loss depends on the nature of the scatter. Rayleigh-type scatter results in a more or less equal loss of CS at all spatial frequencies. Scatter by larger particles (more common in the eye) tends to affect CS for higher spatial frequencies more than for the lower. In this case, high-contrast acuity is slightly reduced, but because sensitivity is also reduced at lower spatial frequencies, the overall quality of vision will be worse than indicated by high-contrast acuity.

For example, consider the CSF for a patient with a refractive error and a patient with increased light scatter (*Figure 1.9*). These two patients would have approximately the same high-contrast acuity, but the 'quality' of vision would be worse for the patient with increased light scatter.

In some patients with cataracts, the loss is primarily at high spatial frequencies. In these cases, high-contrast acuity tends to correlate well with the patient's reported visual disability. However, when there is also a loss of sensitivity at lower spatial frequencies, high-contrast acuity tends to underestimate the degree of disability. In

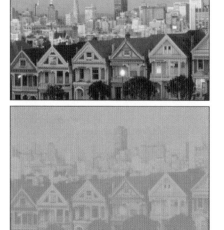

Figure 1.7
The effect of light scatter on a real-world scene

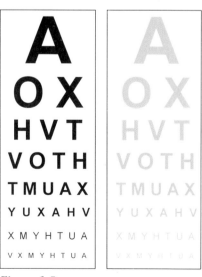

Figure 1.8
Light scatter reduces the contrast of the retinal image, but it has surprisingly little effect on high-contrast visual acuity

these patients, measurements of CS at lower spatial frequencies can be useful. For example, the two patients illustrated in *Figure 1.10* will have the same high-contrast visual acuity, but will have different low-contrast acuities and different results on the Pelli–Robson chart.

Glare

The effects of light scatter become particularly troublesome when there are large differences in the light level between different parts of the visual field at the same time, as when the sun is low in the sky or when facing oncoming car headlamps at night. The light from the bright source is scattered by the ocular media and forms a veiling luminance over the retina, thus reducing the contrast of the image. This is known as disability glare.

Patients with increased light scatter in the eye therefore have particular difficulties in these situations. However, under the subdued lighting conditions of a consulting room, this aspect of a patient's vision is seldom apparent.

Various tests have been devised to assess glare sensitivity. The simplest of these involves placing a bright light source next to or around a letter chart. Patients with increased scatter tend to record poorer acuities with the glare source than without, particularly for low-contrast letters.

The Brightness Acuity Tester (BAT) provides a more elegant solution. It consists of an internally illuminated hemispherical bowl with a hole in the middle. The patient holds the instrument to his or her eye and views the test chart through the hole. This provides a bright uniform glare source that can be used in conjunction with acuity and CS tests.

Summary

While visual acuity measured with a high-contrast letter chart is a sensitive test for refractive error, it may overestimate the visual capability of some patients with media opacities and various neural problems. In these cases, measurements of contrast sensitivity and/or low-contrast acuity provide the clinician with a better understanding of the patient's visual capability.

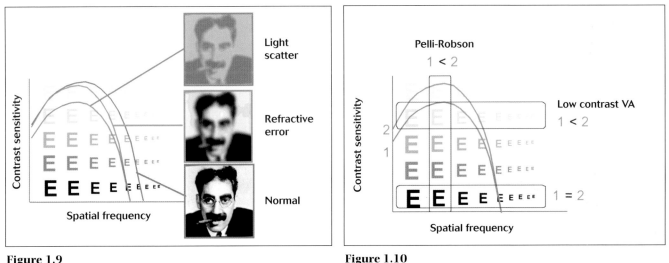

Figure 1.9
Contrast sensitivity functions for a patient with increased light scatter and a patient with a refractive error. Both patients would have a similar high-contrast acuity, but a very different quality of vision

Figure 1.10
Patients 1 and 2 will have approximately the same high-contrast visual acuity (VA), but different low-contrast acuities and Pelli–Robson contrast sensitivities

References
1 Snellen H (1862). *Scala Tipografica Measurae il Visus* (Utrecht).
2 Bailey IL and Lovie JE (1976). New design principles for visual acuity letter charts. *Am J Optom Physiol Opt.* **53**, 740.
3 Campbell FW and Green DG (1965). Optical and retinal factors affecting visual resolution. *J Physiol.* **181**, 576–593.
4 Ginsburg AP (1984). A new contrast sensitivity vision test chart. *Am J Optom Physiol Opt.* **61**, 403.
5 Pelli DG, Robson JG and Wilkins AJ (1988). The design of a new letter chart for measuring contrast sensitivity. *Clin Vis Sci.* **2**, 187–199.

Further reading (articles)
Arden GB (1978). The importance of measuring contrast sensitivity in cases of visual disturbance. *Br J Ophthalmol.* **62**, 198–209.
Bennett AG (1965). Ophthalmic test types. *Br J Physiol Optics.* **22**, 238–271.
Campbell FW and Robson JG (1968). The application of Fourier analysis to the visibility of gratings. *J Physiol.* **197**, 551–556.
Green DG and Campbell FW (1965). Effect of focus on the visual response to a sinusoidally modulated spatial stimulus *J Opt Soc Am.* **55**, 1154.
Hess R and Woo G (1978). Vision through cataracts. *Invest Ophthalmol Vis Sci.* **17**, 428–435.
Regan D and Neima D (1983). Low-contrast letter charts as tests of visual function. *Ophthalmology* **90**, 1192–1200.
Schade OH (1956). Optical and photoelectric analog of the eye. *J Opt Soc Am.* **49**, 425–428.

Further reading (books)
Bennett AG and Rabbetts RB (1984). *Clinical Visual Optics*, Chapter 3 (London: Butterworth Heinemann).
Edwards K and Llewellyn R (1988). *Optometry*, Chapters 2 and 8 (London: Butterworth Heinemann).
Nadler MP, Miller D and Nadler DJ (1990). *Glare and Contrast Sensitivity for Clinicians* (Berlin: Springer-Verlag).

2
Use and development of computer-based test charts in the assessment of vision

David Thomson

The Snellen chart is an old and trusted friend, but clinicians should be aware of a number of flaws in its design (see Chapter 1). Modern chart designs have overcome most of these problems, but as a result of over 100 years of inertia the clinical community are reluctant to accept them.

Over the past few decades, major advances have been in the methodology available to assess various aspects of vision and visual function. The literature is laden with examples of tests that have been shown to provide valuable information about the integrity of the visual system and the quality of its function, yet very few of these tests have found their way into clinical practice. Indeed, most clinicians have a remarkably small armoury of tests available for the assessment of vision and some of the tests that are used are based on outdated and flawed design principles.

Why has clinical practice lagged so far behind the 'cutting-edge' of vision research in this respect? Combinations of practical, educational, economic and political factors have certainly played a part. It is also fair to say that the research community has not been good at taking tests that have been proved in the research environment through to a stage of development that allows them to be implemented in clinical practice. As a result, clinicians have been limited to the restricted and outdated battery of tests available on test chart units (and projectors) and an *ad hoc* mixture of either hand-held or wall-mounted charts.

Recent developments in computer graphics and display technology are set to change all this. Modern PCs, coupled with high-resolution displays [particularly thin-film transistor (TFT) liquid crystal flat-panel displays], are able to generate an

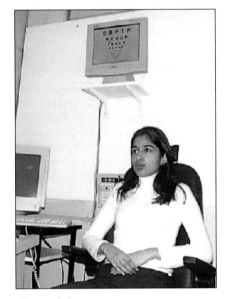

Figure 2.1
Computerised test chart in use

almost infinite variety of test stimuli on a single screen. This gives the clinician access to a much wider range of tests and facilitates the transition of tests from the research laboratory to the consulting room (*Figure 2.1*).

Computer displays

The simplest method for producing test charts is to print the test stimuli on paper or card. This method is very versatile and, with modern printing and photographic methods, the contrast, colour and spatial configuration of the charts can be controlled very precisely. The main disadvantage of these reflective charts is that they

require external illumination and it can be difficult to ensure that the illumination is adequate and uniform across the chart.

This problem can be overcome to some extent by printing the test stimuli onto a diffusing material, which is then back-illuminated. However, it is more difficult to vary the contrast and colour of charts produced in this way.

A disadvantage of both types of chart is that they can only be used at one predetermined distance (unless an adjustment is made to the scoring). In addition, the range of tests that can be incorporated is limited by the size of the test chart unit (also see Chapter 1).

Projection charts overcome many of the disadvantages of printed charts and can present a wide range of test stimuli. However, with projection systems it is difficult to achieve high contrasts, particularly in rooms with high ambient illumination. While projection systems can present a wider range of test stimuli, they offer little scope for the clinician to change stimulus parameters or customise the charts.

The potential of computer monitors for the display of visual test stimuli has been recognised for many years. Computer displays have been used extensively in vision research since the late 1960s.

A number of computer-based test charts have been developed for use in the consulting room, but (until recently) the high cost and limitations of the hardware limited their uptake to a few enthusiasts and specialist clinics.

However, over the past few years the quality of computer displays has improved dramatically and a standard PC is now able to generate high-resolution images of suitable quality for use as test stimuli. The one remaining hurdle in the past was the monitor. Conventional computer monitors use a cathode ray tube (CRT) to generate images. In CRTs, images are formed by sweeping electron beams across the phosphor-coated screen in a series of horizontal lines, from the top to the bottom of the screen, a technique known as raster scanning. To avoid flicker, this process is repeated between 60 and 120 times per second (the refresh rate). An image displayed on a CRT screen is therefore a complex form of spatial and temporal modulation.

When viewed from a distance of 50–100cm, this scanning is too rapid for the visual system to detect and flicker is not usually perceived. However, from longer viewing distances, eye movements can interact with the raster scan, which results in the perception of bursts of flicker on the screen. This phenomenon makes conventional CRT monitors less than ideal for displaying distance test-charts, unless very high refresh rates are used. Furthermore, the luminance of CRT monitors takes a while to stabilise when first turned on and CRTs cannot generally generate contrasts comparable to those of printed test charts. There is also the practical problem of mounting a bulky monitor above the patient's head.

Most of these problems are overcome by flat panel displays (FPDs). These monitors employ a variety of display technologies, but the most promising in terms of displaying test stimuli are the thin-film transistor liquid-crystal displays (TFT LCDs). These displays consist of a thin layer of liquid crystal material sandwiched between a vertical and a horizontal polariser. The liquid crystal material is made up of long crystalline molecules. The individual molecules are arranged in a spiral fashion such that the direction of polarisation of light passing through is rotated by 90°. Light entering through the vertical polariser is thus rotated by 90° and passes through the horizontal polariser. However, when an electric field is applied to the crystals, they all line up and lose their polarising characteristics. Without the polarizing effect of the liquid crystal layer, the vertical and horizontal polarisers attenuate most of the light.

Conventional LCDs use horizontal and vertical grids of wires to generate a matrix of electric fields. Individual cells within the matrix can then be turned on or off by applying a current across specific elements in the grid.

TFT (active matrix) LCD panels have a transistor for each cell in the matrix. The transistors allow the state of the crystals to be changed more rapidly, which enables images to move without smearing. The transistors also allow the degree of polarisation to be varied, which gives a range of grey levels between on and off. The transistor also serves as a memory for the cell, allowing it to stay on without being refreshed. TFT LCD panels are therefore virtually flicker-free.

Colour displays are possible by dying the liquid crystals and juxtaposing red, green and blue cells. The individual coloured cells are too small to be resolved by the eye. Therefore varying the relative intensity of the red, green and blue cells in each triad can produce a wide gamut of colours.

TFT LCD FPDs are used by most laptop computers and are becoming increasingly popular for desktop PCs as an alternative to CRT monitors.

FPDs are light, have excellent resolution and contrast (typically 250:1) and are flicker free (see *Figure 2.1*). They are also able to produce adequate luminance ($200cdm^{-2}$), good uniformity across the screen and are very stable over time. They are therefore ideal for presenting test stimuli when assessing vision and visual function. With the popularisation of TFT LCD screens, the final hurdle has been removed and computer-based test charts are now a viable and cost-effective alternative to conventional test charts and projectors. An example of such a system developed by the author and his colleagues is described in the following sections. It is outside the scope of this chapter to compare and contrast each of the computer-based charts that are commercially available.

Test Chart 2000

Test Chart 2000 is a computer-based test chart and is discussed in the following sections. It is a *Windows*-based program that will run on any PC supporting this platform; it can also be installed on a laptop computer, which is particularly useful for domiciliary examinations.

The monitor may be viewed directly or via a mirror (all optotypes can be reversed). The program can be configured for any viewing distance, but in practice viewing distances of less than 3 metres are not advised because the smaller letter sizes do not reproduce well on the monitor and some refractive compensation for the viewing distance may be necessary.

The program works with most monitors and graphics cards. However, the best results are obtained using a 15 or 17 inch monitor that can operate at a resolution of 1024×768 or higher. Adequate results are obtained at lower resolutions provided that viewing distances of 4 metres or more are used.

To reproduce the various colours and contrast levels used by the program, the graphics card must be able to generate 'true colour' (16 or 32 bit). For CRT monitors the refresh rate should be set as high as possible to avoid flicker. The British Standard stipulates that test charts should have a luminance of $120cdm^{-2}$, which is well within the range of most modern monitors.

Standard CRT-based monitors are generally adequate to display test stimuli, although some flicker may be apparent even at high refresh rates because of the interaction between eye movements and the raster scan. FPDs are particularly suited for this purpose.

Within the consulting room, it is useful to have one monitor for the patient to view and a second monitor beside the practitioner. Most laptop computers provide support for a second monitor. Unfortunately, most desktop PCs do not. However, a second monitor can be added by using a splitter device, which come in two forms:

- Passive splitters are simply cables that take the signal from the graphics card and split it into two plugs. This generally causes some loss of luminance and image quality on both monitors.
- Active splitters buffer the video signal before splitting it to ensure that there is no loss of luminance or quality. Active splitters are therefore preferred for this purpose.

However, with both of these solutions, the two monitors display the same image. To view other programs (e.g., practice management software) on the practitioner's monitor and the test chart on the other, a graphics board that can support two independent displays must be installed.

The tests

The program can be controlled using the keyboard, the mouse or an optional infrared remote control unit.

There are 11 primary display modes:
- LogMAR chart;
- Snellen chart;
- Single-letter chart;
- Duochrome test;
- Fan-and-block test;
- Cross-cyl targets;
- Fixation-disparity test;
- Fixation targets;
- Number-plate test;
- Phoria test;
- Contrast sensitivity test.

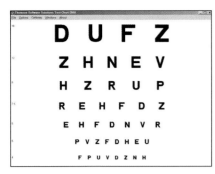

Figure 2.2
Snellen chart display

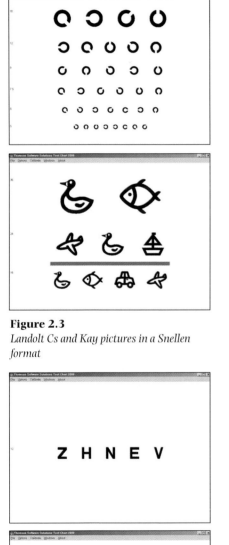

Figure 2.3
Landolt Cs and Kay pictures in a Snellen format

Figure 2.4
Single row and column displays

Visual acuity tests

Visual acuity measured using high-contrast optotypes is still a useful measure of visual performance (also see Chapter 1). It is very sensitive to refractive error and, in most cases, shows a good correlation with symptoms. Despite the well-documented problems with its design, the Snellen chart format is still the most widely used in clinical practice (*Figure 2.2*).

In Test Chart 2000, the letters can be randomised. Letter size can be increased or decreased using the cursor control keys, mouse or remote control. A range of optotypes in the Snellen format, including Landolt Cs, tumbling Es and Kay pictures (*Figure 2.3*) can also be displayed.

A red line can be placed under any row of optotypes by clicking on the row. A single row can be displayed by double clicking on the row, while a single column of letters can also be displayed (*Figure 2.4*).

While the Snellen chart is perfectly adequate for refraction purposes, a number of flaws in its design affect its accuracy as a test of visual performance (see Chapter 1).

The only significant disadvantage of the LogMAR chart is that it is wider than a Snellen chart, and so manufacturers of conventional test chart units tend to prefer the Snellen format. However, this is less of a problem with computer displays, as the whole screen can be used.

The scoring of a LogMAR chart is also a little more complicated to the uninitiated. To overcome this, Test Chart 2000 incorporates an automated scoring module.

A variety of optotypes can be displayed in the LogMAR format (see *Figure 2.5*).

It is sometimes useful to test acuity using single characters, particularly with children and those with learning difficulties. Test Chart 2000 allows all of the optotypes (letters, Landolt Cs, tumbling Es and Kay pictures) to be displayed singly, with or without crowding bars (*Figure 2.6*).

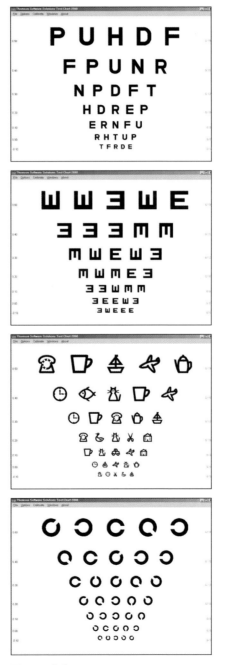

Figure 2.5
A range of optotypes arranged in a LogMAR format

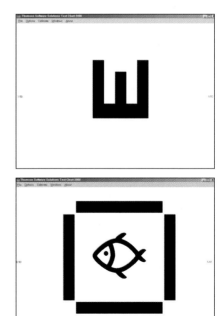

Figure 2.6
Single characters can be displayed with and without crowding bars

Contrast sensitivity

Conventionally, the technique involves measuring the response to sine-wave gratings. The patient is shown a grating of a certain spatial frequency (spacing) and the contrast is adjusted until the bars can only just be seen (i.e., the contrast threshold). This is usually repeated for at least five different spatial frequencies. The resultant contrast sensitivity function (CSF; *Figure 2.7*) provides information about how well a patient sees across a range of spatial frequencies.

Visual acuity is a measure of the highest spatial frequency that can be detected at a high contrast (usually >90 per cent). It can be shown to relate (approximately) to the intersection of the CSF with a horizontal line at a corresponding contrast (*Figure 2.8*, and also refer to Chapter 1). Therefore, visual acuity is sensitive to conditions that produce a loss of contrast sensitivity at high spatial frequencies (such as refractive error), but it is not so good at quantifying the quality of vision when there is a loss of sensitivity at lower spatial frequencies (as may occur in some neurological conditions, cataracts, corneal disturbances, contact lenses, etc).

Contrast sensitivity is a good example of a test that has been used extensively in vision research, but that has failed to find a place in the routine assessment of vision despite its proven value. This is probably because conventional methods of testing contrast sensitivity are time consuming and, until recently, required specialised and expensive equipment. However, with the introduction of computer test charts, contrast sensitivity testing has become a viable proposition in optometric practice.

To measure a full CSF is, indeed, time consuming and rather tedious, but Pelli and colleagues introduced an alternative approach.[1] The Pelli–Robson chart consists of rows of letters of the same size, but decreasing contrast (*Figure 2.9*). The chart is usually viewed from a distance of 1 metre,

from where the letters equate to approximately one cycle per degree. Thus, the Pelli–Robson chart gives a measurement of contrast sensitivity at one spatial frequency.

Another approach is to measure visual acuity at a lower contrast, for example 10 per cent. This method also provides a second point on the CSF (*Figure 2.9*).

The Pelli–Robson and low-contrast acuity charts only provide a single point on the CSF. However, visual acuity measured with a high-contrast chart provides a second point on the CSF and these two

measurements are usually adequate to predict the shape of the entire CSF and therefore provide a powerful description of a patient's visual capability.

Test Chart 2000 provides both options. The contrast of the Snellen, LogMAR and single-letter charts can be varied, which allows visual acuity to be measured at any contrast level from approximately 0.1 per cent to 95 per cent or more.

Alternatively, triplets of letters of the same size but decreasing contrast can be displayed. The contrast of the letters is decreased until the patient can no longer identify at least two out of the three letters. This procedure can be repeated for different letter sizes, and so the CSF is sampled at different spatial frequencies (*Figure 2.10*).

Duochrome test

A variety of targets can be displayed against the duochrome background, including rings, dots and a variety of optotypes (*Figure 2.11*).

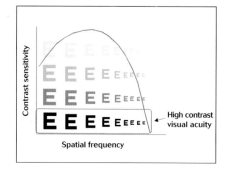

Figure 2.8
Relating visual acuity to the contrast sensitivity function

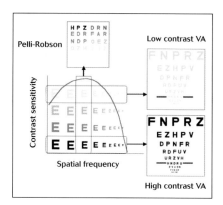

Figure 2.9
Relating high- and low-contrast visual acuity (VA) and Pelli–Robson contrast sensitivity to the contrast sensitivity function

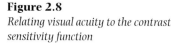
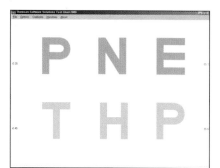

Figure 2.10
Contrast sensitivity test

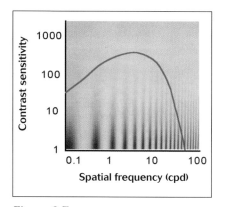

Figure 2.7
The contrast sensitivity function

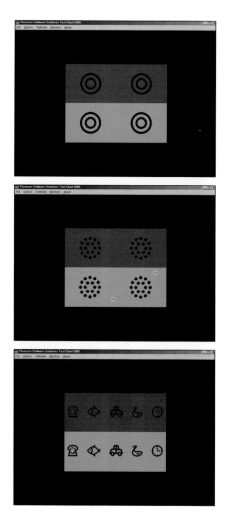

Figure 2.11
A range of stimuli presented on the duochrome background

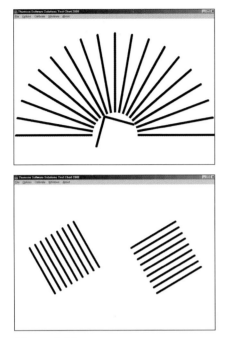

Figure 2.12
The fan-and-block test

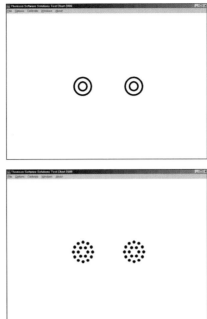

Figure 2.13
Cross-cyl test

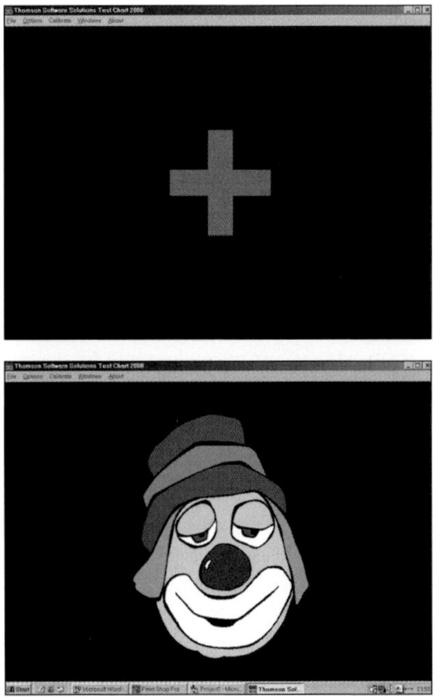

![Figure 2.14 fixation targets]

Figure 2.14
A wide range of fixation targets is available

The fan-and-block test

The fan-and-block test continues to be popular among some clinicians. This test can be replicated well on a computer screen (*Figure 2.12*).

Cross-cyl targets

Test Chart 2000 includes a variety of targets for the cross-cyl test (*Figure 2.13*).

Fixation targets

Computer-generated programs allow a variety of fixation targets to be generated for use during retinoscopy, ophthalmoscopy or the distance cover test. The ability to produce dynamic and moving images provides greater scope for maintaining the patient's attention. For example, a fixation cross can be made to change colour gradually, a clown's nose can be made to flash or the expression on the clown's face can be changed (*Figure 2.14*). Other favourite images can be imported for this purpose, including movies.

Phoria test

To measure phoria, the patient wears red-and-blue goggles, the room lights are extinguished and aligned red and blue bars are presented on the screen. If the patient has a phoria, the bars do not appear to align. To measure the phoria, prisms may be used to align the bars or the bars themselves can be moved until they appear to be aligned. The displacement of the bars can then be displayed on the screen to give an accurate measure of phoria.

Fixation-disparity test

The program incorporates a fixation-disparity test similar to the Mallett test. However, it is not possible to use polarised targets and therefore red-and-blue dissociation is used (*Figure 2.15*). This is not ideal as it tends to induce some degree of retinal rivalry, which may cause individuals with fragile binocularity to suppress. In these situations it is advisable to use a standard Mallett test to assess fixation disparity. However, laboratory tests suggest that, provided patients do not suppress, the fixation disparity measured using this test correlates well with the standard Mallett test.

Number-plate test

The number-plate test remains the only statutory test of vision required for driving in the UK. The law states that an individual should be able to read a number plate in good daylight (with spectacles or contact lenses if worn) that contains letters and characters 79.4mm high at a distance of 20.5m. From this distance the characters subtend an angle of 13.3 minutes of arc, which equates to a Snellen letter size of approximately 6/16. However, the font used for number plates is different to that used on test charts and the spacing of the letters is much less. These factors increase the difficulty of the task, and Drasdo and Haggerty[2] found that, in fact, the test equates to a Snellen acuity of approximately 6/9–2.

Although some test chart units do include a number-plate test, the font and spacing of the characters used rarely conforms to that of actual number plates. As a result, the clinician is often required to advise the patient on the basis of the extrapolated Snellen equivalent. Computer-based test charts are able to replicate exactly a series of front and rear number plates using the exact fonts and character spacing. The number plates can

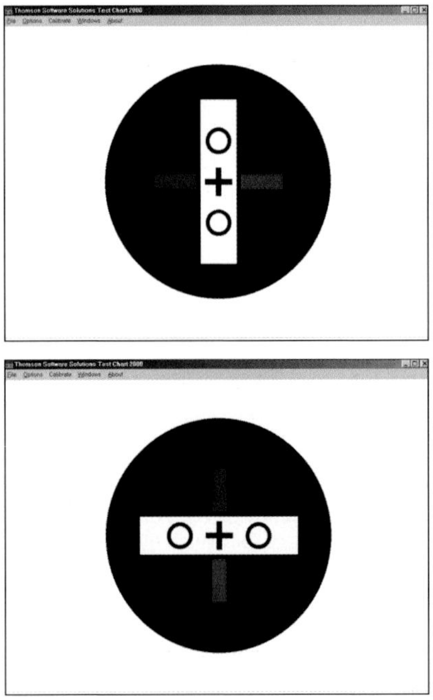

![Figure 2.15 fixation-disparity test targets]

Figure 2.15
Fixation-disparity test

also be presented against a variety of backgrounds to simulate real-world conditions. This allows the practitioner to give a more realistic appraisal of a patient's vision in relation to their ability to pass the numberplate test.

Split-screen displays

During an eye examination, it is often useful to be able to display more than one test at the same time. For example, during refraction it may be useful to display the duochrome alongside some small letters. Computer-based charts, such as Test Chart 2000, allow the screen to be split horizontally. Different tests may be then be displayed in each part of the screen (*Figure 2.16*).

Programmable keys

Computer-based charts provide considerable scope to customise the program according to users' preferences. For example, various display configurations can be assigned to specific keys. This allows the user to select quite complex display configurations by pressing a single key on the keyboard or remote control unit.

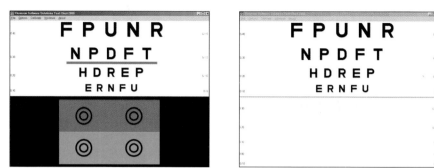

Figure 2.16
Any combination of tests can be displayed in split-screen mode

Summary

Computer-based test charts offer many advantages over conventional test charts and projection systems. An almost infinite variety of test stimuli can be presented on a compact display, giving the clinician access to the normal battery of tried-and-tested stimuli plus a variety of tests that have hitherto been confined to research laboratories.

The theoretical advantages of computer-based test charts have been acknowledged for many years, but they have not been widely used in optometric practice because of the cost, size and relatively poor performance of the hardware. However, recent advances in computer and display technology have now made computer-based test charts a very attractive and cost-effective alternative to conventional test charts and projection systems. In particular, the popularisation of TFT LCD FPDs provides an ideal medium for the display of test stimuli in the consulting room. For the cost of a FPD, a standard PC can be turned into a powerful consulting-room tool for assessing many aspects of visual performance. Furthermore, the benefits of new tests of visual function can be readily passed on to clinicians as software modules, without requiring any change in the hardware.

The inclusion of Kay pictures and the Mallett test in Test Chart 2000 is subject to contract.

Acknowledgement
Images of Test Charts 2000 are reproduced with kind permission of 100 Marketing.

References
1 Pelli DG, Robson JG and Wilkins AJ (1988). The design of a new letter chart for measuring contrast sensitivity. *Clin Vis Sci.* **2**, 187–199.
2 Drasdo N and Haggerty CM (1981). A comparison of the British numberplate and Snellen vision tests for car drivers. *Ophthalmol Phys Opt.* **1**, 39–54.

Further reading
Arden GB (1988). The importance of measuring contrast sensitivity in cases of visual disturbance. *Br J Ophthalmol.* **62**, 198–209.
Augsberger A, Sheed, JE and Schoessler JP (1979). Reflectance of visual acuity screens. *Am J Optom Physiol Opt.* **56**, 531.
Bailey IL and Lovie JE (1976). New design principles for visual acuity letter charts. *Am J Optom Physiol Opt.* **53**, 740.
Bennett AG (1965). Ophthalmic test types. *Br J Physiol Optics.* **22**, 238–271.
Campbell FW and Green DG (1965). Optical and retinal factors affecting visual resolution. *J Physiol.* **181**, 576–593.

French CN (1997). The UMIST eye system. *Spatial Vis.* **11**, 91–93.
Hess R and Woo G (1978). Vision through cataracts. *Invest Ophthalmol Vis Sci.* **17**, 428–435.
Kay H (1983). New method for assessing VA with pictures. *Br J Ophthalmol.* **67**, 131–133.
Kay H (1984). A new picture VA test. *Br J Orthoptics.* **41**, 77–79.
Regan D and Neima D (1983). Low-contrast letter charts as tests of visual function. *Ophthalmology* **90**, 1192–1200.
Thomson WD and Saunders JE (1997). The perception of flicker on raster-scanned displays. *Hum Factors.* **39**, 48–66.

3

Colour vision examination

Jennifer Birch

Introduction

Colour deficiency is caused by inherited photopigment abnormalities. There are three different types of colour deficiency and differences in severity in each type. Colour-deficient people have different practical difficulties with colour recognition and variable hue-discrimination problems. All colour-deficient people see fewer separate colours in the spectrum and in the environment. Some colours, which look different to people with normal colour vision, appear to be the same and are confused. Relative colour lightness and contrast are also changed because of alteration in the relative luminous efficiency of the eye. Colours are only confused if there is no perceived lightness difference.

The characteristics of different types of colour deficiency were documented over 50 years ago, but the origin of inherited photopigment abnormalities was established only recently. Gene analysis shows that hybrid genes, at key positions in the X-chromosome gene chain, tune the spectral sensitivity of the resulting photopigment, which causes anomalous trichromatism. Alternatively, a gene may be lost or a mis-sense mutation may have occurred so that no photopigment is produced, which results in dichromatism. Molecular genetic studies show how cone photopigments have evolved. Only primates are routinely trichromatic, but the colour vision of New World primates is polymorphic and determined by an unknown mechanism of gene suppression. Many species are colour deficient in human terms. The mechanism of gene suppression in humans is also unknown, and it is not always possible to predict the phenotype from the genotype.

All colour-deficient people are excluded from occupations that require accurate colour matching and colour-quality control, or in which connotative colour codes are used without redundancy. For example, incorrect or slow identification of connotative transport signals is a safety hazard. People with a slight colour deficiency are accepted for other occupations, such as fire-fighting, for which detailed task analysis has established that safety is not compromised. In such cases it is necessary to use both a screening test, to identify colour deficiency, and a 'grading' test to determine the severity and type.

Screening

Pseudoisochromatic tests, such as the Ishihara plates, are used to identify red–green colour deficiency. These tests have a simple visual task and are easily understood. Hue-discrimination tests that comprise Munsell colour samples are frequently used in grading tests. The visual task is more complex and the examiner requires more expertise to administer the test. The colour-difference steps determine the pass/fail level of grading tests. People with a slight colour deficiency 'pass' and those with a moderate or severe colour deficiency 'fail'. Tests composed of pigment colours are unable to distinguish dichromats and anomalous trichromats.

It is essential that all clinical colour-vision tests fulfil the needs of quality audit and are shown to be 'fit for the purpose'. A spectral anomaloscope, such as the Nagel anomaloscope, is the 'Gold Standard' reference test for red–green colour deficiency. The sensitivity and specificity of the intended screening tests must be compared with anomaloscope results. A large group of colour-normal subjects

and a representative group of diagnosed colour-deficient subjects are needed in the study. Screening tests must have 100 per cent specificity. This ensures that no one with normal colour vision is identified incorrectly as 'colour deficient' (no false positives). At least 95 per cent sensitivity is desirable. In such cases, 5 per cent of the colour-deficient population are not identified (false negatives). The anomaloscope data must show that those not identified have a very slight colour deficiency. Failure to identify people with severe colour deficiency is not desirable. The pass/fail level of grading tests is compared with the anomaloscope matching range. The audit is based on the documented chromaticities and colour-difference steps employed in the design. These can be obtained for Munsell colours from published spectrophotometric data. Grading tests intended to select people for a particular occupation should employ the smallest colour difference that needs to be discriminated in the work environment. Good test–retest consistency is needed and confirms that the visual task does not unduly affect test performance.

Types of inherited colour deficiency

Types of inherited colour deficiency have been described since the 18th century. John Dalton (1798) investigated his own colour deficiency and noted that pinks appeared 'sky blue', 'greens inclined to brown', and crimson fabric was like 'dark drab' or 'mud'. To Dalton, spectral red, orange, yellow and green all looked 'yellow' and the remainder of the spectrum was 'blue', gradually changing to 'purple'. He concluded, reasonably enough, that he lacked the ability to see long-wavelength red light. Dalton bequeathed his eyes to the

Table 3.1 Classification of congenital colour deficiency

Number of colour-matching variables needed to match all spectral hues	Number of cone pigments	Type	Denomination	Hue-discrimination ability
1	None	Monochromat	Typical (rod) monochromat	None
1	One	Monochromat	Atypical, incomplete (cone usually blue cone) monochromat	Limited discrimination in mesopic viewing conditions
2	Two	Dichromat	a) Protanope b) Deuteranope c) Tritanope	Severely impaired
3	Three	Anomalous trichromat	a) Protanomalous b) Deuteranomalous c) Tritanomalous	Continuous range from slight to severe impairment, depending on the characteristics of the abnormal photopigment

Manchester Philosophical Society and it was a surprise when molecular genetic analysis showed that he was a deuteranope, not a protanope.[1] Dalton did not think that colour naming was a good screening method and devised a matching test with coloured ribbons. A colour-sorting test consisting of over 300 coloured papers was introduced by August Seebeck in 1837. Seebeck's results showed that there were two distinct types of red–green colour deficiency, with differences in severity in both types. Reduced sensitivity to red light was found in only one type. A framework for interpreting Seebeck's results was provided by John William Strutt, the second Baron Rayleigh, in 1881. Rayleigh developed a spectral colour-matching test and showed that some colour-deficient people could be classified as dichromats and others as anomalous trichromats (*Table 3.1*). A Rayleigh match presented in a spectral anomaloscope, such as the Nagel anomaloscope, remains the reference test for identifying and diagnosing types of red–green colour deficiency.

Normal trichromatic colour vision is derived from three classes of cone photopigment. These have maximum spectral sensitivity at about 420, 530 and 560nm. Three colour-matching variables are required to match all the spectral hues. The terms used to describe different types of colour deficiency are based on the number of photopigments present and hence the number of colour-matching variables needed. The retina may lack all functioning cone photopigments or there may be only one or two photopigment classes instead of the normal three. The majority of colour-deficient people have three photopigments and are trichromatic, but the spectral sensitivity of one photopigment is abnormal. Molecular genetic analysis has shown that amino-acid substitutions at a small number of specific points in the X-chromosome gene sequence have the effect of tuning the spectral sensitivity of the photopigment. All or some of these substitutions may be present and result in different amounts of spectral tuning. Differences in severity of colour deficiency in anomalous trichromatism are derived from the range of abnormal photopigments produced.

In protan colour-deficiency, absence or abnormality of the photopigment sensitive to long wavelength ('red') reduces long-wavelength spectral sensitivity and shifts the relative luminous efficiency of the eye towards shorter wavelengths. Shortening of the red end of the spectrum reduces the visibility of red warning lights and signals. Protans are excluded from occupations in which this is a safety hazard.

Monochromats see only lightness differences in the spectrum and are truly 'colour blind'. Typical (rod) monochromats have no functioning cone receptors and poor visual acuity, 6/60 or 6/36, photophobia and nystagmus. Most rod monochromats lack all cone photopigments and have no cone-mediated responses. In rare cases, cone photopigments are present and absence of colour vision results from an abnormality in the visual pathway. At least three different gene abnormalities, on chromosomes 2, 8 and 14, have been found to produce typical rod monochromatism in different families. Mis-sense mutations in these genes appear to prevent transcription of enzymes that are key components of the cone phototransduction pathways. In Pingelap (see below) the abnormality is identified at 8q 21-22.

Atypical 'incomplete' (cone) monochromats have the photopigment sensitive to short wavelength ('blue' cone) only. Residual colour discrimination is possible in mesopic light levels when both rods and cones are functioning. Visual acuity is reduced in the range 6/9–6/24 and only people with acuity less than 6/18 have photophobia and nystagmus. Some blue-cone monochromats develop a slowly progressive central retinal degeneration and visual acuity declines with age.

The group terms protan, deutan and tritan (derived from Greek words meaning first, second and third) are used to describe colour deficiency that involves a particular photopigment type. Each term includes dichromatism and anomalous trichromatism. Characteristic colour-matching functions, which show the range of colours confused by protans and deutans, were documented in the 1930s using visual colorimetry. These measurements established isochromatic (same colour) zones in the Commission Internationale d'Eclairage (CIE) 1931 system of colour measurement. Colours specified within an isochromatic zone look the same in each type of colour deficiency and are confused if there is no perceived lightness difference (see *Figure 3.1*).

Lightness contrast enables areas of colour to be distinguished as different even if there is no difference in the perceived hue. Isochromatic data for tritans were established in 1952 after a number of tritanopes came forward for investigation following publication of a specially designed pseudoisochromatic plate in the magazine *Picture Post*. The chromaticities of coloured light sources, filters and pigment colours can all be analysed and specified in the CIE system of colour measurement. These data can be compared with isochromatic zones. Colours in connotative and denotative codes, and in colour vision tests, can be evaluated in this way. If the colours in pseudoisochromatic designs are not within appropriate isochromatic zones, or if there is a perceived lightness difference, the design will not fulfil the intended purpose.

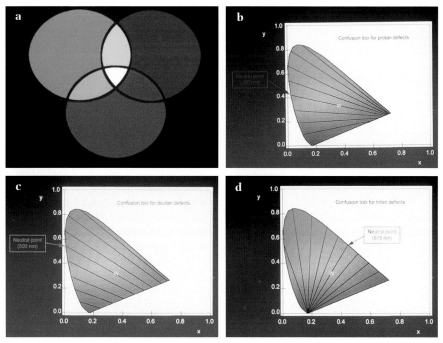

Figure 3.1

(a) Venn Diagram of primary colours. Isochromatic zones for (b) protans, (c) deutans and (d) tritans shown on the CIE 1931 chromaticity diagram. Colours specified within isochromatic zones look the same to colour-deficient people in each class and are confused, as long as there is no perceived lightness difference

Both protans and deutans make similar colour confusions in the red–yellow–green part of the spectrum. These colours are used in pseudoisochromatic screening tests to identify both types of red–green colour deficiency. Achromatic or 'neutral' colours, which are confused with grey, are different in protans and deutans and these colours are used in pseudoisochromatic designs to distinguish, or classify, protan and deutan colour deficiency. Dichromats confuse bright, fully saturated colours. Anomalous trichromats confuse pale, less saturated colours (*Table 3.2*). Loss of long wavelength red sensitivity results in significant practical consequences for protans, so it is important that the correct classification is obtained.

Pseudoisochromatic designs are camouflage patterns. Spots or patches of colour are selected to break up the outline of a figure and conceal its shape. Hue discrimination grading tests present a number of colours selected from a hue circle of equal lightness. These tests have different pass/fail levels depending on the number of colours and the saturation level.

Prevalence of inherited colour deficiency

Large population surveys, using reliable screening methods, show that the prevalence of red–green colour deficiency is about 8 per cent in men and about 0.4 per cent in women (*Table 3.3*). Similar figures were obtained in the most recent survey carried out in secondary schools in Tehran.[2]

A large population sample and an efficient screening method are needed to give an accurate figure for the prevalence of colour deficiency. The surveys listed in *Table 3.3* included men and women in the same population and all the data show characteristics of an X-linked relationship. The large survey carried out in Greece in1975 used the Nagel anomaloscope to diagnose the type of red–green colour deficiency.

Table 3.2 Colours confused in protan, deutan and tritan colour deficiency

Colour confusion	Type of colour deficiency		
	Protan	Deutan	Tritan
Red/orange/yellow/green	*	*	
Brown/green	*	*	
Green/white threshold saturation discrimination	*	*	
Red/white threshold saturation discrimination	*	*	
Blue–green/grey/red–purple	*		
Green/grey/blue–purple		*	
Red/black	*		
Green/black		*	
Violet/yellow–green			*
Red/red–purple			*
Dark blue/black			*
Yellow/white			*

Table 3.3 Prevalence of red–green colour deficiency obtained from large population studies

Country	Year	Men			Women		
		Number examined	Number colour deficient	Percentage	Number examined	Number colour deficient	Percentage
Germany	1936	6863	532	7.75	5604	20	0.36
France	1959	6635	594	8.95	6990	35	0.5
Norway	1927	9049	725	8.01	9072	40	0.44
Greece	1975	21,231	1687	7.95	8754	37	0.42
		Average percentage 8.14			Average percentage 0.43		

Table 3.4 Approximate prevalence of different types of red–green colour deficiency

Type of colour deficiency	Prevalence in men (%)	Prevalence in women (%)
Protanopia	1	0.01
Protanomalous trichromatism	1	0.03
Deuteranopia	1	0.01
Deuteranomalous trichromatism	5	0.35
Total prevalence	8	0.40

This study confirmed that deuteranomalous trichromatism is the most common type, with a prevalence of about 5 per cent in the male population (*Table 3.4*).

Careful reading of the literature does not support the idea that the prevalence of colour deficiency varies in different ethnic groups or is associated with geographic latitude and cultural development. The prevalence of genetic disorders is always different in populations that are isolated geographically or by religious practice, because the gene pool is restricted. Geographic isolation and intermarriage between people who share a common ancestor is responsible for the high prevalence of typical rod monochromatism in the Pacific Island of Pingelap. In large randomly mating populations the prevalence of non-fatal genetic traits remains constant. Examining small groups of isolated unsophisticated non-verbal subjects presents similar problems to those encountered in examining young children.

Adapting the visual task to one that is easily understood may significantly reduce screening accuracy and give a false estimate of prevalence. Results that do not show an X-linked prevalence ratio suggest that the screening method is inappropriate. The small number of colour names used by some primitive peoples is because names for these colours have developed by association, such as 'coloured-like spring', and there has been no need to define subtle differences.

Congenital tritan defects are inherited as an autosomal dominant trait and there is equal prevalence in men and women. Results of the *Picture Post* survey suggested that the frequency of congenital tritanopia is not more than 1 in 10,000. However, a population survey in the Netherlands using a spectral test to measure short-wavelength thresholds suggested that the prevalence of incomplete tritanopia (tritanomalous trichromatism) may be as high as 1 in 500.

Inheritance and molecular genetics

A large pedigree showing red–green colour deficiency (deuteranopia) inherited as an X-linked recessive trait through six generations was published by Horner in 1876. The most usual transmission is from maternal grandfather to grandson. In each generation there are four possible combinations of X- and Y-chromosomes (genotypes) that children inherit from their parents (*Figure 3.2*). All the daughters of a colour-deficient father inherit his X chromosome with the gene abnormality and are heterozygous (carriers) of colour deficiency. They transmit the same abnormal X chromosome to 50 per cent of their sons, who are colour deficient, and 50 per cent of their daughters, who are heterozygous. Brothers of a colour-deficient man have a 50 per cent risk of being similarly affected. Women are only colour-deficient if they inherit abnormal X-chromosome genes for the same photopigment from both parents. Women who are mixed-compound heterozygotes, with an abnormal gene coding for a protan defect on one X chromosome and for a deutan defect on the other, have normal colour vision.

The long- and medium-wavelength photopigment genes are positioned in a tandem 'head-to-tail' array near the distal end of the long (q) arm of the X chromosome (Xq28) and have almost identical amino-acid sequences. Both genes consist of 364 amino acids and are different at only 15 sites. This suggests that two genes evolved from a single gene sensitive to middle waves fairly recently on the evolutionary time scale. During meiosis, homologous paired chromosomes can exchange parts of their genetic material. The close proximity and similarity of photopigment genes means that crossover of genetic material during meiosis can readily occur. If the genes are slightly misaligned and crossover takes place with the break point between the two genes, one chromosome will lose a gene and the other gain one. A man who inherits an X chromosome that lacks a photopigment gene will be a dichromat. If the break point is within the gene a hybrid is formed, which combines regions of the long and middle wavelength genes into a single gene. The hybrid may be 'red–green' or 'green–red' with the larger gene fragment dominating the spectral sensitivity of the resulting photopigment. A man who inherits a hybrid gene will be an anomalous trichromat.[3] Amino-acid changes at three of the 15 possible sites have been found to have the greatest effect on the sensitivity of the resulting photopigment. Two of these,

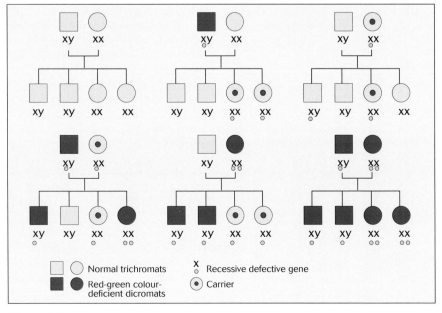

Figure 3.2
Examples of X-linked inheritance

at sites 277 and 285 on exon 5, are close together. The third site is at position 180 on exon 3. On crossover sites 277 and 285 will normally remain together and the spectral sensitivity of the photopigment will largely depend on whether this fragment is derived from the long or middle wavelength gene.[4] Site 180 is polymorphic in both long- and -medium wavelength genes. Serine instead of analine is found in about 40 per cent of men with normal colour vision and produces a visual pigment with a slightly greater long-wave sensitivity.

Explanation of different types of colour deficiency in terms of lost or hybrid genes is very attractive, but appears to be an oversimplification. Most normals have a large number of X-chromosome photopigment genes (as many as 10 is not unusual). These are positioned in sequence from the locus control region at the head of the gene array. Gene expression is governed by the 'down stream' order. Colour normals usually have only one copy of the long wavelength gene and multiple copies of the medium wavelength gene, possibly followed by a number of hybrid genes.[5]

Cones can be filled with any pigment and the identity of an individual cone is dictated by the gene order. (This explains how dichromats have normal visual acuity even though they lack a photopigment.) Only the first two genes have a significant role. The first gene, normally long-wavelength sensitive, is expressed at the highest level and occupies about 60–70 per cent of cones. The second gene, normally medium-wavelength sensitive, is expressed in most of the remaining 30–40 per cent of cones. Genes further along the array are either not expressed or expressed in progressively smaller and smaller numbers of cones. A hybrid gene only produces anomalous trichromatism if it is in either

the first or second position downstream of the locus control region. Some protanomalous males have different hybrid genes in the first two positions in the gene array. Although a gene required for normal colour vision is usually absent in dichromats, this is not always the case, which shows that more than one mechanism produces dichromatic colour vision.[6] A mis-sense mutation that prevents transcription of the photopigment has been identified at position 203. There may be other hidden mutations within the gene structure or abnormalities in the locus-control region that result in a gene being by-passed and not expressed (*Figure 3.3*). An abnormality in the region of the locus-control gene has been identified in X-linked blue-cone monochromatism. This apparently prevents expression of all X-chromosome photopigment genes. The gene that codes the photopigment sensitive to short waves is on chromosome 7 at 7q 31-32. Three different mis-sense abnormalities, involving amino-acid substitutions, at key sites in the gene sequence have been identified in families with congenital tritan colour deficiency.[7] Incomplete manifestation or penetrance is a characteristic of autosomal dominant inheritance and results in differences in gene expression in affected family members. Some affected family members are tritanopes and others are incomplete tritanopes (tritanomalous trichromats). No paired homologous photopigment gene on chromosome 7 can recombine to form a hybrid gene. Some tritanopes are found to have cones sensitive to short wavelengths outside the foveal region. This interesting finding emphasises that the mechanism that transcribes photopigment into each cone cell and determines its identity is not yet understood.

Colour vision examination

The efficiency of screening tests can be analysed in terms of specificity and sensitivity. Specificity is the percentage of normals correctly identified as normal, and sensitivity is the percentage of abnormals correctly identified as abnormal in comparison with a 'Gold Standard' reference test. The reference test for red–green colour deficiency is the Nagel anomaloscope. In general, specificity and sensitivity over 90 per cent are considered to indicate a good screening test. However, 90 per cent specificity results in an unacceptable 10 per cent false-positive rate in the large colour-normal population. Specificity of 100 per cent must always be obtained so that no person with normal colour vision is incorrectly identified as colour deficient. Ideally, sensitivity should be greater than 90 per cent. Raising the sensitivity from 90 per cent to 95 per cent halves the number of false negatives from 10 per cent to 5 per cent. A small number of false negatives (colour-deficient people not identified) is satisfactory only if they have very slight (minimal) anomalous trichromatism.

It is not easy to design efficient colour-vision screening tests. Knowledge of isochromatic zones and accurate colour reproduction is the essential first step. Visual display units appear to offer an ideal medium for the design of colour-vision tests and several examination techniques have been developed in research institutions that have the necessary equipment to calibrate the screen phosphors. Calibration is needed to ensure that the desired CIE chromaticities are reproduced. The equipment is very expensive and efficient colour-vision examination using personal computers is not yet an option.

Nagel anomaloscope
The Nagel anomaloscope was introduced in 1907 and is no longer manufactured. The instrument consists of a Maxwellian view spectroscope in which two halves of a 3° circular bipartite field are illuminated, respectively, by monochromatic yellow (589nm) and a mixture of monochromatic red and green wavelengths (670 and 546nm). A system of reciprocating slits keeps the luminance of the mixture field constant for any red–green mixture ratio. The aim of the examination is to determine the exact matching range of the subject. Normal trichromats make a precise colour match within a small range of red–green mixture ratios. The matching ranges of protanomalous and deuteranomalous trichromats are outside this

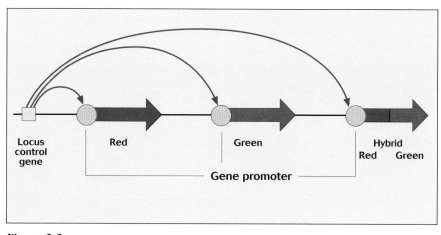

Figure 3.3
An example of a photopigment gene array

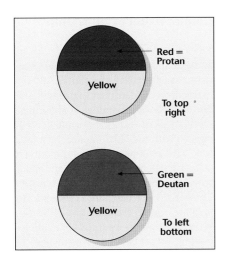

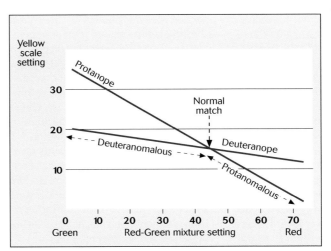

Figure 3.4
Graphic representation of diagnostic results obtained with the Nagel anomaloscope showing different matching ranges and yellow luminance values in protan and deutan colour deficiency

range and form two separate distributions. Protanomalous trichromats require significantly more red light in their colour mixture and deuteranomalous trichromats require more green. The extent of the matching range shows the severity of the discrimination deficit and, by inference, the alteration in sensitivity of the affected photopigment. Protanopes and deuteranopes have only one photopigment in the spectral range provided by the instrument and are able to match any red–green mixture ratio with yellow. The luminance of the yellow test field can be altered to obtain an exact match. Protanopes are distinguished from deuteranopes by the yellow luminance value for matches with pure red and pure green. Protanopes set the yellow luminance very low when matching pure red, but deuteranopes match pure red and pure green with approximately the same yellow luminance values (*Figure 3.4*). Quality audits, which compare performance with results obtained using the Nagel anomaloscope, have been carried out for the Ishihara plates, Ishihara test for Unlettered Persons, American Optical Company (HRR) plates, Farnsworth D15 test, City University test 2nd edition, the Farnsworth Munsell 100-hue test, Holmes–Wright Lanterns (A and B) and the Farnsworth Lantern.

Ishihara pseudoisochromatic plates

The Ishihara pseudoisochromatic plates were introduced in 1917. A large number of other pseudoisochromatic screening tests for red–green colour deficiency have been produced since that date, but none have achieved the accuracy of the Ishihara plates. The Ishihara test is currently used worldwide.

There are a number of different editions. The first fifteen editions are ranked in numerical order, but those published after 1962 are identified by the year of publication. The quality of colour reproduction varies slightly in different editions, but this does not affect the overall screening accuracy.[8] The full test has 38 plates (*Table 3.5*). Twenty-five plates have numerals and thirteen plates contain pathways. There is an Abridged test with 24 plates and a Concise test with 14 plates. The 38-plate test is preferred. A test for 'Unlettered Persons' is available; it has circles, squares and simplified pathways and is intended for the examination of children between 3 to 7 years of age.

Only about 50 per cent of colour-deficient people (usually protans) are able to see figures in 'hidden digit' designs. These plates can be omitted and only the 16 'transformation and vanishing' number plates used for screening (*Table 3.6*).[9] Transformation designs provide positive and vanishing designs provide negative evidence of colour deficiency. Almost 90 per cent of colour-deficient people make at least 12 errors on these 16 plates. Although the test is not intended to grade the severity, people with very slight colour deficiency make fewer than eight errors.

The serif design of the Ishihara numerals causes misreadings by some normals, who 'fill in' partial loops in the design. For

Table 3.5 Design and function of the 25 numeral plates of the 38-plate Ishihara test

Plates	Function	Intended design
1	Introduction	Seen correctly by all observers; demonstrates the visual task; identifies malingering
2–9 Transformation	Screening	A number is seen by colour normals and a different number is seen by red–green colour deficient; sometimes colour deficient see no number
10–17 Vanishing	Screening	A number is seen by colour-deficient, but cannot be seen by red–green colour deficient
18-21 Hidden digits*	(Screening)	A number cannot be seen by normals, but can be seen by red–green colour deficient
22-25 Classification Only used when screening plates identify colour deficiency	Classification of protan and deutan deficiency	Protans only see the number on the right side of each plate and deutans only see the number on the left If colour deficiency is identified by screening plates and both numbers are seen, classification can be obtained from comparing the relative contrast of the paired numbers; interpretation is as if the less clear number cannot be seen People with severe red–green colour deficiency, especially protanopes, cannot see either classification number

* These plates have poor sensitivity and specificity and should be omitted.

Table 3.6 Sensitivity, specificity and screening efficiency of the 16 transformation and vanishing plates of the Ishihara test

Number of misreadings by normals	Specificity (%)	Screening efficiency (overall predictive value)	Sensitivity (%)	Number of errors by red–green colour deficient
8	100	90.2	80.5	8
6	95.4	94.7	90.4	6
3	94.1	96.4	98.7	3

example, 5 may become 6, or 3 become 8. Misreadings on vanishing designs are not errors and should not be interpreted as a failure of the plate. However, completing partial loops on transformation designs may give an ambiguous result if the reported number is an amalgamation of the correct and transformed numerals. This type of misinterpretation is sometimes referred to as a 'partial error' and can be made by both normal and colour-deficient observers. Colour-deficient people invariably make clear errors on other plates and there is no uncertainty in the overall result. If misreadings and misinterpretations are placed in context, 100 per cent specificity and over 90 per cent sensitivity can be achieved.

The intended function of the Ishihara protan/deutan classification plates is not always realised. About 40 per cent of colour-deficient people identified by the screening plates are able to see both classification numerals. This result suggests a slight anomalous trichromacy. The correct classification is obtained, in 94 per cent, by asking the subject to compare the clarity of the numerals. Classification is obtained by assuming that the less clear numeral had not been seen. Severe colour deficiency, usually protanopia, is present when neither classification numeral can be seen.

Each plate of the test is exposed for a few seconds only and the subject must make an immediate verbal response. Undue hesitation suggests slight colour deficiency. In the 38-plate test, plates 26–38 contain pathways that are intended for the examination of non-verbal subjects. Drawing over these pathways takes too long for the design to be effective and these plates are not recommended. The Ishihara Test for Unlettered Persons is the recommended alternative. Good screening efficiency is also achieved with the Color Vision Testing Made Easy Test. This pseudoisochromatic test for very young children has vanishing geometric shapes, but can only be purchased in the USA.[10]

It is possible to shorten the 38-plate test to achieve more rapid screening using a minimum of six of the most efficient screening plates. The plates recommended are four transformation plates (plates 2, 3, 5 and 9) and two vanishing plates (plates 12 and 16). The introductory plate and a classification plate should also be included, to make eight plates in all. A different selection of plates is recommended for young children who have the ability to respond verbally to low numbers (*Table 3.7*). When the design has two numbers, a card can be placed over one side of the plate, so that these can be identified individually.

The American Optical Hardy, Rand and Rittler (AO HRR) plates (second edition)
The AO HRR plates were printed in 1954. The second edition is a re-release of the original test. The test is intended to identify protan, deutan, tritan and 'tetartan'

colour deficiency and to grade their severity. 'Tetartan' colour deficiency was first thought to originate from abnormalities of a fourth yellow-sensitive photopigment, but this type of colour deficiency does not exist and 'tetartan' designs are not needed. There are 24 plates with paired vanishing designs that contain geometric shapes (circle, cross and triangle). The shapes are printed in neutral colours on a background matrix of grey dots. The saturation of the neutral colours increases in successive plates to produce designs with progressively larger colour-difference steps. There are six plates for screening (four red–green and two tritan), 10 plates for grading the severity of protan and deutan defects and four plates for grading tritan defects.

The red–green screening plates of the HRR test have unacceptably low specificity and sensitivity. The value of the test is in confirming the classification of protan and deutan defects and in grading the severity of red–green colour deficiency when the Ishihara test is failed. Moderate and severe tritan colour deficiencies are also identified. However, only two grades of colour deficiency can be distinguished with certainty: slight (comprising the intended minimal and slight categories) and severe (comprising the intended moderate and severe categories). Protan/deutan classification is correctly realised for 95 per cent of colour-deficient subjects who fail the test.[11]

A third edition of the HRR plates was printed in 1991. Unfortunately, the original colours, particularly the deutan neutral colours, have not been correctly reproduced.

Hue-discrimination grading tests

A continuous range of severity occurs in anomalous trichromatism and there are no distinct subcategories. Identifying categories of severity therefore depends on the test design. Grading is achieved either by utilising ranked colour-difference steps, as in the HRR plates, or by designing tests with large colour differences that identify people with severe colour deficiency, but enable people with slight colour deficiency to pass without error. People with moderate colour deficiency often obtain borderline results and may either pass or fail 'on the day'. Grading tests incorporate different colour differences and different visual tasks and the pass/fail rate for people with moderate colour deficiency should not be expected to agree precisely.

Table 3.7 Recommended plates from the 38-plate Ishihara test for examining children

Plate	Design	Normal response	Red–green colour-deficient response
1	Introduction	1, 2	1, 2
6	Transformation	5	2
7	Transformation	3	5
10	Vanishing	2	–
14	Vanishing	5	–
24	Classification	3, 5	Protans see 5, deutans see 3

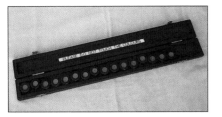

Figure 3.5
The Farnsworth D15 test

The Farnsworth D15 test

The Farnsworth D15 was introduced in 1947 and is used throughout the world as a grading test for occupational selection. The test is composed of Munsell hues of value 5 and chroma 4 from an almost complete hue circle. The subject has to arrange the 15 moveable hue samples into a natural colour sequence starting from a reference colour (*Figure 3.5*). The test divides people into two groups. The first group consists of people with normal colour vision and a slight colour deficiency who pass, and the second group consists of people with moderate and severe colour deficiency who fail. Farnsworth considered that the former would be able to use industrial colour codes safely and that the latter would be 'unsafe'. One transposition of adjacent colours is normally allowed as a pass. A single error of two or more colour steps is a fail. The colour arrangement made by the subject is drawn on a circular diagram that represents the hues. Isochromatic colour confusions give rise to lines that cross the diagram, showing that colours from opposite sides of the hue circle have been placed next to each other in the arrangement. The colour-difference steps are not uniform across the hue circle and isochromatic confusions with smaller steps are made more frequently. Two grades of deficiency (moderate or severe) can therefore be identified from the number of isochromatic confusions made (*Figure 3.6*).

Two desaturated versions of the D15 test are available. These have hues with Munsell value 5 and chroma 2 (Adams test) and Munsell value 8 and chroma 2 (Lanthony test). These tests are usually used to evaluate acquired colour deficiency.

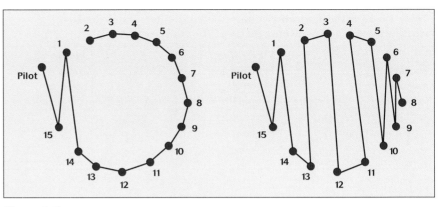

Figure 3.6
Examples of D15 results obtained in moderate and severe protan colour deficiency

The City University test (first and second editions)

The first and second editions of the City University test (TCU or CU test) are derived from the D15 test. Use of this test is mainly confined to the UK. There are 10 plates. Each plate displays a central colour and four peripheral colours. Subjects select the peripheral colour that looks most like the one in the centre. Three peripheral colours are typical isochromatic confusions with the central colour in protan, deutan and tritan deficiency. The fourth colour is an adjacent colour in the D15 sequence and is the intended normal preference. Like the D15, the CU test identifies moderate and severe colour deficiency only. People with slight colour deficiency pass without error.

The second edition has six of the original designs and four designs that contain desaturated Munsell colours. The desaturated designs do not effectively identify people with moderate colour deficiency who fail these plates only. A design problem of the CU test results in ambiguous protan/deutan classification in more than 60 per cent of people who fail the test. This is not 'mixed' colour deficiency as suggested in the test manual. The majority classification result gives the correct classification in 80 per cent of cases.[12] The number of errors is related to the severity of colour deficiency in deutans, but not in protans. Deutans who make five or more errors have severe colour deficiency (*Table 3.8*).

Similar colours are used in the D15 and CU tests, but the visual task is different. About the same percentage of colour-deficient people fail each test, but only 60 per cent of these subjects fail both.[12] More protans fail the D15 and more deutans fail the CU test. In spite of some limitations, the CU second edition is useful for identifying moderate and severe colour deficiency when a format other than the D15 is required.

The CU test third edition (1998) has different aims and includes entirely new designs intended for colour-vision screening. The visual task of the screening plates is to identify colours that look the same or different, and is not used in any other test. The parameters of the test design have not been published and there has been no audit of test performance. Only four of the six grading plates are reproduced from the first and second editions.

Vocational tests and colour-vision standards

Vocational tests aim to show practical hue-discrimination skills or the ability to identify colours correctly by name. Normal colour vision with good hue-discrimination ability is needed for work in colour-quality control in manufacturing industries and printing. Colour-vision standards are in place in other occupations for well-defined safety reasons, and when

Table 3.8 Grading severity of colour deficiency with the AO HRR plates, Farnsworth D15 test and the CU test

Ishihara plates	AO HRR plates (second edition)	Farnsworth D15 test	City University test (second edition)	Severity of red–green colour deficiency
Fail	Slight	Pass	Pass	Slight
Fail		Fail with partial errors	Fail with four* errors or less	Moderate
Fail	Severe	Fail with complete errors	Fail with five* errors or more	Severe
*Effective for deutans, but not protans.				

Table 3.9 Occupational colour-vision standards in the UK

Careers and occupations known to require normal colour vision

- Some branches of the Army and Royal Air Force (pilots, engineers, signals personnel) (*under review*)
- Royal Navy Officers and Watch Keepers; all submarine personnel
- Merchant Navy Officers and Watch Keepers
- Customs and Excise Officers
- Commercial airline pilots, aircraft engineers, airport technical and maintenance staff, air traffic controllers (NB: colour-vision standards in aviation and related industries are currently *under review*)
- Train drivers, rail-track engineers and rail-track maintenance staff
- Electrical and electronic engineers
- Hospital laboratory technicians, histopathology technicians and hospital pharmacists
- Workers in industrial colour-quality control (colour matchers, printers, workers in paper and textile manufacture)

Careers and occupations that have a colour vision entry standard

- Some branches of the Army, Royal Air Force and Royal Marines (*under review*)
- Fire service: slight deutans able to pass the D15 test are accepted
- Merchant Navy engineers: ability to pass the D15 test
- Police Service: people who obtain seven correct answers on the 10 plates of the CU test second edition are accepted (*under review*)
- Non-detailed electrical work: people able to pass the Farnsworth D15 test are usually accepted

accurate recognition of connotative, or important denotative, colour codes is needed.[13] Delayed reaction to a connotative colour code may be a safety hazard.

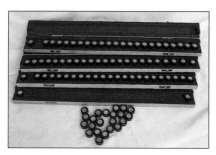

Figure 3.7
The Farnsworth–Munsell 100 hue test

Protans are particularly at risk because red lights and printed warnings have low visibility and the response time is significantly increased. Even so, all colour-deficient people have a right to expect that their needs are considered when new colour codes are introduced, if this can be achieved without compromising the performance of colour normals. For example, the red–green–black colour code for domestic electrical wiring was changed in the 1960s to be safe for all users. The CIE also selects the chromaticities of signal lights to give as much assistance as possible to colour-deficient users. Recent legislation also ensures that employment restrictions must be justified if challenged on the grounds of unequal employment

opportunity. This has prompted task analysis and review of vision standards in a number of occupations. Detailed investigation is needed to establish the level of hue discrimination required in the workplace. For example, a study was undertaken by the UK Home Office in 1996 to establish the colour-vision requirement for firefighters. This study investigated all the colour-coded material likely to be encountered by firefighters and set an appropriate revised colour-vision standard based on the evidence obtained. Other occupational colour-vision standards are currently under review (*Table 3.9*).

The Farnsworth–Munsell 100 hue test (F–M 100 hue)

The F–M 100 hue test was introduced in 1943 to examine hue-discrimination ability and to select people for work in colour-quality control. There are 85 Munsell hues selected from a complete hue circle. These are distributed in four boxes (*Figure 3.7*). Isochromatic colour confusions cannot be demonstrated because colours from opposite sides of the hue circle are not available at the same time. Hue-discrimination ability is estimated from the total error score and the type of colour deficiency is determined from the graphic representation of the results. Characteristic F–M 100 hue plots in congenital protan, deutan and tritan defects show concentrations of errors in two well-defined positions, which are nearly opposite in the polar diagram that represents the circle of hues where the hues are within an isochromatic zones. These positions occur where isochromatic zones are tangential to the hue circle (*Figure 3.8*). The combined effect is of an axis of confusion centred around particular caps (*Table 3.10*). The axis of confusion is more prominent in severe colour deficiency, which produces a higher error score. Protan and deutan error clusters tend to overlap and

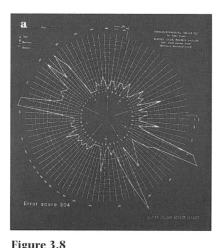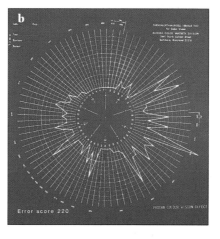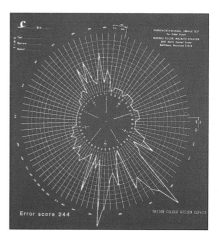

Figure 3.8
Examples of F–M 100 results in severe (a) protan, (b) deutan and (c) tritan colour deficiencies

Table 3.10 Position of the centre caps defining the axis of confusion on the Farnsworth–Munsell 100 hue test for congenital dichromats

Type	Mean position of the centre cap	Range
Protanopes	17	15–26
	64	58–68
Deuteranopes	15	12–17
	58	53–60
Tritanopes	5	4–6
	45.5	45–46

classification of the type of colour deficiency may be difficult to determine. Poor general hue discrimination is shown by random errors without an axis of confusion. Some recruitment personnel set an acceptable error score as the colour vision standard for the occupation. The F–M 100 hue test is widely used to evaluate acquired colour deficiency. The design is not based on typical colour confusions found in congenital colour deficiency and overall loss of hue discrimination can be identified. The scoring system enables changes in acquired colour deficiency to be monitored with time.[14]

Lantern tests

Lanterns were introduced in the 19th century as vocational tests to select applicants for occupations in the transport industries that required signal-light identification. Lanterns are well accepted by potential recruits because they appear to reproduce the visual task necessary in the occupation. Lanterns used in different countries are based on different design principles. Only the Holmes–Wright lanterns display specified signal-light colours. Safety considerations are paramount. The CIE currently approves use of the Holmes–Wright lanterns (UK), the Beyne lantern (France) and the Farnsworth lantern (USA). Only the Holmes–Wright lanterns and the Farnsworth Lantern (Falant) have been subjected to audit and the results validated in clinical trials.[15,16]

The Holmes–Wright lantern Type A shows nine pairs of colours separated vertically. The subject must name the colours seen. The colour pairs are separated horizontally in the Type B lantern. Both lanterns have two reds, two greens and white, which are CIE-specified signal-light colours. The lanterns are viewed at 6m (20ft). Detailed operating instructions are provided. The lanterns are no longer manufactured, but are robust and are likely to remain in service for the foreseeable future. These tests are carried out in specific examination centres.

The Holmes–Wright Lantern (Type A) is used by the UK Armed Services and the Civil Aviation Authority (CAA). There are two operational luminance settings and the test can be given in normal room illumination (approximately 200 lux) or following dark adaptation. Examiners can select either high or low luminance according to the occupational requirements. No errors are permitted. Low luminance in the dark is the most exacting visual task and some people with normal colour vision make errors because of night myopia. Effective colour-vision screening with 100 per cent specificity is obtained with high luminance in room lighting and in the dark. Sensitivity is slightly less than that obtained with the Ishihara plates.[15]

The Holmes–Wright lantern (Type B) is used by the Marine Coastguard and Safety Agency (previously the Board of Trade) to select personnel for the merchant marine service. The colours represent ships' lights at a distance of 2 miles and exactly match the recognition task undertaken by marine watch keepers. The Ishihara plates are the standard test for occupational selection and a lantern test is only given on appeal.

The Ishihara plates and the Holmes–Wright Lantern (Type A) are currently used to categorise colour perception in the UK armed services (*Table 3.11*). Colour-perception requirements vary with the branch of service. Aircraft pilots must obtain CP1. Engineers, signals officers, naval officers and submarine personnel require CP2. Young people considering a service career are strongly recommended to write to recruitment offices before they begin basic training and obtain written confirmation that they fulfil the requirements of the intended service.

The Farnsworth lantern (USA) shows larger pairs of colours than the Holmes–Wright Type A. The colours shown are desaturated red and green and yellow–white. These colours are not within the specifications for signal lights, but are selected specifically to be within isochromatic zones that promote colour confusions. There is only one luminance level and the lantern is viewed in room illumination. A score is derived from the number of errors made, which allows some people with moderate-to-slight colour deficiency to pass. The pass/fail level is poorly related to the performance on other grading tests, such as the Farnsworth D15.[16] A new version of the Farnsworth lantern, the Optec 900, is now available.

The Beyne lantern (France) shows single colours, derived from narrow wavelength bands, and white. The presentation is programmed and the viewing time is very short (about 2 seconds). No audit is available for this lantern. A new version of the Beyne lantern, the TriTest L3, is now available.

Table 3.11 Colour-perception (CP) classification for occupations in the armed forces

Colour-vision classification		Standard
CP1	Superior colour vision	No errors on the Holmes–Wright A lantern at low luminance in complete darkness at 6m (20ft)
CP2	Normal colour vision	Army and RAF: correct recognition of all the transformation and vanishing plates of the Ishihara test
		Royal Navy: correct recognition of 13 of the 16 transformation and vanishing plates of the 38-plate Ishihara test
CP3	Slight colour deficiency	No errors on the Holmes–Wright A lantern at high luminance in complete darkness at 6m (20ft)
CP4	Moderate colour deficiency	Army and RAF: unable to obtain CP3
		Royal Navy: correct recognition of coloured wires
CP5	Severe colour deficiency	Royal Navy only: unable to obtain CP4

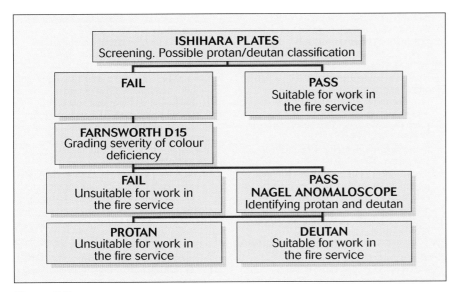

Figure 3.9
Colour-vision examination protocol to fulfil the standard for firefighting

International occupational colour-vision standards for transport

CIE recently revised the recommended colour-vision standards for national and international transport services (*Table 3.12*).[17] There are three standards based on the use of the Ishihara plate, lantern and Farnsworth D15 tests. Standard 2 suggests that people with a slight colour deficiency are able to pass a lantern test. This is not the case with the Holmes–Wright lantern Type A, unless a scoring system similar to that used with the Farnsworth lantern scoring is applied.

Protans are specifically excluded from occupations in transport because the delayed recognition of red is considered to be a safety hazard in all environments.[13]

Electronics and electrical industries

Colour coding is widespread in the electronics and electrical engineering industries and its correct use is needed for safety. There is no general colour-vision standard. Employers base their policies on the complexity of the work and either exclude all colour-deficient people who fail the Ishihara plate test or accept applicants who pass the D15. Considerable data support the intended use of the D15 test to select personnel for routine electrical work. However, it is important to consider career flexibility at the recruitment stage. An electrician with a slight colour deficiency may be required to undertake more detailed work, or may wish to transfer to another company, but be prevented from doing so because normal colour vision is needed. Applicants should be counselled about these limitations. No formal 'resistor wire test' exists, but some recruitment personnel make their own. While some tests, such as the one used by the Royal Navy, are carefully designed, others are not. No quality audit is possible. Poorly designed 'resistor wire tests' are ineffective for identifying a significant colour deficiency.

The police force

There is no national colour-vision standard for police forces in the UK. Individual forces have their own requirements, which reflect the ease of local recruitment. At present it is possible for candidates with a slight colour deficiency to 'shop around' for acceptance. This may cause problems if an officer wishes to transfer to another force. Police vehicle drivers, officers licensed to carry firearms and drug-enforcement officers must have normal colour vision. The Ishihara plate test is used for screening. In some forces candidates who are able to obtain correct results on seven out of 10 plates on the City University test (second edition) are accepted for training. This policy is currently under review. Severe colour deficiency is unacceptable in the police force because conflict of evidence, regarding the colour of clothing or vehicles, may prevent convictions in criminal cases.

The fire service

A new colour-vision standard was introduced for firefighters in 1996 as a result of a Home Office review.[18] Colour-deficient applicants are accepted if they pass the Farnsworth D15 test without error and have deutan colour deficiency. The standard is implemented with the Ishihara plate test (for screening), the D15 test and the Nagel anomaloscope. The anomaloscope is needed to confirm that people who pass the D15 are not protan (*Figure 3.9*). Protans are not accepted as firefighters because of possible difficulties identifying red traffic lights at night and because oxygen (black) and acetylene (maroon) gas cylinders may be confused in poor viewing conditions.

Table 3.12 CIE standards for colour vision in transport[17]

Standard 1: Normal colour vision

Normal colour vision is required for people in high-risk activities in which recognition of distant coloured signal lights and other codes is critical to safe operation; the Ishihara plate test is the recommended test

Standard 2: Slight colour deficiency

This standard applies to people in low-risk activities and people with deutan colour deficiency who demonstrate the ability to recognise signal colours at moderate distances; the recommended tests are the Ishihara plates, an approved colour-vision lantern and an anomaloscope to exclude protans

Standard 3: Slight–moderate colour deficiency

This standard passes people in low-risk activities who demonstrate the ability to recognise pigment colours; applicants who fail the Ishihara plate test must be able to pass the Farnsworth D15 test

REFERENCES

1 Mollon JD, Dulai KS and Hunt DM (1997). Dalton's colour blindness: An essay in molecular genetics. In *John Dalton's Colour Vision Legacy*, p. 15–33, Eds Dickinson C, Murray I and Carden D (London: Taylor and Francis).

2 Moddarres M, Mirsamadi M and Peyman GA (1996/7). Prevalence of congenital colour deficiency in secondary school children in Tehran. *Int Ophthalmol.* **20**, 221–222.

3 Neitz J, Neitz M and Jacobs GH (1991). Spectral tuning of pigments underlying red–green colour vision. *Science* **252**, 971–974.

4 Neitz J, Neitz M and Kainz PM (1996). Visual pigment gene structure and the severity of human color vision defects. *Science* **274**, 801–804.

5 Neitz J, Neitz M and Jacobs GH (1993). More than three different cone pigments among people with normal colour vision. *Vision Res.* **33**, 117–122.

6 Neitz M, Neitz J and Jacobs GH (1995) Genetic basis of photopigment variations in human dichromats. *Vision Res.* **35**, 2095–2103.

7 Weitz CJ, Went LN and Nathans J (1992). Human tritanopia associated with a third amino acid substitution in the blue-sensitive opsin. *Am J Hum Genet.* **51**, 444–446.

8 Birch J and McKeever LM (1993). Survey of the accuracy of new pseudoisochromatic plates. *Ophthalmol Physiol Opt.* **13**, 35–40.

9 Birch J (1997). Efficiency of the Ishihara plates for identifying red–green colour deficiency. *Ophthalmol Physiol Opt.* **17**, 403–408.

10 Cotter SA, Lee DY and French AL (1999). Evaluation of a new color vision test: 'Color Vision Testing Made Easy. *Optom Vis Sci.* **76**, 631–636.

11 Birch J (1997). Clinical use of the American Optical Company (Hardy, Rand and Rittler) pseudoisochromatic plates for red–green colour deficiency. *Ophthalmol Physiol Opt.* **17**, 248–254.

12 Birch J (1997). Clinical use of the City University test (2nd Edition). *Ophthalmol Physiol Opt.* **17**, 466–472.

13 Cole BL (1993). Does defective colour vision really matter? *Documents in Ophthalmology Procedings Series* 56, p. 67–86, Ed B. Drum. (Dortrecht: Kluwer).

14 Dain SJ and Birch J (1987). An averaging method for the interpretation of the Farnsworth Munsell 100 hue test. *Ophthalmol Physiol Opt.* **7**, 267–280.

15 Vingrys AJ and Cole BL (1983). Validation of the Holmes–Wright lanterns for testing colour vision. *Ophthalmol Physiol Opt.* **3**, 137–152.

16 Cole BL and Maddock JD (1998). Can clinical colour vision tests be used to predict the results of the Farnsworth Lantern test? *Vision Res.* **38**, 3483–3485.

17 CIE (2001). *International Recommendations for Colour Vision Requirements for Transport.* Technical Report (CIE 143-2001).

18 Margrain TH, Birch J and Owen CG (1996). Colour vision requirements of firefighters. *Occup Med.* **46**, 114–124.

Multiple-choice questions, Section 1

There is one correct answer per question. The answers are given at the end of the book.

1 A patient reads all the letters on a logMAR chart down to the 0.1 line and two letters on the line below. Their logMAR score would be:
A 0.3
B 0.12
C 0.06
D 0.14
E −0.2

2 The logMAR equivalent of 6/9 is:
A 0.176
B 0.214
C 0.182
D 0.122
E 0.163

3 Visual acuity obtained using a letter chart (90 per cent contrast) can be estimated from the contrast sensitivity function (CSF; see *Figure 1.4*) by examining:
A The intersection of the CSF with the *x*-axis.
B The peak of the CSF.
C The intersection of the CSF with the *y*-axis.
D The intersection between the CSF and a horizontal line passing through 1.11 on the contrast sensitivity scale.
E The intersection between the CSF and a horizontal line passing through 0.90 on the contrast sensitivity scale.

4 The contrast of a sine wave grating (as defined by the Michelson equation) ranges from:
A 0 to 10
B 0 to 1
C 1 to 100
D 0 to 100
E 0 to 1000

5 The Pelli–Robson chart measures:
A Visual acuity at low contrasts.
B Contrast sensitivity for one spatial frequency.
C A contrast sensitivity function.
D Contrast sensitivity for one contrast.
E Two points on the contrast sensitivity function.

6 A contrast sensitivity function shows a loss of sensitivity at low spatial frequencies and normal sensitivity at high spatial frequencies. State which of the following is true:
A High-contrast visual activity (VA) and Pelli–Robson contrast sensitivity (CS) will be reduced.
B High- and low-contrast VA will be reduced.
C High-contrast VA will be reduced, but low-contrast VA will be normal.
D High-contrast VA will be reduced, but Pelli–Robson CS will be normal.
E High-contrast VA will be normal, but Pelli–Robson CS will be reduced.

7 State which of the following statements is true:
A Cathode ray tube (CRT) monitors are capable of producing 100 per cent contrast.
B Eye movements cause raster-scanned screens to appear to flicker.
C The luminance of CRT monitors is not high enough to present test-chart stimuli.
D CRT monitors do not have adequate resolution to present test-chart stimuli.
E CRT monitors cannot display coloured images.

8 State which of the following statements is true:
A Thin-film transistor (TFT) flat panel liquid-crystal displays (LCDs) are raster scanned.
B TFT flat panel LCDs can only produce low contrast images.
C TFT flat panel LCDs do not flicker.
D TFT flat panel LCDs cannot display coloured images.
E Eye movements cause TFT flat panel LCDs to appear to flicker.

9 The logMAR equivalent of 6/6 is:
A 0
B 1
C 0.1
D −1
E 0.6

10 A patient reads all of the letters on the 0 logMAR row and three letters on the line below. Their logMAR score would be:
A 3
B 0.6
C −0.03
D 0.06
E −0.06

11 A patient has reduced contrast sensitivity (CS) for high spatial frequencies, but normal CS for low spatial frequencies. State which of the following statements is true:
A High-contrast visual acuity (VA) will be normal and Pelli–Robson CS will be reduced.
B High-contrast VA will be normal and Pelli–Robson CS will be normal.
C High-contrast VA will be reduced and Pelli–Robson CS will be reduced.
D High-contrast VA will be reduced and Pelli–Robson CS will be normal.
E High-contrast VA will be normal, but the patient will report poor vision.

12 **Patients with various neurological conditions, such as glaucoma, optic neuritis and multiple sclerosis, sometimes show a reduction in contrast sensitivity to low and intermediate spatial frequencies while maintaining good sensitivity to high spatial frequencies. In these cases, state which of the following statements is false:**

- A High-contrast visual acuity (VA) will be normal.
- B Low-contrast VA will be normal.
- C Pelli–Robson contrast sensitivity will be reduced.
- D Low-contrast VA will be reduced.
- E High-contrast VA will be normal, but the patient will report poor vision.

13 **What is the prevalence of protan colour deficiency in females?**

- A 0.01 per cent.
- B 0.03 per cent.
- C 0.04 per cent.
- D 0.10 per cent.
- E 0.30 per cent.

14 **Which combination of colour vision tests are recommended to implement CIE colour vision Standard 3?**

- A The Ishihara plates and the Farnsworth D15 test.
- B The Ishihara plates and the Holmes–Wright Lantern Type A.
- C The Farnsworth D15 test and the Holmes–Wright Lantern Type A.
- D The Ishihara plates and the Holmes–Wright Lantern Type B.
- E The Farnsworth Munsell 100-hue test and the Holmes–Wright Lantern Type.

15 **Which of the following colour combinations are not confused by protanopes?**

- A Yellow and red.
- B Purple and grey.
- C Brown and green.
- D Orange and yellow.
- C Green and violet.

16 **Which of the following statements is false?**

- A Women who are mixed-compound heterozygotes have normal colour vision.
- B Specificity is the percentage of normals correctly identified as normal.
- C Typical monochromats rarely have nystagmus.
- D John Dalton was a deuteranope.
- E Neutral colours are used to classify types of colour deficiency.

17 **Which of the following statements is true?**

- A The Farnsworth Lantern shows pairs of signal colours.
- B Congenital tritan defects are inherited as an autosomal recessive trait.
- C The majority of fovea cones contain middle wavelength sensitive (green) photopigment.
- D Colours specified within a specific isochromatic zone are confused.
- E Fifty percent of the daughters of females who are heterozygous for X-linked traits are also heterozygous.

18 **Which of the following statements concerning the Nagel anomaloscope is untrue?**

- A The Nagel anomaloscope is used to grade the severity of colour deficiency.
- B The Nagel anomaloscope is the reference test for diagnosing all different types of colour deficiency.
- C The Nagel anomaloscope is used in clinical trials to ensure that colour-deficient people taking part are representative of the colour-deficient population as a whole.
- D The Nagel anomaloscope is sometimes used as part of a battery of colour vision tests used to select recruits to the UK fireservice.
- E The Nagel anomaloscope presents a Rayleigh match (red + green = yellow).

Section 2

ASSESSMENT OF THE EYE

4

Principles of the slit-lamp biomicroscope

Kamlesh Chauhan

Introduction

Of the instrumentation available to the optometrist, the slit lamp is arguably the most adaptable. Fitted with the appropriate attachments, all the ocular structures of the eye can be clearly viewed. Measurements of the thickness of ocular structures and intraocular pressure can be made, corneal sensitivity can be assessed and ocular photography can be performed. In ophthalmology, the slit lamp is used in the delivery of laser therapy for various eye disorders. It is necessary that the principles and use of this most versatile instrument be well understood by the clinician. This chapter attempts to explain the basic principles of the instrument and gives an idea of common viewing techniques.

Principles

A compound binocular microscope, an illumination system and the mechanics that link the two make up the modern instrument (*Figure 4.1*). In normal usage the illumination system and the microscope should be focused in the same plane. The slit lamp in its current form has changed little, in principle, since 1933, when Goldmann devised a method of mechanically linking the observation and illumination system on a common pivot and stage. This was a critical progression since, prior to this, the illuminating system and microscope had to be directed and focused independently.

A few moments spent considering the difficulties of this should enable the reader to appreciate the significance of this progression. Key clinicians and scientists in ophthalmology had developed, prior to this, several important aspects of this evolution that are taken for granted. Perhaps the most significant of these was the use of the Koeller illumination system to image accurately and focus a uniformly bright slit on the eye.

The microscope

Slit lamps use binocular microscopes with magnifications of between about 5 and 40×. Ideally, the microscope should have excellent resolution and a good depth-of-field (DOF). Unfortunately, however, these two factors are inversely linked, so that good resolution leads to poor DOF. Therefore, a compromise has to be reached. Note that although magnification is an important aspect of the microscope, it is by no means the most important. A greatly magnified but unclear image is of little benefit. The resolution of the microscope is perhaps the most important factor, although resolution and magnification beyond the resolution capability of the eye yield no greater benefit. Increasing the magnification to very high levels is counter-productive, since small, involuntary eye movements will render the image too unstable to view. The resolution of the microscope is governed by its numerical aperture (NA), which in turn depends on the:

- diameter of the objective (the bigger the better);
- working distance (the shorter the better);
- refractive index of the medium between the objective lenses and examined eye (the higher the better); and
- wavelength of light (the shorter the better).

Improving the NA appears to be a simple option, so that the above factors are increased or decreased accordingly. Unfortunately, doing this has negative effects as well:

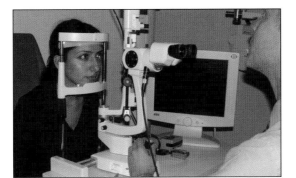

Figure 4.1
Slit-lamp examination is an integral part of a full eye examination and it is essential to set up the instrument correctly

- increasing the diameter of the aperture leads to aberrations at the edge of the lens, but improving the optics to reduce this helps considerably;
- decreasing the working distance means that the patient might feel very uncomfortable with such proximity and, additionally, the positioning of supplementary equipment (e.g., a Volk lens) between the microscope and the eye will be hindered;
- it would be impractical to place a fluid such as oil (to increase the refractive index) between the patient's eye and the microscope objective; and
- using short-wavelength light is possible, although this affects the colour-rendering properties of the eye.

The illumination system

The illumination system is a short-focus projector. The system projects a uniform bright image of a mechanical slit on to the plane of focus. This is not a simple task, since the quality of the slit formation is paramount to the quality of the instrument. The ability to project a very sharp and very thin undistorted slit is crucial to obtaining a *bona fide* view of some of the structures of the eye.

The spectral transmission of the source is also important. The higher the colour temperature of the source the better it is to view small particles, for example the flare from aqueous cells or the endothelium in a corneal section. This is because the scatter of light from these structures (scatter of light is the principal method by which they become visible) is related to the inverse of the wavelength of light. So the shorter the wavelength the greater the scatter and the more visible the structures. Clearly, the light used has to be within the visible spectrum. As the structure to be observed becomes progressively larger, the scatter becomes less dependent on the wavelength. It must also be remembered that the light must give a good colour rendering, since some diseases lead to subtle colour changes that would be missed if the colour rendering of the source was poor.

Focusing and setting up

The slit lamp consists of two systems that should have a common focal plane lying in the same plane as the mechanical pivot of the two systems. In most slit lamps this is the centre of the hole in the pivot (*Figure 4.1*). The illumination system has a fixed focus that cannot normally be altered by the user, whereas the focus of the microscope can be varied by adjusting the eyepieces. This is useful to practitioners who wear spectacles because they may choose to remove them when using the microscope, a recommended practice as moving closer to the eyepieces gives a greater field of view (FOV). However, if this leaves large amounts of uncorrected astigmatism it may be better to keep the spectacles on. Some users might have anisometropia, which will require the user to reflect the degree of anisometropia when focusing the eyepieces. Even users who consider themselves emmetropic should appreciate that the 'zero' settings on the eyepieces will not take into account instrument myopia, which could leave the slit lamp inaccurately focused. It is therefore recommended that all users focus the eyepieces prior to use, rather than adjusting the eyepieces to their known refractive error.

Ideally, the slit lamp should be focused by placing the focusing rod in the hole of the pivot (*Figure 4.1*), switching the lamp on and then rotating the eyepieces so that they produce maximum plus. The focused slit should be viewed through the eyepieces one at a time. The true grainy appearance of the focusing rod will be blurred initially, but as the amount of plus power in the eyepieces is reduced it will become clear. As soon as it becomes clear the eyepieces should not be rotated further, as this just causes the user to accommodate. To increase the accuracy of focusing, the magnification of the microscope should be set high, as this requires a greater amount of accommodation to make the rod surface clearer and therefore the critical point of focus can be determined more accurately.

When both eyepieces have been focused, their separation should be adjusted to allow a comfortable and clear binocular view of the focusing rod surface. It has been suggested that it is quicker and simpler to focus the eyepieces on the patient's eyelid. Although this is a useful method in the absence of a focusing rod, it is fraught with inaccuracy and is a lengthier process. The inaccuracies initially result from having to move the entire slit lamp forward and backward until the slit is focused correctly. The point of accurate focus is judged when no parallax is achieved by rotating the illumination system from side to side.[1] This can be a hard point to judge because the eyelid is curved and so the plane of focus of the slit will be accurate only on a portion of the lid. Furthermore, if the slit lamp is accidentally moved or the patient moves once the slit has been focused, it will go out of focus and therefore the microscope will be focused incorrectly.

In a correctly focused and coupled instrument, rotating the microscope or illumination system about the pivot results in neither going out of focus with respect to each other. This means that the angle (the separation angle) between the systems can be altered without loss of focus (*Figure 4.2*). The instrument can be uncoupled so that the two systems can be directed at different areas of the observed eye. This means that they will no longer both be focused at the plane of the pivot, as shown in *Figure 4.2*. The ability to uncouple a slit lamp is useful and is discussed later in this chapter.

The slit-lamp routine

A slit-lamp routine is something that a practitioner develops over time and varies according to the particular patient and the presenting history and symptoms. A general routine, however, or perhaps one that an inexperienced practitioner should initially follow, is described below. It is by no means prescriptive and may be used in part or adapted to individual taste. As a rule-of-thumb, though, it is best to start off with an overview of the eye and then follow with the finer details.

An overview of the eye

It is possible to obtain an overview of the eye by using a relatively broad slit and scanning across the eye in a zigzag fashion, starting with the upper lid and lashes, then across the bulbar conjunctiva and cornea, and finally across the lower lid and lashes. This is fine, but still presents a sequential view of the eye. A more elegant method is to use a diffuser and sufficient magnification so that the whole eye and immediate adnexa can be viewed at the same time. The diffuser enables uniform illumination over the whole eye and allows the practitioner to ask the patient to look in different directions to view the entire eye. Diffuse illumination is also a good technique with which to assess the fit of contact lenses, as the movement of the whole lens can be viewed with equal clarity. Additionally, if relatively low magnification is used, for example approximately 5×, this allows a large DOF and ensures all areas of the contact lens are in focus as well. Any features of interest noted by using diffuse illumination can then be viewed with more 'specialised' techniques to enhance the view of the particular feature. Another technique that allows an overview of the clarity of the cornea is sclerotic scatter, which could be the next technique to use in a routine.

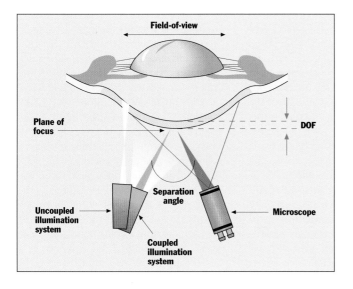

Figure 4.2
The basic set-up of a slit lamp. The observation and illumination systems are focused at the same point and plane, and the point of focus lies directly above the pivot of the two systems. The shaded illumination system shows how, when the instrument is uncoupled, it can be directed and focused at a different point from the microscope. The figure also illustrates the field-of-view (FOV) – the extent of the eye seen through the microscope – and the depth-of-field (DOF), which indicates the depth over which adequate focus of the viewed structure is possible. Note that the DOF and FOV reduce as the magnification is increased

Sclerotic scatter

The principle of this technique is that of total internal reflection.[2] A focused slit of about 1–2mm is directed at the temporal limbal area at an angle of about 40–60° to the normal to the patient's corneal apex. The height of the slit should be around 4mm or 5mm. This ensures that most of the light striking the limbus enters the cornea, rather than impinges on the sclera. Further, the 'extra' light that strikes the sclera serves as a glare source and reduces the contrast of any detail seen on the cornea. The light enters the corneal–limbal boundary and then reflects within the cornea. Total internal reflection occurs throughout the cornea, and only when the light strikes the relatively opaque limbus does it emerge from the cornea. This means that a halo of light is seen around the cornea. If there is a significant local change in the refractive index of the cornea the light is scattered from this region. Oedematous areas or scarred areas of the cornea scatter light, which facilitates their detection. The scattered light appears bright against the dark background of either the pupil or iris, although this will, to a degree, depend on the colour of the iris. If the area of differing refractive index is small it is difficult to notice the minor scatter. To maximise the ability to see any scatter the ambient illumination (room lights, etc.) should be kept as low as possible. This darkens the appearance of the iris and pupil and thus allows greater contrast if light is scattered from within the cornea.

It can be argued that the sclerotic scatter should be viewed from the side of the microscope with a naked eye rather than through the microscope. Looking through the microscope results in an inaccurate focus, since the viewer might be looking at the apical area of the cornea, while the microscope, in a coupled and correctly focused slit lamp, will be focused at the level of the limbus. Although this is undeniably true, if the magnification of the microscope is low, then the DOF might be sufficient to allow a clear view of the apical area as well as the limbal area.

If higher magnification is to be used in this technique, then uncoupling of the slit lamp is required. To do this, firstly a slit with a width of about 1–2mm is directed at the apex of the cornea and focused. The separation angle should be between 40 and 60°. Accuracy of focusing can be checked by asking the patient to blink and ensuring that the tear debris is visible as it floats up and down in accordance with the lid movements. Once this has been achieved, and ensuring that the microscope and patient do not move, the illumination system is uncoupled and the slit directed towards the limbus. When the slit strikes the limbus, a halo of light becomes apparent. Viewing through the microscope now allows an accurate focus on the apex of the cornea. The limbal area will be relatively out of focus. Ideally, this technique should be used with low magnification and with the microscope focused at the apex of the cornea, and the instrument uncoupled. Remember, however, that the limbal area might be out of focus. Since oedema is more prevalent at the apex of the cornea, this bias can be justified. If a corneal lesion has been noted by sclerotic scatter or diffuse illumination, or indeed a lesion in any part of the eye, the use of direct illumination might be appropriate.

Direct illumination

This is a simple method of viewing, in which the object of interest is illuminated by the slit and viewed through the microscope. This method is good for relatively high-contrast objects, for example the puncta or eyelashes, but for low-contrast objects, for example corneal scarring, it is difficult to view the object because of glare from the relatively bright reflection from the corneal surface. In this instance, it is usually better to have the beam of light to one side of the object of interest and view it illuminated by light scattered by the cornea. Provided the FOV is large enough to allow this, and the plane of the object to be viewed is not very different from the focused slit, a good indirect view is obtained. This indirect method of viewing is also useful in many other types of illumination.

A derivative of direct focal illumination is to view sections of the cornea and lens (*Figure 4.3*). This involves directing a thin slit of light at an angle into the cornea. The differing surfaces of the cornea, depending on their refractive indices, scatter light to

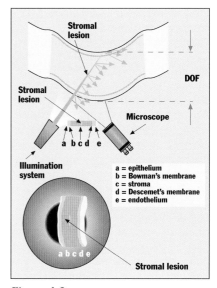

Figure 4.3
Formation of a corneal section

corresponding degrees. This scattered light is viewed through the microscope and is seen as a section through the cornea (*Figure 4.3*). In the case of the crystalline lens, the different layers have different refractive indices and they also scatter light accordingly. Since older lenses have more layers, a greater number of surfaces at which the scatter occurs are visible. In a cataractous lens, there is a very large change in refractive index and, as a result, the cataract is easily differentiated from the rest of the lens. This is by far the best way to classify a cataract in terms of its location within the lens.

The clarity of a section is determined predominantly by the width of the slit. The thinner that the slit is, the better the quality of the section. The reduction in slit width requires the brightness of the slit to be increased. Depending on the make of slit lamp, the slit width might have to be increased to counter-balance the reduction in brightness, even if the brightness of the bulb has been increased to its maximum. The quality of the slit lamp determines how accurately and brightly a thin slit can be formed without distortion occurring at its edges. To view the section at its best it is advisable to increase the brightness of the lamp to its maximum when the slit width has been minimised. After this, increasing the separation angle enables a broader section to be viewed. Additionally, particularly at high magnification, and therefore low DOF, not all of the section is in focus. Since the cornea is curved, either the apex is in focus or the limbal area is in focus. It is best, then, to reduce the height of the slit to about 4mm when viewing the section under high magnification. Additional benefits of this are that it reduces glare from the out-of-focus portions and reduces the amount of light that enters the patient's eye.

Although all the layers of the cornea can be seen in one view, at high magnification and with a large separation angle, slight focusing movements of the instrument might be needed to focus on the different layers. With the considerably thicker crystalline lens it is unlikely that all the layers will be in focus simultaneously, except at small separation angles and low magnifications. This is particularly the case if the observer has a relatively small amplitude of accommodation. It is likely that focusing movements of the slit lamp will be necessary to view the different layers. Each boundary is seen as a bright layer, and the cataractous layers are particularly bright, as they represent boundaries with the greatest change in refractive index. To produce a section, the slit is

focused at the cornea, which automatically puts the slit into approximate focus. The slit may then be viewed through the microscope and focused accurately by viewing the tear-film debris. The separation angle at this stage should be about 30°. Once focused, the slit width should be reduced to its minimum and the brightness increased, at which point the section should be visible. To improve the view the height of the slit should be reduced, the separation angle increased and the magnification increased. Fine focusing movements will be required depending on how still the patient keeps and whether slightly different layers of the cornea need to be observed.

If a section of the crystalline lens needs to be viewed, the magnification and separation angle should be reduced. If the corneal section is still in view and the FOV allows the pupil to be visible, a dull grey, out-of-focus section of the lens should be visible within the pupil. To focus the lens, the instrument needs to be moved towards the patient. Adjustments to the separation angle might be required to keep the section in view. The separation angle required is dependent on the size of the pupil and whether the front or back portion of the lens needs to be in focus. The smaller the patient's pupil, the narrower the separation angle required. The further posterior the section needs to be, the smaller the separation angle required.

Sometimes it is useful to be able to obtain a view of the section and gain an idea of the surface features on the cornea or lens. This may be achieved by widening the slit width once a good section has been established. A loss in detail of the layers of the cornea or lens results, but gives an impression of the surface quality of the structure. A three-dimensional view of the structure is obtained and is called a parallelepiped. This is a good way to scan across the cornea, as it enables the viewer to assess the approximate depth of any feature seen on either corneal surface. A quick reduction in the slit width allows a more accurate assessment of depth, if required. The technique, although possible to perform with the crystalline lens, is perhaps less useful

Specular reflection
Occasionally when a section is formed an annoying bright reflex is observed superimposed on the section. In fact, if a corneal section is formed to the side of where the illumination system lies, a reflex off the cornea is seen (1st and 2nd Purkinje images). If the section of the cornea is moved, by moving the entire instrument

across towards the side of the illuminating system, the section can be made to lie on top of the reflex (*Figure 4.4*). Alternatively, a section can be made and then the illumination system rotated towards the microscope, without moving the microscope, until the Purkinje images fall on the section. When this occurs, a bright light is seen on either side of the corneal section. The one on the epithelial side is a bright white light and the one to the endothelial side is a more yellow-to-golden colour. The second of these reflections represents the reflection off the endothelium. As a quick check it can be noted that these bright reflexes are only visible from one eyepiece of the microscope.

To view the reflection of the endothelium in more detail, the slit width can be widened (a corresponding reduction in brightness is advised and a reduction in the slit height is a good idea as the endothelium will not be visible along the entire height of the slit). Once the slit has been widened the magnification may then be increased to permit a better view of the endothelial surface. Slight adjustments of the illuminating system position and to-and-fro movements of the instrument will be required to keep the view clear. The ability to see surfaces by specular reflection

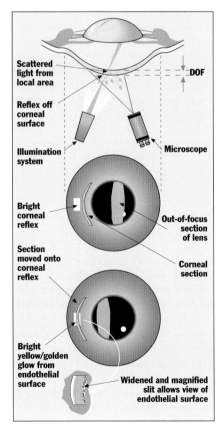

Figure 4.4
Method for obtaining specular reflection of the endothelium

occurs because the reflecting surface is not perfectly smooth. Light is reflected at different angles, which allows the integrity of the surface to be assessed. Clearly, light that is not reflected back towards the microscope gives the impression of dark areas compared to those areas that reflect light into the microscope objective.

A procedure commonly used when attempting to view the endothelium or the anterior surface of the crystalline lens is to place the microscope and illuminating systems on either side of the centre of the eye (*Figure 4.5*). Although it is possible to do this, it is by no means necessary. It is not true that this is the only method to ensure that the angle of incidence (angle of the illuminating system) is equal to the angle of reflection (angle of the microscope). Although these angles do have to be equal, and this is indeed the reason why only one ocular can collect the light reflected from the surface, this straight-ahead position is not the only way to achieve this. Since the cornea is a curved surface, the normal to the cornea alters and the angles around the normal also change. It is thus possible to achieve specular reflection of the endothelium while the microscope is directly in front of the eye (*Figure 4.5*).

The anterior capsule of the crystalline lens may also be viewed in this way. This generates the so-called 'orange-peel effect'. The procedure for viewing the capsule surface is the same as that for the endothelial surface, except that the section of the crystalline lens has to be established rather than that of the cornea, and the reflection from the anterior surface of the lens has to be viewed. The separation angle has to be narrow compared to that when the endothelium is viewed. This reduction in angle is dependent on the size of the pupil (the smaller the pupil, the narrower the separation angle) and is also necessitated by the refraction at the cornea. The posterior capsule may also be viewed in this way when the reflection from it has to be examined. The separation angle in this case is narrower still, this time because of the additional refraction of the lens. This is quite a good technique for examining the capsule for signs of opacification, which is particularly disruptive to vision owing to its proximity to the nodal point. In some eyes the surface of the anterior vitreous may also be seen in this fashion.

Retro-illumination

On occasions it is useful to view objects illuminated from behind rather than from directly in front, such as when viewing the corneo-limbal vasculature (*Figures 4.6* and *4.7*) and the corneal nerves. Viewing these structures with direct illumination can be difficult because of the glare caused by the source of light. Although indirect viewing might be of benefit in such instances, another method is also available: retro-illumination. As the name suggests, this technique involves illuminating the object of interest from a light source behind it. It is not possible to place a source in the eye to illuminate any structures in front of it. However, the reflective nature of some structures of the eye can be used to generate a secondary diffuse source of illumination from within the eye. The most obvious structure is the fundus. We have all experienced the orange glow seen within the pupil when using the slit lamp. Here the light that enters the eye strikes the retina and is diffusely reflected back through the pupil. Any structure that does not allow the light to pass back out of the eye creates a shadow that is seen as a dark area against an orange background. Hence cataracts appear black against the orange background.

During a slit-lamp examination the diffuse reflector is often the iris. Light is directed onto the iris and the reflected light is used to view objects, typically the cornea, anterior to it. It is a misconception that when performing retro-illumination the slit lamp has to be uncoupled. Uncoupling is necessary only when the area of the cornea being viewed is towards the apex, the separation angle is large, high magnification is used and the beam width is narrow (*Figure 4.7*). For small separation angles and areas close to the limbus, the cornea can be viewed in retro-illumination without uncoupling. In

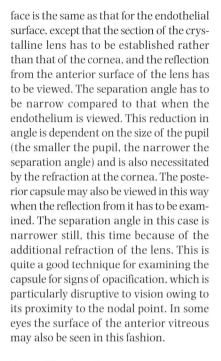
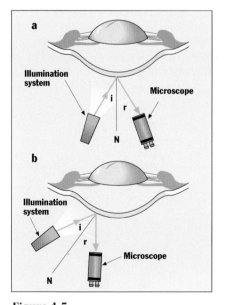

Figure 4.5
Positioning of the microscope and illumination system in specular reflection. (a) Required position if the apical area of the cornea is to be viewed. (b) Move the system round to view other areas. Note how the reflection angle (r) and incident angle (i) remain equal

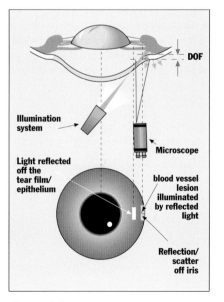

Figure 4.6
Retro-illumination to view corneal vasculature near the limbus. In this area, uncoupling of the limbus is not necessary

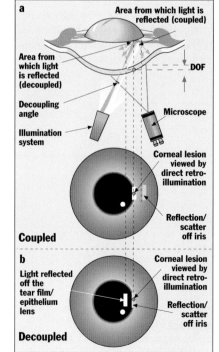

Figure 4.7
Retro-illumination to view an object away from the limbal area of the cornea

Figure 4.7, in which the light from the source is directed towards the edge of the cornea as it strikes the iris, the light is reflected diffusely and scattered. This secondary source then illuminates that area of the cornea from behind. Since the distance from the iris to the cornea is small in this area, the DOF of the microscope, with the accommodation of the observer (if available), enables the cornea to be in focus. This can be further facilitated if the microscope is focused at the level of the cornea and indirect viewing is used to view the object. For areas close to the apex of the cornea and with large separation angles there is a need to uncouple the instrument.

Figure 4.7 shows how this can be achieved. Initially the microscope, and therefore the slit in a coupled instrument, is directed at the object of interest (*Figure 4.7a*). At this stage, if a narrow slit is used, light reflected from the cornea is seen (on the object of regard) and a further light is seen reflecting off the iris. Now, keeping the microscope in the same position, the instrument is uncoupled and the illumination system re-directed so that the position at which the corneal reflex was initially seen is taken by the reflection off the iris (*Figure 4.7b*). The microscope is still focused on the object of interest, but now the object is illuminated from behind. Retro-illumination is also a useful technique with which to discover the nature of any foreign body within the cornea. If it is relatively opaque, then when light is shone directly at it, it reflects light. When it is illuminated from behind, the reflected light is not able to pass through and the foreign body appears dark. If the refractive index of the foreign body is similar to the surrounding tissue, the light passes through it and thereby it appears relatively light. This gives an idea of how solid or opaque the body is.

Retro-illumination is also a useful technique with which to view the limbal and/or corneal vasculature. The method is described above and depicted in *Figure 4.6*. Note that the technique is easier to perform on light-coloured irides, particularly green. The reason for this is that the reflected light is predominantly green, and therefore approaching red-free, thereby improving the contrast of the blood. Further, since the background against which the blood vessels are being viewed is also green the contrast is further enhanced. If the same is attempted with a brown iris, the contrast of the blood vessels is comparatively poor.

Further techniques

Assessment of the anterior chamber angle and depth

This assessment is usually carried out using van Herick's technique[3] or the less well-known Smith's technique,[4] both of which are covered in more detail in Chapter 6.

Conical beam and conic section

This technique basically directs a conical volume of light into the eye. In essence it is not dissimilar to forming a section, except that a broader width but shorter height of slit is used. This technique is useful to check for aqueous flare that might occur, for example, in anterior uveitis. When the ambient lighting is as low as possible the cone of light is directed into the eye. A bright reflex off the cornea is seen and a reflex off the lens or iris is also present. The area between the two reflexes should be dark. If any scattering of light is seen, rather like the sparkle that occurs in the beam of a cinema projector, this indicates inflammatory materials within the aqueous. This scatter from particles is termed Tyndall's effect. When performing this technique the slit height should be about 3–4mm. Rather than a slit, a circular aperture is used. The beam should come into focus somewhere within the anterior chamber, which means that in a coupled instrument the microscope should be focused in this plane.

Provided a good balance between magnification and DOF is used, the entire depth of the chamber should be in focus. The entire area of the anterior chamber may then be scanned to check for inflammatory material, although it is likely (because of gravity) that it will, predominantly, be in the inferior portion. It might, in fact, be wise to ask the patient to look up and then straight ahead, as this causes the settled material to rise from the bottom and then resettle. The resettling material is easier to detect.

Summary

The principles of the slit lamp are described here and a guide to performing the common techniques is given. As with many clinical techniques, it is best to practice the methods shown and to develop one's own routine in using the slit lamp. More specific applications of these techniques in clinical situations are discussed in Chapter 5.

REFERENCES
1   Morris J and Stone J (1997). *The Slit-lamp Biomicroscope in Optometric Practice.* (Fleet: Association of Optometrists/Optometry Today).

2   Freeman MH (1990). *Optics*, 10th edn (Oxford: Butterworth–Heinemann).
3   van Herick W, Shaffer R N and Schwartz A (1969). Estimation of width of anterior chamber. Incidence and significance of the narrow angle. *Am J Ophthalmol.* **68**, 626–629.

4   Smith RJH (1979). A new method of estimating the depth of the anterior chamber. *Br J Ophthalmol.* **63**, 215–220.

5

Clinical use of the slit-lamp biomicroscope

Andrew Franklin

The slit-lamp biomicroscope has become increasingly important in recent years. They were rarely found in practice 20 years ago, and even 10 years ago contact lenses were being fitted without recourse to the instrument. To do so now would be regarded as eccentric at best, and the widespread use of indirect binocular ophthalmoscopy with the Volk lens has made the slit-lamp biomicroscope arguably the most important instrument in the practice of optometry.

It is therefore unfortunate that many candidates for optometry professional examinations appear to have only a rudimentary grasp of the principles and skills involved. The purpose of this chapter is to examine the use of the slit-lamp biomicroscope in optometric practice. Traditionally, first the various types of illumination that can be set up are considered, and then applications for which a particular type of illumination is used are examined. The intention here is to approach from the opposite viewpoint, from application to technique, by considering various contexts in which biomicroscopes are used. The chapter considers the examination of the ocular surface and adnexa, which is similar in both general and contact lens practice, and the examination of the cornea with particular reference to contact lens practice. Other topics covered include examination of the anterior chamber, the lens and the anterior vitreous.

Basic design

As discussed in more detail in Chapter 4, the slit-lamp biomicroscope consists of an illumination system and an observing system linked in such a way that they normally share a focal point and a coincident centre of rotation. Horizontal traverse, both forwards and backwards and side to side, is controlled by a joystick. The joystick may also control vertical traverse (which allows the observer a free hand for the manipulation of eyelids or supplementary devices) or a separate control may be provided.

The illumination system

Nearly all slit lamps employ the Koeller (Vogt's) illumination system, developed from Gullstrand's original design.[1] They are, in effect, short-focus versions of the 35mm slide projector, and project an image of an illuminated slit aperture (rather than the coiled lamp filament).

The slit-lamp beam must be evenly illuminated, and the edges must be sharply delineated, or the tissues observed may appear to be irregular even when they are not. The beam must also be bright enough to allow subtle variations to be seen in what are, essentially, transparent structures. Modern lamps employ halogen or xenon lamps which, while expensive to replace, are brighter than the tungsten lamps used previously, and produce approximately 600,000 lux. Colour rendering is also better with the more modern lamps, and they produce less heat. They also are supposed to last longer, though the reader may be less convinced of this.

The brightness of the beam may be controlled by a multi-position switch or rheostat, which is used to balance the needs of clear visibility and patient comfort.

Bear in mind that modern slit-lamps do emit a lot of light, and the Food and Drug Administration (FDA) document *Slit lamp guidance* contains food for thought.[2] When light is directed to the retina, the exposure dose is a product of the radiance and exposure time. Slit lamps produce considerably more irradiance than direct ophthalmoscopes (up to 15 times more),[3] which can be particularly important when using indirect biomicroscopy to view the retina.

Damage to the macula has been reported after slit-lamp photography to the anterior segment.[4] Long-wavelength (infrared) light can cause thermal injury when absorbed by the pigment epithelium and choroid, and the blue end of the visible spectrum can cause photochemical damage. Children, aphakes and patients with pre-existing macular pathology are particularly at risk. This risk can also increase if the patient has had exposure during the previous 24 hours (i.e., the patient is brought back for another look). Based on safety guidelines for lasers, the 'safe viewing time' for a patient with clear media and a dilated pupil has been calculated for a Haag–Streit instrument at various illumination settings.[5] At the lowest setting the safe time was 21 seconds. At the highest setting this was reduced to eight seconds.

The FDA document recommends:

> Because prolonged intense light exposure can damage the retina, the use of the device for ocular examination should not be unnecessarily prolonged, and the brightness setting should not exceed what is needed to provide clear visualisation of the target structures. This device should be used with filters that eliminate UV radiation (<400nm) and, whenever possible, filters that eliminate short-wavelength blue light (<420nm).

When examining the anterior eye, too much light causes patient discomfort, lacrimation and blepharospasm; it also shortens the bulb life drastically. However, too little light results in important clinical signs being missed, so a balance between these considerations is one of the principal skills involved. Neophytes tend on the whole to err towards employing less than optimal light levels, and one of the most common ways to fail professional examinations for contact lenses is too miss fluorescein staining because of this (*Figures 5.1a* and *5.1b*). The slit beam may be adjusted in several ways:

- *Slit width*. This is usually continuously variable. In instruments towards the top of the range this variable is between zero and 12–14mm. Some slit lamps have a graduated slit width, which is very useful for measurement of the size of a lesion.
- *Slit height*. Usually a series of stops, but may be continuous, and also may be graduated for measurement.
- *Slit orientation*. By rotating the lamp housing, the slit may be rotated from the vertical. A scale may be included either on the lamp housing, or in one of the eyepieces of the observing biomicroscope, to enable accurate measurement of the rotation. This is particularly useful when assessing the rotation of a toric contact lens, as the slit beam can be aligned with reference marks on the lens.
- *Slit focus*. Under normal circumstances the illumination and observation systems rotate about a common centre, which also coincides with the focal point of both systems. The ability to 'decouple' the two components and move the focal point of the illumination system sideways makes indirect illumination techniques easier. Originally, two main designs were used in illumination systems; both were first seen in instruments by Zeiss and Haag–Streit and have been extensively copied. In instruments that employ the Haag–Streit design, the illumination system can be decoupled vertically as well as horizontally, by tilting the whole system. This is useful for gonioscopy and indirect biomicroscopy.

The nature of the light emitted may be modified by the use of filters incorporated in the illumination system:

- *Heat-reducing filter*. These absorb long wavelengths (>700nm) capable of thermal damage, and are sometimes incorporated into the basic system rather than as an optional extra. They are usually employed to enhance patient comfort.
- *Neutral density (ND) filters*. These allow crude control of the illumination levels, and supplement the rheostat or switch.

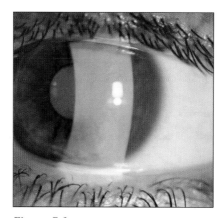

Figure 5.1a
Fluorescein stain observed with low illumination level

- *Polarising filters*. These can be used to reduce unwanted specular reflections.
- *Red-free filters*. These green filters make red objects appear black, and thus increase contrast when observing vascular structures or rose bengal staining (*Figure 5.2*).
- *Diffusing filters*. These defocus and diffuse the light over a wide area, which gives the effect of a much larger light source. This is useful for general viewing of the anterior eye and adnexa under low magnification. The filter often takes the form of a ground-glass screen, which can be flipped up. Alternatively, there may be a reversible mirror with bright and ground-glass surfaces for direct focal and diffuse illumination, respectively. If the slit lamp has no diffuser, a single sheet of tissue makes a functional, if precarious, substitute.
- *Cobalt-blue filter*. This allows long-wavelength light and is normally used in conjunction with fluorescein stain (see below), frequently in conjunction with a yellow filter incorporated into the observation system to reduce reflected blue light. In keratoconus, an annular deposition of iron (Fleischer's ring) occurs at the base of the cone. This is often seen in greater contrast if the cobalt-blue filter is in place.

The observation system (biomicroscope)

The microscope should ideally allow a series of magnifications up to 40–50×, to enable the detection of subtle ocular changes (e.g., microcysts), which are clinically significant in contact lens wearers. The variability may be provided through a series of objective lenses or by a zoom lens system that has the advantage of

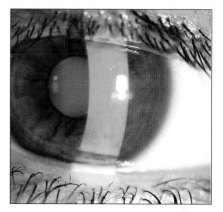

Figure 5.1b
Fluorescein stain at higher illumination level shows greater detail

maintaining the object in view while the magnification is changed. In addition, most microscopes have a choice of eyepieces. These days the higher magnification eyepieces are the most useful for contact lens practice. Clinically, magnification much over 40× is less useful than it might appear, as small involuntary eye movements make the image too unstable without restraints, which are not feasible in routine practice. This can mean that the view obtained in real life of, for example, the corneal endothelium can be rather disappointing to practitioners who are comparing them with textbook illustrations.

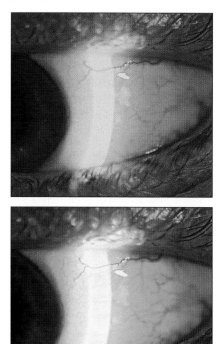

Figure 5.2
Green filters make red objects appear black, and thus increase contrast

Magnification is not the only important characteristic. The ideal biomicroscope would have excellent resolution and depth of field, while allowing the use of various supplementary devices to be placed between the patient's eye and the objective. Unfortunately, these goals tend to compete and this, as well as economic factors, means that the microscope must be the product of compromise.

Controls

The slit lamp and biomicroscope rotate about a common point, which in normal use is also the common focal point of both systems. This point may be moved forwards and backwards to focus at various depths on the patient's eye, and laterally to traverse the eye, by means of a joystick. The point of focus may be raised and lowered by a screw thread, either separate to or, more usually, incorporated into the joystick.

The horizontal position can be locked, which can help when setting up some types of illumination on the cornea (e.g., thin sections). The angle between the two systems can be varied manually and they can usually be locked into position.

Setting up the instrument

Before using the instrument it is essential to ensure that it is set up correctly. Patients co-operate better if they are comfortable and subtle clinical signs are picked up only if the microscope is correctly focused. The PD of the instrument should be set for the observer, who should also check that the instrument is parallel on the runners of the instrument table. The appropriate method for setting the eyepieces is covered in Chapter 4.

Principles of biomicroscope examination

The most important property of the slit-lamp biomicroscope is its ability to make visible the transparent media of the eye. This depends on the Tyndall effect. John Tyndall (1820–1893), a British physicist, used floating particles of dust to reveal the path of light beams. Any transparent medium that is uniformly of the same refractive index will appear optically empty, as does the normal aqueous humour. As the cornea, lens and vitreous are heterogeneous, light is reflected and scattered when focal illumination is directed upon them, rendering the tissues visible. This is a phenomenon known as relucency. Particles within the heterogeneous medium scatter some of the light. The scattered light from any one particle is focused as a diffraction disc in the image plane of the microscope. The increased intensity of light and apparent increase in size that the formation of the diffraction disc achieves render the particles visible. The cornea, lens and vitreous all exhibit the Tyndall effect under normal circumstances, and it is enhanced in pathological conditions.[6] The aqueous may show the phenomenon when inflammatory products disrupt its homogeneity.

Aside from the heterogeneity of the individual layers of the ocular media, the whole array can be considered as a series of layers of different refractive index, with polished curved surfaces. Where light travels across the interface of two materials of different refractive index a number of optical phenomena occur, including regular reflection. The interface acts as a curved mirror and obeys Snell's law, which states that 'the angle of reflection equals the angle of incidence'. A specular (Latin *specularis*, meaning 'mirror-like') reflection of the light source is formed at an equal angle to the angle of incidence that the beam makes with the corneal surface. This specular reflection may be used to study the regularity of the various interfaces (notably that between the corneal endothelium and the anterior vitreous), which is considered in more detail later in this chapter.

It also follows that if the lamp and microscope are aligned so that their optical axes coincide, then these reflexes, some of which are rather bright, reflect straight back at the observer, obscuring the detail that the observer wishes to see. Some angle between the lamp and microscope is therefore desirable. If this angle is small the specular reflections are still close enough to be obtrusive, and part of the illumination system may physically block the view of one of the eyepieces and so render the binocular nature of the microscope somewhat redundant.

Furthermore, as the beam passes through the cornea, the illuminated surfaces of the epithelium and endothelium more or less coincide, and the former masks the detail from underlying tissues (*Figure 5.3*). The wider the beam the more this will occur. It follows, therefore, that the angle between the lamp and the microscope should be sufficient to separate the epithelium and endothelium wherever practical. This is in marked contrast to the technique employed by many beginners to the instrument.

An angled beam also helps to estimate the depth of opacities within the cornea as

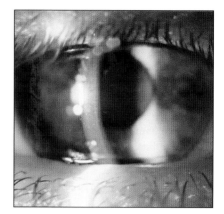

Figure 5.3
Parallelepiped with narrow angle between beam and microscope showing overlap of front and back surfaces

the trailing edge of the parallelepiped can be seen. The extreme case of this is when a thin optical section is employed. Although it is rarely necessary in routine practice, it is worth considering what the ultimate thin section involves. The lamp brightness should be at its maximum setting, and the beam should be as fine as the instrument permits without losing the image altogether. The slit beam should impinge on the cornea normal to its surface, and the angle between the lamp and microscope should be as near to 90° as is practical (the nose tends to get in the way when observing from the nasal side; *Figure 5.4*). The use of an angled narrow beam, either thin section or narrow parallelepiped, enables visualisation of the elevation and depression relative to the surrounding structures. An elevation deflects the beam towards the light source, and a depression deflects it away. The greater the angle between the lamp and microscope, the greater the deflection.

From the above considerations, an angle of 45–60° between the lamp and microscope when using direct focal illumination would appear to be optimal. Such an angle allows easy visualisation of the limbus in

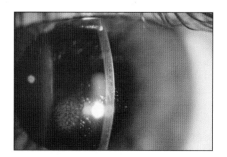

Figure 5.4
Thin section with wide angle showing enhanced view in depth

cross-section. In practice, experienced observers tend to vary the angles of both the illumination and observation systems more or less continuously to optimise the view. Neophytes, in contrast, often forget to switch the direction of illumination even when crossing the corneal midline. A further advantage of using a substantial angle between illumination and observation is that more than one type of illumination can be used at once.

Structures may be illuminated either directly by the light beam, or indirectly using light reflected from surrounding tissue. By angling the lamp, it is possible to examine the cornea with both simultaneously. The portion of cornea on which the beam strikes is seen in direct illumination. If the observer looks to the side of this bright area a darker area of cornea is seen. Opacities within this band are illuminated indirectly and the light scatter produced produces a bright image against the dark background. Adjacent to the band in indirect illumination, on the side away from the light source, is an area on which the cornea is backlit by light reflected from the iris. Opacities appear dark against the light background afforded by the iris. By sweeping the angled beam across the cornea, opacities may 'flash' dark and then light as they pass through the retro and indirect zones, which helps to draw attention to them.

General examination of the eye

Slit-lamp examinations can be divided into general examinations, which are usually conducted on a patient assumed to be normal, and specific examinations that are directed by history, symptoms or findings in the general survey.

The context for such a general examination might be a patient who presents for a preliminary contact lens appointment. Such a patient may well be asymptomatic and have no previous relevant history, so we must survey all we can to eliminate possible sources of future trouble.

A similar sequence of observations may be made during the aftercare examinations, but here there may be symptoms and/or history that direct our attention to specific areas. For example, a long-term soft-lens wearer might require particular attention to the upper lids, to look for contact lens associated papillary conjunctivitis (CLPC), and to the limbal region in search of neovascularisation. Where specific observations are indicated, the general ones are usually still appropriate, but the order and emphasis might change. In either case, optometrists screen the patient

for ocular surface disease, looking for inflammation and degeneration.

Initially, let us consider examination of the lids, conjunctiva and the tear layer.

Illumination

General observation of the eye and adnexa with a low magnification setting may be conducted with focal illumination and a wide beam, but often a far better view can be obtained with diffuse illumination. The diffuser gives the effect of a much larger light source, and gives the eye a more natural appearance, as well as allowing more of the eye to be illuminated at one time. Shadows tend to be minimised, which enables detail to be seen. On the other hand, some loss of information on texture and topographical variation may occur, as the shadows provided by tangential focal illumination may highlight this. A combination of the two forms of illumination is required.

Magnification

To some extent the illumination and the magnification employed interact to channel the attention of the observer. With diffuse illumination and low magnification attention is spread widely, to encompass the whole field of vision. This is ideal for a general survey of the area. As the beam width narrows and the magnification rises, greater detail can be seen, but of a correspondingly more limited area. If we performed only the high-magnification examination, we would probably miss something significant while our attention was focused on some tiny detail elsewhere. We should therefore look at the eye in the same way as we would look for a set of keys, with a general reconnaissance of every room before we demolish the sofa!

Assessment of the lids

Initially, wide diffuse illumination and low magnification are used to look at the external aspect of the lids. We seek signs of inflammation, redness and swelling, either localised or more general. Styes, chalazion and dermatitis might be seen. The lid position should be noted, as ptosis may be significant, both as a neurological manifestation and as a contact lens complication. The way that the lids behave throughout the blink cycle should be observed. The lashes should be observed for signs of ectropion, which may be associated with poor drainage, or ectropion and trichiasis.

When viewing the lid margins, we are essentially looking for signs of blepharitis, which can be associated with changes in both conjunctiva and cornea, and may cause an unstable tear film that could affect contact lens wear. Chronic blepharitis may be encountered as the anterior form, either staphylococcal or sebhorrhoeic.[7] There is a posterior type as well, which is also known as meibomian gland dysfunction.

The staphylococcal form tends to be seen in patients with atopic eczema and is more common in females and young patients. The lid margins are hyperaemic and show telangiectasis (dilated, tortuous blood vessels). There is also scaling – the scales are brittle, and form collarettes around the bases of the lashes. Where these have been removed, small bleeding ulcers may be seen. This condition is caused by chronic staphylococcal infection of the bases of the lashes, so any patient with it has an increased bacterial load. It should be eliminated before contact lens wear is allowed.

Complications that may be observed include whitening or complete loss of the lashes and trichiasis. The lid margins may become scarred and notched. If the infection spreads to the glands of Zeis and Moll, a stye may result. If the meibomian glands become involved, there may be an internal hordeolum. Acute bacterial conjunctivitis may appear, and recur. Apart from these direct bacterial effects, the exotoxins released by the bacteria may cause hypersensitivity reactions. A mild papillary conjunctivitis, marginal corneal infiltrates or, rarely, phlyctenulosis and pannus may occur. About half of all sufferers also have an unstable tear film. Management consists of lid scrubs and referral to a general medical practitioner for antibiotics and, possibly, anti-inflammatory agents.

The sebhorroeic version tends to be associated with sebhorroeic dermatitis, which can affect the scalp, face and chest. There is an oily type in which the scaling is greasy, and also a dry type (dandruff). The symptoms are similar to, though milder than, the staphylococcal form. The hyperaemia and telangiectasia of the lid margins are also more moderate, and the scales are greasy, yellowish and do not leave an ulcer when removed. The lids may be greasy and stuck together. There may be a moderate papillary conjunctivitis and punctate keratitis that tends to favour the middle third of the cornea, whereas the staphylococcal form often affects the lower third of the cornea. Management usually involves lid scrubs, using sodium bicarbonate as a degreasing agent.

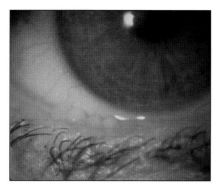

Figure 5.5
Meibomian gland dysfunction showing meibomian glands capped by oily material

Posterior blepharitis may be divided into meibomian seborrhoea and meibomitis. Meibomian seborrhoea causes hypersecretion from dilated meibomian glands. The lid margins may show small oil globules or waxy collections. The tear film may be oily and foamy, and in severe cases there may be a frothy discharge at the inner canthus (meibomian foam). The patient complains of burning eyes on first waking, and signs of inflammation may be few, so this is easy to miss. If the lid margins are gently squeezed copious discharge may be elicited. Remember that the lid margins are sensitive and the expression of meibomian contents usually hurts, especially when attempted by the inexperienced. It is therefore not a procedure to be recommended on an asymptomatic patient.

Primary meibomitis involves inflammation centred round the orifices of the meibomian glands, which may pout and be capped by domes of oily material (meibomana; see *Figure* 5.5). Expressed meibomian contents are thickened and may contain more solid particles, which in some cases resemble toothpaste and require firm pressure to express. If the contents become trapped, meibomian cysts may form.

Papillary conjunctivitis and punctate epitheliopathy may be secondary effects. About one-third of these patients have tear-film instability. Meibomitis may also occur with secondary sebhorroeic blepharitis, associated with sebhorroeic dermatitis; the meibomian involvement is usually relatively mild and patchy. Management involves lid scrubs and referral to the general medical practitioner for oral antibiotics, typically tetracycline. Treatment may take three months or more.

Assessment of the conjunctiva

To examine the conjunctiva, broad-beam diffuse illumination is used initially, with the emphasis on assessing the degree, depth and location of hyperaemia. This may be followed by more detailed examinations using focal illumination. Dyes, stains and filters may be used to reveal areas of damage.

A grading scale may be used to indicate severity. Several grading systems are published, but correlation between them is a little hit and miss, and none is accepted universally. I tend to favour a simple intuitive scale for all observations, as it does not waste time trying to fit the observation to the photographs or diagrams used in the published versions. As a patient, I am not sure I would be very impressed if my practitioner constantly referred to charts. The intuitive scale used is similar to the one described by Woods (*Table 5.1*).[8]

If the observations do not quite fit the gradings, we can use plus and minus increments to convert the scale into a nine-point one, which should be sensitive enough for even the most pedantic observer.

The distribution of hyperaemia may be recorded similarly in terms of numbered subdivisions of the conjunctiva (or lid or cornea), but a diagram is much easier to interpret, particularly as more than one numerical system exists, which could lead to confusion. Distribution is important. A

discrete leash of dilated blood vessels on the bulbar conjunctiva may point to a phlycten. Interpalpebral redness may be associated with drying or with a hypersensitivity reaction to an airborne irritant. Where the hyperaemia is greater under one or both lids, we may be dealing with 'innocent bystander' (secondary hypersensitivity) reactions from inflamed palpebral conjunctiva. Perilimbal flush may suggest a hypoxic cornea, a tight lens in a soft lens wearer or, if deeper, uveitis.

The depth of hyperaemia is important to differentiate mere conjunctivitis from episcleritis, scleritis and uveitis (*Figure* 5.6). The injection associated with conjunctivitis tends to be bright red and greatest towards the fornices. The vessels appear irregular and, if friction is applied through the eyelids (as in the push-up test, but without the contact lens), they can be made to move. Deeper vessels do not move, and do not blanch with either palpation or mild topical decongestants. Going deeper, the hyperaemia associated with episcleritis tends to be salmon pink and wedge shaped, with the apex towards the limbus because of the radial arrangement of the vessels, although the 20 per cent of cases that have the nodular form show a more circumscribed area of redness.

Scleritis produces a purplish hue, which is diffuse and present all the way to the fornices. While conjunctivitis and episcleritis may have some corneal involvement, scleritis tends to be associated with stromal keratitis, and with anterior chamber activity, so flare and cells might well be seen (see later). Secondary uveitis is common. Uveitis itself produces deep injection that is most intense around the limbus.

In general, examination of the bulbar conjunctiva proceeds in three sweeps, taking in the upper, middle and lower thirds, with the lids pulled back to see what lies below. To view the palpebral conjunctiva,

Grade	Appearance	Significance
0	Normal	None
1	Slight	Note but no action
2	Moderate	May require action
3	Severe	Requires action
4	Very severe	Refer for medical action

Table 5.1 Simple intuitive scale for grading observations

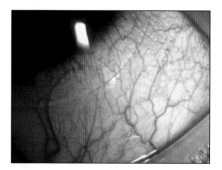

Figure 5.6
Bulbar conjunctiva showing superficial (red) and deeper (purplish) injection. Courtesy of Brian Tompkins

the lids must be everted. It is common for practitioners to use cotton buds for this purpose, but with practice many patients can be everted using the fingers alone. The ubiquitous cotton bud is not an ideal tool for the purpose anyway. The end tends to be too bulbous, but teasing out the fibres often results in a more useful implement that is easier to insert behind the tarsal margin. In the days when smoking was a social accomplishment, matches were the weapon of choice.

The pattern of any hyperaemia should be noted, particularly if CLPC is suspected, as it tends to favour the upper lid. Internal hordeola and concretions, which appear as discrete yellowish dots, may also be encountered. These are of little significance unless they break through to the surface, in which case they are easily removed medically, using a needle.

The other main focus of attention is towards follicles and papillae. Reading case records, it would appear that for many practitioners the two terms are more or less interchangeable, and it must be admitted that I practised for a number of years with only the vaguest idea of the distinction. Essentially, follicles are lymphatic in origin, so they themselves are avascular. They appear as multiple, discrete, slightly elevated bodies that are translucent and shaped rather like a rice grain (arborio rather than basmati; *Figure 5.7*). As they grow they displace the conjunctival vessels, so they can appear with a vascular capsule surrounding the base. They are generally small, but can measure up to 5mm in severe or unusually prolonged disease.

Papillae, on the other hand, have their origin in the palpebral conjunctival tissue and consist of a central vascular tuft surrounded by a diffuse infiltrate, largely composed of white blood cells. They can only occur where the conjunctival epithelium is attached to the underlying levels by fibrous septa. This restricts them to the palpebral conjunctiva and limbal area.

Giant papillae occur when these septa are ruptured (*Figures* 5.8 and 5.9). The size of papillae can vary considerably and, contrary to what was believed earlier, those associated with contact lens wear (CLPC) are rarely 'giant', except in the very late stages. Furthermore, papillae may appear anywhere on the upper palpebral conjunctiva, including the transitional areas (i.e., those areas to either side that do not overlie the tarsal plate).[9]

Finding either does not indicate a firm diagnosis, since follicles may be caused by viral and chlamydial infections, Parinaud's syndrome and hypersensitivity reactions to topical medication; they also occur in asymptomatic children. Papillae are even less specific, being associated with chronic blepharitis, vernal disease, bacterial infection, contact lens complication and superior limbic keratoconjunctivitis. The presence of either (or both, since they can co-exist) is more a wake-up call to investigate the cause further. Initially, white-light examination is required to look for hyperaemia, but focal illumination, directed tangentially, is useful to show the texture, as the shadows are more obvious. With fluorescein installed, surface texture is enhanced as the dye collects in the channels between the swellings.

The tear film

When fluorescein is installed, it largely clears in two minutes or so, though the tear prisms next to the lid margins may continue to fluoresce for some time. Older patients may take a little longer because of the stenosis of the punctae, which normally tends to offset the reduced aqueous production.

Should the fluorescein take a longer time to clear, or should there be a significant difference in the time each eye takes to clear (assuming equal amounts of fluorescein installed), blockage of the

drainage mechanism may be suspected. Placing an optical section through the lower tear prism may corroborate this further. In the literature, the normal height of the tear film is quoted at anything between 0.2mm and 1.0mm, but in general it can be said that it is 0.2mm to 0.4mm in the centre, thinning to about half this at the periphery.[10] It may be higher if the drainage is compromised, which may be a useful indicator that a patient is prone to epiphora, for example if fitted with contact lenses.

Attention should also be given to the punctae. Pouting of the opening suggests canaliculitis. The position of the lid margins and punctae during the blink cycle is worth noting. Further evidence may be gathered by applying what is usually referred to as the Jones test. The full Primary Jones dye test involves the use of 4 per cent cocaine,[11] so what is done in practice is a slightly modified version. Essentially, fluorescein is installed into the conjunctival sac. Two to four fluorets are used, so care must be taken that the patient's face and clothes do not receive an unscheduled colour change. After blinking, normally for five minutes, the patient occludes the nostril on the unaffected side (or occludes each eye in turn if the problem is bilateral) and blows his or her nose into a white tissue. If fluorescein can be detected on the tissue with the cobalt filter the drainage pathway is patent. If no fluorescein is recovered, further tests may be performed to determine the site of the obstruction, but these are probably best avoided by the inexperienced practitioner. A more detailed description of the procedures involved is given by Elliott.[12]

Excessive tearing is of significance, but insufficient tears tend to give rise to more problems, especially in contact lens wearers. A clue may be gained by observing the tear prism in section. As previously mentioned, the normal tear prism is about 0.2 to 0.4mm in height, and it appears convex in section. A scanty tear film has a low

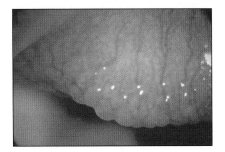

Figure 5.7
Follicles: note the absence of central vasculature

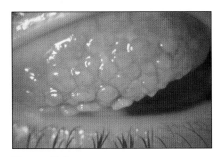

Figure 5.8
Giant papillae showing vascular cores surrounded by infiltrate

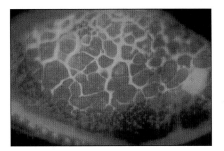

Figure 5.9
Giant papillae: fluorescein makes the outline of the cobblestones much easier to see

meniscus (less than 0.2mm), which appears concave. Irregularity of the prism along the lid edge suggests a poor tear film.

It is also worth observing the movement of dust particles and bubbles within the lower rivus under high magnification. In the normal tear film, particles on the surface move more slowly than deeper ones, as a result of surface tension. If the movement of particles is too fast, a thin, watery tear film is indicated. Immobile particles reveal excessive viscosity in the tear film. Such a tear film may show interference fringes under specular reflection. As the patient blinks these emerge, like waves, from the lower lid margins. As the lids close, the fringes come together, and then open out again as the eye opens.[13]

The tear volume can be investigated using Schirmer's strips or similar tests, though the results are inconsistent. The tear break-up time (TBUT) may be assessed by installing fluorescein, and then waiting for a few seconds for the tear film to stabilise while the patient blinks. The eye is illuminated with a broad beam and a cobalt filter. The patient is instructed not to blink, and the time noted for dark spots or streaks to appear in the tear layer as it breaks up. Normally, this would take 15–20 seconds, and anything below 10 seconds is probably abnormal. Where the same area consistently breaks up rapidly, the cause is a surface irregularity rather than a dry eye.

TBUT may also be measured without the use of fluorescein, which may destabilise the tear film and so give artificially low results.[14] Keratometer mires can be used for this, or a Keeler Tearscope-Plus may be used to project a grid pattern on to the eye's surface, which is then observed for distortion as the tear film breaks. Typical non-invasive break-up times for normal patients are around 40 seconds by this method.[15] The original Tearscope was designed to allow specular reflection over the whole cornea. The later Tearscope-Plus has a range of inserts, which enable a range of observations on the tear film and ocular surface. It uses a cold cathode light and the design of the instrument allows the light to be positioned away from the corneal surface, eliminating induced evaporation through heat transfer. The Tearscope can also be used to observe interference patterns in the tear film, allowing an estimate of the tear thickness to be made. This is a useful, though expensive tool for diagnosing tear film anomalies, but a detailed description is beyond the scope of this chapter. Guillon is a good source for more detail on this attachment.[16,17]

If a Tearscope is not available, some idea of the quality of the tears may be obtained if the first Purkinje image of the slit beam is observed, especially if the illumination is reduced and the beam narrowed. Coloured fringes around the Purkinje image, seen in conjunction with an irregular tear prism, strongly suggest a poor tear film.[13]

The patient with dry eye often has, as an early sign, mucus strands and debris in the tears. This occurs as the mucin layer becomes contaminated with lipid as the tear film breaks up. In more severe cases, mucin may also combine with cellular debris to form filaments, which are attached to the epithelial surface and move with each blink. Mucous plaques, whitish–grey translucent lesions of varying shape, may appear in concert with the filaments. Fluorescein reveals punctae epitheliopathy, either in the inferior portion of the cornea or in the interpalpebral area.

Damage may also be revealed with rose bengal stain. This stains dead and devitalised cells and mucus red. Typically, dry-eye patients show staining of the interpalpebral bulbar conjunctiva, with two triangular areas of stain either side of the cornea, with their apices towards the inner and outer canthi. Mucus strands, filaments and plaques also show up better with rose bengal.

The drawback to rose bengal is that it is a considerable ocular irritant and, as luck would have it, this quality is rather worse in dry-eye patients. Lissamine Green SF (Wool Green, Light Green SF), which stains dead cells and mucus blue–green, and is less of an irritant, appeared in the 1960s as an alternative. It is available in the USA as impregnated strips, but is at present unavailable commercially in the UK.[18]

Fluorescein assessment of contact lens fits

On the subject of tear-film assessment, it is appropriate to consider the use of fluorescein to assess the fit of contact lenses, since, in essence, we are assessing the thickness of the tear layer under the lens. Sodium fluorescein is orange–red in colour and, when in dilute concentration in an aqueous solution, is excited by short-wavelength light (peak absorption 485–500nm) to emit a green light (maximum intensity 525–530nm). The cobalt-blue filter on the slit lamp allows this process to occur while eliminating wavelengths that have little effect. This reduces veiling glare. To improve contrast, a yellow barrier filter (e.g., Wratten No 12) may be placed before

the observation system,[19] either in a custom-made attachment or as a cardboard-mounted accessory widely available from contact lens manufacturers. This filters out the reflected blue light from the eye. Fluorescein has long been used to assess the fitting characteristics of rigid contact lenses, both scleral and corneal. Traditionally, this was done using a Burton lamp that employed a pair of 'Blacklight Blue' miniature fluorescent tubes.[20] Unfortunately, some rigid gas-permeable materials are formulated to absorb light in the UV-A band (315–400nm) with the result that the fluorescein under such a lens does not fluoresce sufficiently to allow an accurate estimation of the fit. The cobalt-blue filter of the slit lamp emits light of longer wavelength, so the fitting characteristics of the lens may be better visualised.

The appearance of silicone hydrogel lenses has created another application for fluorescein. The relative rigidity of these lenses compared to conventional hydrogel lenses, plus the resistance to fluorescein spoilation of the materials, allows fluorescein to be used to visualise edge stand-off. Silicone hydrogel lenses absorb little fluorescein (*Figure 5.10*), as their hydrogel content is low, but conventional hydrogel lenses take up fluorescein enthusiastically. Attempts have been made in the past to use fluorescent dyes with a high molecular weight (e.g., fluorexon, also known as Fluoresoft®), but these have not really caught on. This is partly because there is little point in looking at the tear film beneath a modern soft lens, and partly because many practitioners feel that subtle epithelial staining tends not to show up as well as it does with fluorescein. Fluorexon is considerably less fluorescent then fluorescein.[21]

Fluorescein itself is usually installed from sterile, impregnated paper strips (fluorets), because the multidose containers originally used were found to be rather good breeding grounds for *Pseudomonas*.

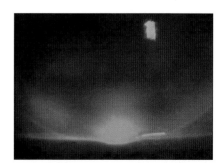

Figure 5.10
Fluorescein used to visualise edge fluting on a silicone hydrogel lens. Courtesy of Brian Tompkins

However, this has led to an exaggerated fear of contamination of soft lenses with fluorescein, to the extent that it is used to justify soft lens aftercare that avoids the use of fluorescein altogether. This is dangerous, since even experienced observers may miss epithelial damage if no fluorescein is used. The chances that sterile fluorescein from a fluoret, bathed in the tear film, which has effective antimicrobials, floating over an intact cornea (or why are they wearing lenses?) or in an effective storage solution, constitutes a significant risk of infection are minimal. If the patient hasn't brought spectacles, irrigation with saline can always be used and, in most cases, a temporary correction can be provided in the form of daily disposable lenses. There really is no longer any excuse for not using fluorescein, if there ever was.

Examination of the Cornea in Contact Lens Wear

The examination of the cornea is essentially the same in both contact lens wearers and non-wearers. It consists of two phases. The first is a general survey conducted at medium magnification with white light, and the second comprises more specific examinations using white light and, after the instillation of fluorescein dye, blue light. The specific examinations occur in response either to findings that come to light in the general examination or to anticipated problems that might not be detected by the general examination. The basic method is the same whether the slit-lamp examination forms part of the initial pre-fitting assessment or the aftercare examination. However, with current or previous wearers the emphasis shifts towards the anticipation of lens-induced complications, rather than merely responding to the findings of the general white light examination.

General white light examination of the cornea

Magnification
The magnification used for the initial examination of the cornea is important. If this is set low, the whole cornea (indeed, half of the patient's face) can be covered in one fell sweep. Unfortunately, very little of clinical significance can be detected. Initially, this may be reassuring for both patient and practitioner, but the longer-term consequences for both are unattractive. An initial examination at too high a magnification takes rather a long time,

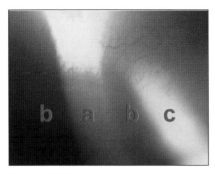

Figure 5.11
Upper limbal vessels with an angled beam. The vessels and cornea are seen simultaneously by direct (a), indirect (b) and retro-illumination (c)

even assuming that the full concentration of both parties can be maintained for the duration. It is also far too easy to become lost if the field of vision is too small to contain reference points to navigate by. Therefore, initially, the cornea is examined with medium magnification, set so that the whole cornea may be seen in three horizontal sweeps. If an anomaly is detected the magnification can be increased to have a closer look.

Beam width and angle
Modern slit lamps allow continuously variable beam width from zero to an upper limit of up to 14mm. A beam set at this upper limit illuminates the entire cornea. Light scattered by those structures near the surface tends to mask that from deeper structures, and only dense opacities are visible. Furthermore, no indication of the depth of the opacity is apparent. In contrast, a very narrow beam illuminates a thin optical section, which, if observed with the microscope set at an angle, enables an observer to assess the depth or elevation of an anomaly.

This angle between the slit beam and the visual axis of the microscope is important for a number of reasons. It allows deeper structures to be observed without an overlay of reflected light from more superficial structures, which enhances clarity considerably. The wider the slit beam the greater becomes the angle between the beam and the microscope required to achieve this separation. Another happy consequence of an angled beam is that it is possible to view the cornea by direct, indirect and retro-illumination simultaneously (*Figure 5.11*). The area of cornea in which the beam strikes is illuminated directly, and if the observer looks to either side of this bright area the cornea may be seen in indirect

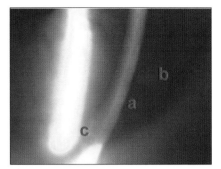

Figure 5.12
Corneal scarring with direct (a) and indirect (b, c) illumination

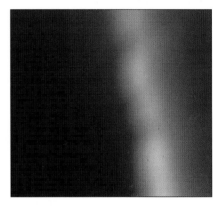

Figure 5.13
Microcysts seen by retro-illumination. Those on the fringes of the illuminated background are showing reversed illumination

illumination. Opacities scatter light and can be seen as light areas against a dark background (*Figure 5.12*). A dark background is essential for this, so the room lighting should be off. To the opposite side of that from which the beam is directed is an area of cornea that is backlit by reflected light from the iris. Opacities here appear in silhouette, dark against a light background (*Figure 5.13*).

For the initial examination of the cornea the beam width should be set at about 2mm or so, which illuminates a thick slice of the cornea, termed a parallelepiped. An angle of 45–60° between beam and microscope allows some appreciation of depth, since the edge of the parallelepiped on the opposite side to that from which the light is coming is, in effect, an optical section of sorts (*Figure 5.14*). The beam is slowly swept from the limbus to the central cornea. Most authorities recommend that the illumination should come from the same side as the hemicornea being examined. Thus, when observing the cornea to the left of the midline, the lamp is positioned to the left of the microscope, with the illumination system

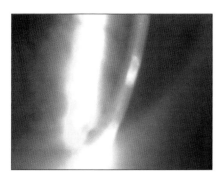

Figure 5.14
Anterior stromal scar seen in a narrow parallelepiped. The scar does not appear on the side face of the parallelepiped, which indicates that it is near the surface

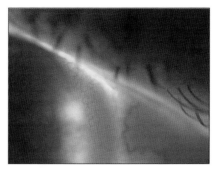

Figure 5.15
Limbal arcades seen in retro-illumination. The light beam is coming from the 'wrong' (left) side

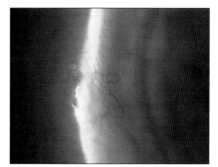

Figure 5.16
Light beam directed on the limbus. The limbal light arcades are seen partly by light internally reflected within the cornea, and partly by light reflected back from the iris

swung round to the other side as the mid-line is crossed. However, I prefer to sweep from limbus to limbus with the illumination from each side in turn. Light bounced from the iris can then be employed to retro-illuminate the limbal arcades on the 'wrong side' (Figure 5.15).

When the beam is directed to the limbus, it may be worth widening the beam momentarily and observing the cornea with the naked eye, particularly if the patient wears polymethylmethacrylate (PMMA) or low permeability (Dk), rigid gas-permeable (RGP) lenses. The light under these circumstances is internally reflected within the cornea and a bright glow may be seen around the limbus. Dense central oedema causes the internally reflected light to scatter and produces a grey glow seen against the dark pupil area. It is possible to decouple the instrument to view the cornea through the microscope, but this is rarely necessary since the demise of PMMA lenses. The technique is referred to as sclerotic scatter, and it is really only a version of indirect illumination. Sclerotic scatter can also be useful when observing the limbal arcades. A 1–2mm angled beam is directed at the sclera immediately adjacent to the limbus. The microscope remains coupled, but the attention is directed to the limbus and the area of the cornea immediately inside it. The limbal arcades can be seen partly illuminated by internally reflected light and partly by light reflected back off the iris (*Figure 15.16*).

The sweeps are performed with the patient looking slightly down, level and slightly up, and new users should be careful to remember all three. It is essential to look at the upper cornea. The area of cornea under the lid is particularly likely to develop anomalies from hypoxia, since oxygen levels are generally lower under the lid, and may also show 'innocent bystander' effects, such as the keratitis

associated with CLPC, caused by close proximity to the lid. For this reason it is a good idea to develop the habit of viewing the upper cornea first every time.

Specific white light examination of the cornea

More detailed examination of the cornea occurs in response to the following two demands:

- The general examination reveals an anomaly (e.g., a corneal opacity or neo-vascularisation).
- The history and symptoms of the patient suggest the possibility of specific clinical findings that may not be detected by a general scan of the cornea (e.g., contact lens wear likely to give rise to microcysts).

Anomalies revealed by general examination

The most typical examples of these are infiltrates and scars often seen on both contact lens wearers and non-wearers. Initially, either may appear as a light grey blob in greyer surrounding tissue, and before we can decide what to do about it, we need to decide what we are looking at, and the likely cause of it.

For the moment, suppose that the general examination has revealed the presence of a greyish-white blob in the lower right side of the cornea. What information do we need?

Exactly where is it?

Location with regard to various landmarks can be determined by widening the beam and, if necessary, reducing the magnification. Accurate recording of the distance from the limbus (or centre) and the clock position not only makes it easier to find the anomaly again, but gives some indication

of its seriousness. Central infiltrates are more likely to be serious than not, since a powerful stimulus is needed for an infiltrate to form so far from the vascular system. However, peripheral infiltrates also might be serious because in contact lens wearers any physical damage to the epithelium, which probably always precedes infection, is more likely near the limbus.

The estimation of distances when the eye is under magnification is a challenge to the inexperienced microscopist, and can cause unnecessary alarm when applied to suspect neovascularisation, for example. Some slit-lamp microscopes have a graticule eyepiece, which can be useful when making quantitative observations. However, some observers (including the author) find the graticule distracting. Reasonable estimates of dimensions may be made with a little practice by comparing the size of the object of attention with a known dimension. The visible diameter of the cornea is 11–12mm, and the amount by which a normal soft lens exceeds this is about a millimetre all round. Alternatively, one can always hold a millimetre rule close to the anomaly (but be careful!).

How big and how many?

With a wide beam and lowish magnification, the size of a large opacity, or the number of multiple opacities, may be determined. Large single opacities may be associated with bacterial infection, or the later stages of herpetic ulceration, whereas multiple smaller ones may be caused by a non-microbial agent, or by a viral or protozoan infection.

Colour and density

Colour and density are best assessed with direct illumination. Though most corneal lesions tend towards the monochrome, a haemorrhage within the cornea gives rise to a red lesion, and a rust stain might betray a ferrous foreign body. Some of the less dense lesions are more or less invisible under direct illumination and may only appear under indirect or retro-illumination, the classic example being ghost vessels (see below). Oscillation of the beam so that the type of illumination alternates may be useful, and can be achieved either with the joystick or by decoupling the instrument and swinging the illumination system independently.

How deep is it?

The depth of an infiltrate or scar tends to correlate with the seriousness of its cause. Intraepithelial infiltrates are usually a response to a non-microbial trigger, although this may include bacterial exotoxins. The deeper, subepithelial and stromal infiltrates are more likely to be associated with infection, and may lead to scarring. Depth perception through a biomicroscope results from a composite impression of a series of observations and improves with practice. Experienced microscopists often appear to fidget with both the illuminator and the microscope, seemingly at random to the casual observer. However, valuable information can be gleaned from these manoeuvres, even though much of it may be subliminal to the microscopist:

- Varying the position of the light source affects the degree to which the scattered light from layers near to the surface interferes with the clear resolution of objects in the deeper layers. Parallax between the object and the leading edge of the parallelepiped is also induced.
- Swinging the microscope also creates parallax between structures at different levels (see below).
- The microscope allows binocular fixation, so stereopsis may be used, provided that the array is sufficiently detailed
- Not all layers of the cornea are in focus at the same time, particularly at high magnification when the depth of focus is small.

However, by far the best way to determine the depth of a lesion within the cornea is to narrow the beam, and observe the resultant thin optical section through a microscope set at a considerable angle to the illuminating system. As discussed in Chapter 4, the best possible section is obtained with the beam directed to strike the cornea normal to its surface, and the microscope set at as near to 90° as is physically possible. Normally, though, it is sufficient that the microscope be set at about 60° to obtain a satisfactory section.

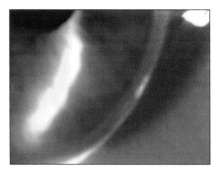

Figure 5.17
Thin section of the cornea with a beam angled at about 60°, showing an anterior stromal scar, and below it a less dense deeper stromal scar

Provided that magnification and illumination are sufficient, and the instrument correctly focused, five distinct layers will, in theory, be visible within the section of the cornea with a good slit lamp. These are formed by the tears, epithelium, Bowman's membrane, stroma and endothelium. In practice, three or four layers can be seen, particularly if the tear film is stained with fluorescein. However, if all we need to know is whether an opacity is stromal or not, the exact number of layers seen is not vitally important (*Figure 5.17*).

The thin section can tell us how deep an opacity is within the cornea, but it can also tell us whether the cornea itself is thinned or thickened and, using a pachometer, the thickness of the cornea may be measured. This has not really caught on in practice, because of the time it takes and doubts about the reliability of measurements; the emergence of high-Dk materials, which tend not to produce corneal thickness changes, probably means that it never will.

The other very useful property of a thin section is that elevations and depressions in an interface or surface deviate the beam. Elevations deviate the beam towards the side that the light beam is coming from, whereas depressions bend it away from the source. Where the cornea is perforated, a gap occurs in the corneal section. To make the most of this effect, an angled beam is essential.

Neovascularisation

Neovascularisation induced by contact lenses may be seen during the general examination of the cornea. It is rarely a surprise, but still would warrant a routine specific investigation in any soft lens wearer. It is most likely to be found in the upper cornea under the top lid, and the angled beam direct–indirect–retro-illumination combination gives the best results. Ghost vessels are nearly impossible to see under direct illumination (hence the name), but readily visible under indirect and retro-illumination.

When looking at superficial neovascularisation, it is important to make sure that all of the vessels are in sharp focus, and to move the lamp and microscope to create parallax. Deep stromal vessels may lurk beneath the superficial pannus, and are very significant. Their subterranean nature can sometimes be confirmed by the use of a thin section across the limbus, but this is much easier in the 3 and 9 o'clock positions than at 12 o'clock, as it is impractical to set up a horizontal, angled beam that is confocal with the microscope.

Microcysts

Microcysts are unlikely to be seen during a general survey of the cornea, as they are too small. To detect them magnification of the order of 25× is required, and rather more than that to be able to identify them for certain. They are best examined using a special technique called marginal retro-illumination. Light reflected from the iris and, to a lesser extent, the lens illuminates the cornea from behind. Irregularities in the cornea can be seen against a bright background of reflected light (so-called direct retro, but actually an indirect technique) or against a dark background (indirect retro) by looking to the side of the area of cornea directly (retro-illuminated). It helps considerably if the illuminating system is decoupled and the beam directed so that the interface between the light and dark areas is positioned in the centre of the field of view, with the microscope focused on the cornea. Under such circumstances under high magnification, microcysts seen at the dark–light interface show reversed illumination. The microcysts show a light side and a dark side, but they are the wrong way round (*Figure 5.18*). This is useful to

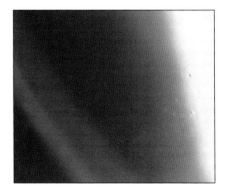

Figure 5.18
Marginal retro-illumination showing microcysts (reversed illumination) and a vacuole (non-reversed illumination, to the right of the picture below the midline)

differentiate microcysts from vacuoles, which do not exhibit reversed illumination under these circumstances. Reversed illumination indicates that the object has a higher refractive index than the surrounding tissue, and is also shown by endothelial bedewing, for example. When looking for microcysts, it is worth considering first where they are likely to be most numerous. As their presence is a good indicator of chronic hypoxia, they are most likely to be found in the part of the cornea that receives least oxygen. In a hydrogel lens, this is under the thickest part of the lens, which varies with the power and design, and under the top lid. In an RGP lens, this depends on the Dk of the material, but a low-Dk lens is more likely to produce a microcyst response under the centre of the lens.

The endothelium

The long-term use of contact lenses may have serious effects on the corneal endothelium, and some way to monitor this is desirable. The method of choice for viewing the endothelium is specular reflection, in which its surface is used as a mirror to reflect an image of the slit aperture. The endothelial cells normally have a flat surface, and reflect light well, whereas their junctions are a little irregular, and reflect it poorly. The whole layer normally forms a regular surface, but disturbances in size or shape to the cells alter the reflex and produce dark irregularities within the it. Blebs, polymegathism and pleomorphism all produce this effect.

Students are often rather disappointed at what they can actually see, once the euphoria of seeing the endothelium for the first time has faded. There is an enduring myth that the endothelium appears as a golden glow, which it may well do using an old slit lamp with a tungsten bulb. While it can look like beaten metal, with modern lamps the colour tends towards a greyish sludge. Those who expect to see the classic honeycomb appearance are also likely to be disappointed. At 25× magnification, the endothelium appears as a rather boring stippled area, like fine emery paper. At 40× individual cells start to appear, but most textbook illustrations are based on twice this and more. The value of monitoring the endothelium in this way is questionable given the limitations of practice instrumentation, although this has improved over time (possibly just in time for super-high Dk lenses to make the debate largely academic).

The technique for viewing the endothelium is simple, but the basics have to be right or no endothelium will be seen. The instrument must be set up correctly, and

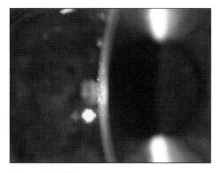

Figure 5.19
Specular reflection set-up. The parallelepiped is close to the Purkinje image, but not yet in contact

the microscope focused on the corneal endothelium. This can be achieved by setting the arms of the instrument at an angle of about 30° with medium magnification and a beam width of about a millimetre. Focus is initially on the front surface of the parallelepiped, and the movement of particles within the tears indicates when this is achieved. The focus is nudged forwards about half a millimetre to focus the endothelium. We now need to ensure that the microscope is at the right angle to collect the specular reflection coming from the endothelial surface. This obeys Snell's law, in that the angles of incidence and reflection are identical. Fortunately, a rather obvious marker is provided by the defocused image of the bulb filament (second Purkinje image), which is also created by reflection from the endothelium. This is seen as a bright patch of light to the side of the parallelepiped in the direction of the light source. In other words, if we examine an area slightly temporal to the midline, with the light coming from the temporal side, the bright Purkinje image is seen temporal to the parallelepiped (*Figure 5.19*). Using the joystick, the focal point of the instrument is moved laterally, which ensures that sharp focus is maintained, so that the parallelepiped and the Purkinje image are brought into coincidence. At this point a very bright reflex is seen where the two images touch, and immediately nasal to it (in this example) is seen the duller, textured endothelium (*Figure 5.20*). The slit width and illumination can now be adjusted to optimise the image, and the magnification taken up to its maximum level. By asking the patient to fixate on an adjustable target, a larger area of endothelium may be examined. A light-blue filter may be employed to cut down reflection from the front surface of the cornea, though on some slit lamps the loss of light intensity outweighs any gain in contrast.

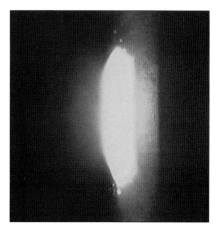

Figure 5.20
Specular reflection. As the beam and the Purkinje image collide, a bright reflex is formed and the endothelium can be seen immediately to the side

Blue light examination of the cornea

The use of fluorescein to examine epithelial integrity is a vital part of every aftercare examination, and there is no valid reason not to do it. If concerned that the patient's hydrogel lenses will be discoloured, the patient can always be given a daily lens to wear home. In the initial assessment of prospective contact lens patients, fluorescein installation is also essential, both to assess the epithelium and to monitor TBUT. Fluorescein may also be installed in response to findings on a general scan of the cornea, or where the symptoms and history suggest that epithelial damage is likely (e.g., a suspected dry eye).

Fluorescein colours the tear film rather than staining the tissue.[20] Normally the lipid membranes of the epithelial cells prevent ingress of the substance, but if this is breached by trauma or disease, the tear layer gains access to deeper layers. The absorption spectrum and the degree of fluorescence depend on pH peaking when the pH is 8. The underlying tissues, because they have a different pH to the surface, fluoresce more, so the defect is shown up as a green area. In the deeper layers, the fluorescein does diffuse sideways and so tends to exaggerate the area of the lesion. This spread of fluorescein in the stroma may be a useful clue in itself when evaluating epithelial defects (*Figure 5.21*). When using the cobalt filter, remember that considerable light has been filtered out, and so

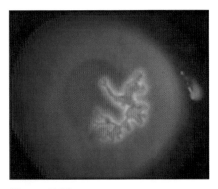

Figure 5.21
Dendritic ulcer, showing the spread of fluorescein in the stroma

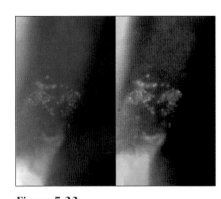

Figure 5.22
Punctate staining with and without the Wratten filter, showing the enhanced contrast when the filter is used. As with any filter, illumination may have to be increased to gain the full benefit

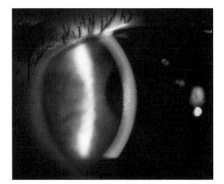

Figure 5.23
Krukenberg's spindle

adjust the rheostat to give a bright beam. Contrast may be considerably enhanced with a yellow filter (Wratten #12 or #15) to eliminate reflected blue light from the cornea (*Figure 5.22*). The magnification should also be appropriate. Fine punctate staining cannot be detected at low magnification and may be significant. Fluorescein in the tear film may make corneal staining more difficult to see. It helps if the instillation is frugal, as fluorescein will dye the patient's face or clothing at least as well as the cornea. A short delay (a minute or two) between installation and observation is useful, to allow the tears to dilute the fluorescein.

Examination of the anterior chamber and the iris

There are two main reasons why we examine the anterior chamber in optometric practice. The first is to assess the risk of angle-closure glaucoma. This involves assessment of the anterior chamber depth (see Chapter 6) and examination of the anterior chamber for signs of pigment dispersion syndrome (PDS). The iris may be scanned for signs of new vessel growth following a venous occlusion, to prevent 30-day glaucoma. The second category of examination is the search for evidence of active or past inflammation, within the chamber itself, or on its limiting structures, that is the corneal endothelium, the iris and the anterior surface of the lens. Additionally, the slit-lamp biomicroscope also lends itself to the investigation of pupil defects, which may be related to uveitis or to lesions remote from the eye. Occasionally, a suspicious lesion must be monitored for evidence of malignancy.

Pigment dispersion syndrome

In PDS, iris pigment granules are translocated throughout the anterior and posterior chambers.[22] The trabecular meshwork is affected, which predisposes the eye to glaucoma. Pigment is shed because of rubbing between the lens and the posterior pigment layer iris, as a result of excessive bowing of the peripheral part of the iris.

PDS may be quite common, with the prevalence recently estimated at 2.45 per cent of the population,[23] though it was previously thought to be rarer. The percentage of those with PDS who develop glaucoma has been variously stated at about 10 per cent,[24] 25.6 per cent[25] and 50 per cent.[26]

The chances of having PDS appear similar for both males and females, but males are five times as likely to develop pigmentary glaucoma. There is an association with moderate myopia, and with lattice degeneration. The age of onset of the glaucoma is early, 20 to 40 years, especially in males.

There is a triad of diagnostic signs associated with PDS:
- Krukenberg's spindle;
- Trabecular meshwork pigmentation;
- Iris transillumination defects.

Krukenberg's spindle is, as the name suggests, a spindle-shaped collection of pigment cells on the corneal endothelium below the centre of the cornea (*Figure 5.23*). The base is often wider than the apex. The shape is probably determined by aqueous convection currents. The anterior lens surface may also show pigment on both anterior and posterior surfaces.

The trabecular meshwork can only really be seen well with gonioscopy (see Chapter 6), but sometimes associated pigmentation may be seen on the corneal endothelium near the limbus. If a circular or square beam is directed through the

pupil, the light reflected back from the retina can be used to retro-illuminate the iris.

The lamp and microscope are positioned directly in front of the eye, aligned and the retina is illuminated by a circular or square beam that will just fit into the pupil without striking the iris. Light is reflected back from the retina towards the observer. Normally, the pigment cells prevent the passage of this light through the iris, but with pigment dispersion the loss of pigment may result in slit-like defects through which the orange glow from the retina is visible (*Figure 5.24*). The pupil should ideally not be dilated for this, as the defects may be obscured. In some cases minimal dilation is required to allow enough light into the eye.

Patients with PDS often show very deep anterior chambers, particularly in the mid-peripheral portion, and an excessive anterior chamber depth to corneal thickness ratio should alert the practitioner to the possibility of finding one or more of the diagnostic signs.

There is also an increased incidence of lattice degeneration in these patients.

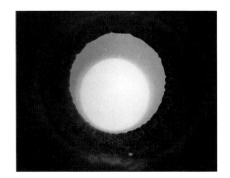

Figure 5.24
Retro-illumination of an atrophic iris

Table 5.2 Common systemic associations with anterior uveitis and possible symptoms

Condition	Patient symptoms
Ankylosing spondylitis	Lower back pain
Reiter's syndrome	Wrist and ankle pain (males 20–40 years of age)
Juvenile idiopathic arthritis	Pain in knees (under 16 years of age)
Crohn's disease	Stomach cramps, vomiting, diarrhoea
Sarcoidosis	Cough (black females 20-40 years of age)
Tuberculosis	Cough
Syphilis	Rash on palms, soles of feet, back
Behçet's disease	Tongue, mouth and genital ulcers

Inflammatory signs

Inflammation that involves the anterior chamber may be acute or chronic. In the former case, detection is rarely a challenge as the patient usually complains of pain and photophobia, and has perilimbal hyperaemia. This alerts the practitioner to the likelihood of further clinical signs that enable the differential diagnosis of uveitis from the other causes of acute red eye.

Many chronic cases of anterior uveitis are asymptomatic and the eye may be white, yet the diagnosis of the disease is no less important. Inflammation may lead to secondary glaucoma, and chronic anterior uveitis may be among the first signs of systemic conditions that have considerable implications for the future well-being of the patient.

The systemic conditions associated with anterior uveitis include collagen–vascular disorders, inflammations and infections, though the precise nature of some of these is speculative. The more common ones are listed in *Table 5.2*, along with symptoms to which the patient may admit when questioned. All patients with signs of uveitis and no diagnosis should be referred for medical opinion, as the underlying pathology may be sight- or life-threatening in the long term and early diagnosis may ameliorate the effects.

Keratic precipitates

Keratic precipitates (KPs) are caused by the deposition of white blood cells on the corneal endothelium. They are usually found on the lower half of the cornea and may form a spindle shape or triangle, though in acute anterior uveitis (AAU) the deposition may be more diffuse.[27]

Small- and medium-sized KPs occur in both acute and chronic non-granulomatous keratitis. Large KPs are often termed 'mutton fat KP' because of their fatty appearance (*Figure 5.25*). These tend to be associated with granulomatous disease, in which nodules are formed within the tissues by cells called granulocytes. The causes of granulomatous disease are varied, and include infection by viruses (e.g., *Herpes zoster*,) bacteria (tuberculosis, leprosy), fungi or parasites like toxoplasmosis and toxocariasis. Non-infectious causes include sarcoidosis.[28]

The presence of KPs in an eye that is otherwise quiet and healthy indicates a previous uveitic episode, though the seriousness of the cause can vary. Fine KPs, termed 'endothelial bedewing', may appear in extended-wear contact lens patients after a sterile inflammatory incident such as contact lens related acute red eye. This can be useful as the bedewing can persist for several months, and its discovery at a routine aftercare appointment may alert the

practitioner to events between aftercare visits. Small and medium KPs are fairly unspecific, but bilateral manifestations and the absence of symptoms point to a chronic, systemic association.

The chronology of the episode may be indicated by the appearance of the KPs. New KPs tend to be discrete, round and white or whitish yellow in appearance, and tend to shrink, flatten and fade with age. Ageing mutton-fat KPs tend to take on a ground-glass appearance. KPs usually take days to form and weeks or months to disappear. They may persist indefinitely, and in time they become entrapped within the endothelium, rather than lying upon it.[29]

KPs are often best seen initially in indirect and retro-illumination, so a fairly wide parallelepiped angled at about 60° is ideal (*Figure 5.26*). When lying upon the surface, they may show 'reversed illumination' at the margins between direct retro- and indirect illumination (*Figure 5.27*). The appearance may be identical to microcysts, but at the endothelial rather than epithelial level. A thin parallelepiped should allow the level to be determined.

Older KPs of all types may become pigmented, and the pigment may form a Krukenberg spindle and/or Arlt's triangle in the lower part of the cornea (*Figure 5.25*), with its base towards the limbus. Very fine pigmented KPs must be differentiated from the 'pigment dusting' associated with the endothelial guttatae in early Fuchs' dystrophy. An inspection of the endothelium using specular reflection is useful in such cases. Pigment dispersion is another possibility if the eye is otherwise quiet.

Cells and flare

KPs arise from white blood cells floating in the aqueous, released from the uveal vasculature in response to an inflammatory stimulus. If patients have cells within the aqueous, they have active anterior uveitis, even if the eye is white. Proteins may also

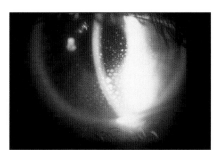

Figure 5.25
'Mutton fat' keratic precipitates in an Arlt's triangle formation

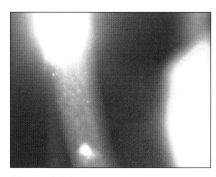

Figure 5.26
Appearance of fine keratic precipitates using retro-illumination

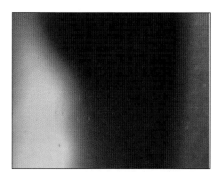

Figure 5.27
Reverse illumination of keratic precipitates using retro-illumination

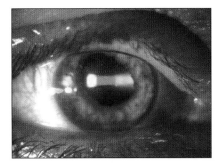

Figure 5.28
Presence of cells and flare in the anterior chamber

Table 5.3 Grading system for cells

Cells	Grade
5–10	+1
11–20	+2
21–50	+3
>50	+4

Table 5.4 Grading system for flare

Flare appearance	Grade
Faint, just detectable, iris clear	+1
Moderate, iris seen clearly	+2
Marked, iris detail hazy	+3
Intense, severe fibrous exudate	+4

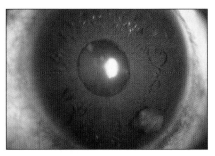

Figure 5.29
Busacca nodules aggregate away from the pupil margin

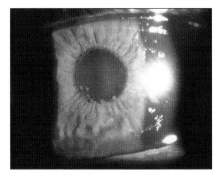

Figure 5.30
Koeppe nodules appear at the pupil margin

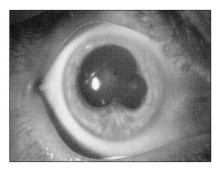

Figure 5.31
Distortion of the pupil margin because of posterior synechiae

leak from dilated or damaged uveal capillaries, to produce the clouding of the aqueous known as flare. Flare may persist beyond the active inflammation, which indicates residual vascular damage.

The traditional method for detecting cells and flare involves the use of a 'conic section' or pin-point illumination. The room illumination should be off, and the practitioner dark-adapted for a few minutes. A narrow circular beam, angled at about 45°, is focused mid-way between the cornea and endothelium, and the point of focus moved either laterally or back and forth with the joystick. This 'oscillation' technique is employed to increase the visibility of cells by alternating direct and indirect illumination. Cells and flare show up because of the Tyndall phenomenon. The normal aqueous is optically empty and cells and flare are revealed by the light they scatter. The effects are similar to those seen in car headlights in winter. Flare resembles fog, and cells look rather like snowflakes moving gently on random gusts of wind (*Figure 5.28*).

It is useful to be able to grade the levels of flare and cells, for which a parallelepiped of known dimensions is employed. Kanski describes a 3 × 1mm parallelepiped.[30] This should be angled at 45–60° and focused between the cornea and the lens. Inexperienced observers may find it useful to focus on each in turn a few times to feel how much joystick travel is needed, and then move it half-distance.

Catania recommends that the slit beam should mostly be directed towards the pupil,[32] but that a small portion strikes the iris. This may help to detect darker cells, which are seen more easily against the lighter background of reflected light from the iris. The cells seem to move slowly upwards or in an irregular direction. Patience is needed in mild cases, and the practitioner should be prepared to continue to look for a minute or so to be sure that there are no cells. The findings may be graded as in *Table 5.3* (after Kanski[30]).

In practice, anything over grade two is uncountable, and grade four resembles a snowstorm.

Flare may be graded with the same slit-lamp set-up (*Table 5.4*).

The vast majority of cells seen in the anterior chamber are white blood cells, but darker cells may also appear. Red blood cells may be released after trauma, and red blood cells may leak through from the vitreous in aphakes, following vitreous haemorrhage or complications with cataract extraction. These cells lose their haemoglobin after two weeks, and become 'ghost cells'. They appear reddish brown or khaki under slit-lamp observation.

Anomalies of the iris
The inflamed iris may show a number of anomalies. Granulomatous diseases are so termed because they produce granulomas, which appear on the iris as iris nodules. These are aggregations of white blood cells that may form on the surface of the iris away from the pupil margin, called Busacca nodules (*Figure 5.29*). However, more commonly they appear at the pupil margin, when they are termed Koeppe nodules (*Figure 5.30*). These accumulate pigment over time. Their presence is indicative both of an increased risk of synechiae and of the presence of systemic disease. The inflamed tissue is sticky, and adhesions may occur between the iris and the anterior lens surface (posterior synechiae), or between the peripheral iris and the cornea near the angle (anterior synechiae, best seen with a goniolens). Posterior synechiae are more likely in the presence of flare, or if Koeppe nodules are seen.[31] They may cause the iris to assume an irregular shape (*Figure 5.31*), either under normal conditions or when dilated.[27] If the adhesion advances, the pupil may become fixed (seclusio pupillae), and bowed forward (iris bombe) and secondary glaucoma may ensue.

Synechiae sometimes come adrift from the lens surface, especially after treatment, and leave characteristic irregular shapes on the lens surface, quite unlike the smaller epicapsular stars, which are often congenital, but these irregular shapes may be the result of pigment deposition after uveitis. Synechiae themselves may be distinguished from the common persistent pupillary membrane (PPM) by origin (pupil margin or posterior iris as opposed to the collarette in the case of the PPM) and by the fact that they are fibrous and resist pupil dilation, whereas PPMs are elastic.[32]

The iris itself may become swollen, and crypt definition may be lost. This condition, rather splendidly termed 'boggy iris', is best observed with a tangential beam, which tends to show the surface texture well. However, dense flare usually accompanies it, so observation may be difficult. In chronic or recurrent uveitis, pigment cells may be lost to the extent that transillumination defects appear. Alternatively, the iris may become lighter in colour than its fellow, as in Fuchs' heterochromic iridocyclitis, though heterochromia may also occur congenitally as part of Horner's syndrome.

The pupil

Apart from the irregular pupil shape produced by adhesions, a number of other pupil anomalies may be observed with the slit-lamp biomicroscope. The brightness of the beam and the magnification allowed by the microscope make the instrument particularly suitable for observations of the pupil, especially when the iris is very dark, or the pupil sluggish. A broad beam, with or without the diffuser, is the most suitable form of illumination, using the rheostat to vary the level of illumination.

Staying with uveitis, in acute attacks the pupil is classically miotic, but this is not always the case. The pupil reactions range from normal to sluggish, and correctopia may appear if the pupil dilates. A further use of the slit lamp in suspected uveitis is the Henkind or consensual pain reflex test. This is performed when active uveitis is suspected, but no cell or flare can be seen. The suspected eye is occluded. The fellow eye is given a bright light stimulus, which produces a consensual pupil constriction in the suspected eye. If uveitis is present, this constriction should produce pain, though false negative results are possible.[33]

A sluggish pupil may be produced by anomalies within the globe, such as glaucoma, or by lesions that affect the nerve supply. Similarly, correctopia may occur when the ciliary nerves are damaged in one sector. Where the pupil appears inactive to the naked eye, the slit lamp often allows the practitioner to distinguish the merely tonic from the completely paretic.

One further technique is useful when the patient shows a homonymous field defect. The afferent pupillary fibres initially travel with the visual fibres within the optic nerve and tract, but leave the visual pathway shortly before the lateral geniculate nucleus. Lesions that occur in the optic tract before the pupillary fibres leave give rise to a form of afferent pupil defect as well as a homonymous field defect. Light that strikes the side of the visual field affected fails to elicit pupil constriction in either eye, whereas light that strikes the visually normal hemifield triggers normal direct and consensual constriction. This is known as Wernicke's hemianopic pupil.[34]

In theory, the technique should be easy, but in practice many of the patients to whom it would be applicable have media opacities that tend to scatter light entering the eye. For this reason, a fine beam of bright light, similar to a conic section, must be used.

Suspicious masses and pigmentation of the iris

Iris melanomas are, for the most part, slow growing and the prognosis is excellent, especially if diagnosed early. They usually present in patients between 40 and 60 years of age and most often appear in the lower half of the iris as a single nodule, pigmented (*Figure 5.32*) or non-pigmented (amelanotic). Some associated vascularisation is possible, but it is not indicative of malignancy as it relates to the size of the pigmented lesion rather than its nature, and in highly pigmented tumours it may be masked, whereas it is more apparent in amelanotic ones.

Suspicion is aroused by large lesions, spontaneous hyphaema, localised lens opacities and distortion of the pupil margin, though naevi can occasionally cause these anomalies if close enough to the pupil.[35] Other bodies that are sometimes mistaken for tumours include granulomas and iris cysts.

Multiple iris freckles rarely cause worry, but a single large naevus must always be monitored carefully. Excessive pigmentation may be secondary to certain medications. The most important sign of malignancy is growth, so measurement and documentation are vital. Photographic evidence is the best, so patients with suspicious naevi should have them photographed if this facility is available. The emergence of higher resolution, and less expensive, digital cameras and more efficient data-storage systems may make photographic recording a common feature in general optometric practice in the future.

Beyond the anterior chamber

The major slit-lamp biomicroscope is usually associated with the anterior part of the eye, yet with suitable supplementary lenses it permits investigation of the internal structures of the eye up to and including the retina. Even without supplementary lenses, both the lens and the anterior vitreous may be examined.

Defects of the transparent media of the eye result in interfaces between materials of different refractive index. This allows anomalies to be detected by their refractive and reflective effects on the light beam. In the case of the lens, useful information may be gained from retro-illumination, using the fundus as a reflecting surface. Anomalies may be detected when they either block the returning light or deflect its path. Direct focal illumination shows up opacities through the Tyndall effect, and the distribution of opacities within an optical section of the lens can reveal the likely onset and cause of the defect. Specular reflection may also reveal interfaces of refractive index, especially at the anterior and posterior surfaces of the lens.

With care, the anterior vitreous may also be examined, both for signs of vitreous anomalies and to detect the inappropriate presence of cells, which can indicate inflammation, haemorrhage, tumour or retinal detachment (*Figure 5.33*).

Pseudoexfoliation syndrome

This is a relatively common cause of open-angle glaucoma, and is seen in elderly patients, often with co-existent cataract. It is bilateral in about a third of cases, though often asymmetric. Where one eye is affected, there is a 20 per cent chance of the other eye becoming affected within 10 years.[36]

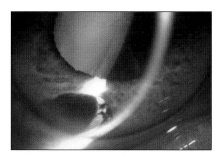

Figure 5.32
Single pigmented nodule in the lower half of the iris. Iris melanoma should be suspected

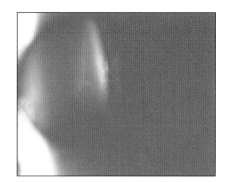

Figure 5.33
Slit-lamp view showing the Y-shaped suture and the retrolental space and anterior uveitis

The characteristic sign is pseudoexfoliative material (PXM) on the anterior surface of the lens. This is whitish and is said to resemble dandruff. It is thought to be the product of abnormal cell metabolism and to arise from the lens capsule, zonules and inner layer of the ciliary epithelium.[37] On the surface of the lens, it is easily seen with direct focal illumination and a parallelepiped section. The movements of the iris dislodge the PXM from the lens capsule surface. This leaves a central disc of PXM with a clear zone that surrounds it and separates it from a peripheral band of PXM, which has numerous radial striations. The peripheral band can only be seen if the pupil is dilated. Rubbing of the iris also dislodges pigment from the iris, and pigment similar to that seen in PDS can be seen in conjunction with the PXM on the corneal endothelium.

Defects of the pupillary frill are common, and PXM may be seen deposited upon the pupil margin. Iris transillumination defects can also occur, similar to those seen in PDS, but confined to the pupil margin. This can be seen by retro-illumination against the red reflex from the fundus.

Pseudoexfoliation syndrome is the leading cause of unilateral glaucoma in the elderly. Some 20 per cent of patients that exhibit pseudoexfoliation have glaucoma at the time of detection. Most are asymptomatic, though pain is possible with greatly elevated pressure. Many patients have advanced field losses by the time they are detected, and the glaucoma is often harder to control than primary open-angle glaucoma. In an ideal world, routine detailed slit-lamp examination would be possible for all patients but, more realistically, any patient over 60 years of age with suspicious pressures, especially if they are asymmetric, should be examined carefully for signs of pseudoexfoliation.

Retro-illumination of the lens

This technique is used to examine the lens and anterior vitreous as well as the iris. Initially, the microscope is placed in the straight-ahead position, with the lamp nearly coaxial and yet allowing binocular viewing. The microscope is focused on the structure under consideration, then the beam is decoupled and swung so that it enters the pupil near the margin. The beam should be moderately wide, and the beam height adjusted to avoid unnecessary reflections from the iris. The red reflex from the fundus can be 'tuned' by making small adjustments in the position and direction of the beam, to maximise brightness. In addition, slight nasal rotation of the subject's eye can bring the beam to reflect from the optic nerve head, which is rather more reflective than the surrounding retinal surface.[38]

When investigating iris transillumination defects, the pupil is normally undilated or only moderately dilated, but lens anomalies are easier to examine with a dilated pupil, particularly as the pupil diameter tends to decrease with age. Opacities of the lens appear dark against the red reflex, but there are also a number of 'non-opaque' defects,[39] which are associated with the formation of cataract, both as precursors to and in association with opacification.

Water clefts are spindle-shaped cavities, filled with fluid, that lie along lens sutures. With retro-illumination, they may appear similar to cataract, as dark radial wedges. Most water clefts, however, are not visible by retro-illumination, but can be seen more easily with a retinoscope. This curious fact may be explained because the retinoscope, which itself uses a form of retro-illumination to produce its reflex, is used at approximately 66cm, whereas the biomicroscope is much closer. The water clefts contain fluid that has a refractive index only slightly different to the surrounding lens material, so only a small deviation of the emerging light is induced. The further back the observer, the more the rays are separated.

To summarise, if a defect can be seen in the retinoscope reflex, but not by retro-illumination with the slit lamp, it is probably a water cleft. At the commencement of ophthalmoscopy, it may be useful to focus on the pupil area from a distance of 1–2 feet, which enables water clefts to be seen against the fundus glow.[40]

Vacuoles are fluid-filled spheres within the lens cortex, and range from 10μm to 1.3mm in diameter. With retro-illumination they have a similar appearance to corneal vacuoles in that they show unreversed illumination, because their contents have a lower refractive index than the surrounding tissue. They are common in patients over 45 years of age, and the incidence increases with age. Individual vacuoles are transient phenomena that disappear in weeks or months. They can appear at any layer in the cortex, but are very unusual in the nucleus.

Retrodots are also small rounded phenomena, which often coalesce into lobulated forms. Individually they range in size from 80–500μm. They are located in the deeper regions of the cortex, and occasionally in the superficial layers of the nucleus. They are thought to consist of crystalline material contained within a membrane, and the crystalline material gives the retrodots the property of birefringence. This ability to rotate the plane of polarised light means that, when observed with polarised light, they appear bright against a dark background. When observed with retro-illumination, retrodots exhibit reversed illumination, which indicates a higher refractive index than the surrounding tissue.

Focal illumination of the lens

The lens may also be investigated using a parallelepiped or thin section. The appearance of a mature adult lens, when first encountered, can be a bit of a shock. The lens of a child, which consists largely of nucleus, is optically rather empty, but in the adult the cortex in section shows bands of differing brightness. These resemble the growth rings of a tree, and are constantly being pushed more centrally by the formation of new fibres. These bands of discontinuity are a normal feature and become most prominent around the age of 45 years. The increased general light-scattering properties of the elderly lens tend to mask these bands in later life. Upon first encountering the bands of discontinuity, it is tempting to see cataract, though the visual acuity will be normal (*Figure 5.34*).

The anterior cortex of the lens tends to have a bluish tinge when seen in section, as long wavelengths of light are scattered selectively. Opacities in the cortex appear white, though those in the posterior cortex may be tinged yellow by nuclear brunescence.

Capsular opacities may occur at either pole of the lens, and are normally congenital and may be associated with PPMs or hyaloid remnants. The most commonly seen is the Mittendorf Dot, which is a white, round opacity found either on or close to the posterior capsule, often

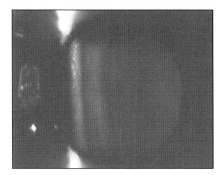

Figure 5.34
The bands of discontinuity ('onion layer') become more prominent with age

attached to a floating hyaloid remnant. A white cone may project from the pole of the lens, termed a pyramidal cataract. Sometimes capsular anomalies are associated with defects of subadjacent cortical fibres. The effect over time is to produce a repeated opacity that resembles a stack of plates. Opacities at the posterior pole tend to have more effect on vision than anterior ones, because of their proximity to the nodal point of the eye. This is particularly so in bright light conditions, as the pupil constricts.

This is also true of subcapsular opacities, which may arise from senile changes or secondary to ocular inflammations or from degenerative conditions such as retinitis pigmentosa or high myopia. The distinction may be made by examining the layers of the cortex below the subcapsular opacity. With senile changes, the underlying layers are normal, as they were when they were subcapsular. With 'complicated' (i.e., secondary to pathology) changes, the underlying fibres were also affected when they were near the surface, so opacities are found in the deeper layers. Thus the position of formerly subcapsular opacities within the cortex can indicate the age of onset of the condition that caused them, in the same way that botanists can deduce the date of climatic change from the growth rings of a tree. If deeper layers are opacified, yet more superficial layers clear, the prognosis is probably good, since whatever was producing the opacity is now resolved.

Subcapsular opacities may also be produced by trauma, and initially may be invisible under focal illumination. Retro-illumination may reveal the presence of vacuolated defects, which later opacify.

Cortical opacities seen in retro-illumination may be cataract or water cleft. An optical section will differentiate the two. In direct illumination, cataract appears whiter than the surrounding tissue, whereas water clefts are dark, optically empty spaces. Cortical opacities commonly appear in the lower nasal quadrant first, which may be related to embryology, as the foetal fissure is situated in this quadrant.

When cortical spoke cataracts are examined with a parallelepiped beam, fine striations are often seen running at right angles to the spokes, which are themselves radial. These are termed fibre folds, and are believed to be a phenomenon produced by reflection from the surfaces of fibres that have become corrugated. The corrugation is believed to be associated with a break in the fibres in the equatorial region of the lens, and produces a crescent-shaped defect that has been termed a circular shade.[41]

This can be seen by direct focal or retro-illumination with the eye looking down and the pupil dilated. The fibre folds are common in the elderly, with 18 per cent of those who are 60–70 years of age having them, usually bilaterally.[39] Fibre folds cannot be seen in retro-illumination and are invisible to retinoscopy, which suggests that they have little effect on the vision.

Nuclear cataract tends to occur in the very young or the elderly. In the child, the defect is initially subcapsular, and it gradually becomes more central with age as new fibres are laid down. If the subsequent fibres are normal, the optical section reveals a lamellar cataract, with an opacified layer with clearer layers above and below it. Genetic, metabolic and infective causes are probable. Senile nuclear cataract appears yellow or brown because of blue-light absorption by lens proteins. It tends to affect colour perception; the artists Rembrandt and Turner used a palette that contained much more orange, red and brown in later life. Monet used yellow-tinted spectacles after cataract surgery, as he hated the increase in blue that the surgery brought in.

Christmas-tree cataract is an uncommon but spectacular lens defect. Despite its name, it is not an opaque phenomenon; it is probably a diffractive phenomenon produced by cystine crystals. Under direct focal illumination it appears as multicoloured 'needles' that criss-cross the fibres of the deep cortex. Retro-illumination may produce a dim outline and the retinoscope reflex may contain a slight dark anomaly. Christmas-tree cataract may be seen in isolation in an ageing lens (when it produces no measurable loss of vision) or coincidentally with other forms of cataract.

Specular reflection

The technique of using specular reflection to visualise the corneal endothelium is described above. Any interface between materials of differing refractive index produces reflections. The easiest to see is that produced by the anterior capsule surface, which has a characteristic shagreen or appearance like an orange peel. Though easy to produce, this is of limited practical value, as even pseudoexfoliation is easy to see in direct illumination. However, where a capsular opacity disrupts the surface, a dark halo may be seen to surround the opacity (Vogt's sign), and this may help to differentiate a capsular from a subcapsular anomaly. Fibre folds are seen by reflection, and water clefts may be seen by light reflected from their posterior walls.

Vacuoles produce a bright reflex from anterior or posterior surfaces, and retrodots appear as round elevations by specular illumination.

Anterior vitreous examination

Examination of the vitreous with the slit lamp is a challenge, as a number of overlying structures scatter the light. The pupil margin may limit the angle between the lamp and microscope, which helps to reduce the masking effect of scattered light. The structure of even the normal vitreous is difficult to interpret with a slit lamp. Indeed, of the early pioneers who examined the vitreous with the slit lamp, 'Gullstrand saw membranes composed of a network of web-like structures, Koeppe described vertical and horizontal fibres arranged in regularly intercrossing systems and Baurmann saw a grill-like pattern of lighter and darker bands representing several layers of chain-link fences'.[42] Even the use of post-mortem dark-field microscopy resulted in confusion, and might be regarded as a little overzealous in optometric practice.

With all this difficulty, the first question to address is not 'How to?', but 'Why bother?' The answer to this question is that the anterior vitreous can provide vital information regarding inflammation and retinal detachment.

The portion of the vitreous accessible without supplementary lenses is normally virtually acellular. The exact dimensions of the accessible area vary with refraction, being deeper with hypermetropic eyes and maximal with aphakic ones. Pupil diameter also limits the visible area and, where possible, observations should be made with the pupil dilated. Anomalies of the vitreous are often subtle and a high level of illumination is required. To avoid reflected light from overlying structures, the angle between the lamp and the microscope should be as high as possible, but the angle obtainable limits the maximum beam width that is practical. The observer should dark-adapt before the examination. Precise focusing is essential.

The vitreous in a young eye is relatively optically empty, though there are structures within the vitreous gel that can reflect light and appear as membranes. The most anterior visible structure is a 'wrinkled, extremely thin and optically reflective limiting layer' according to Vogt,[43] who called it the membrana hyaloidea plicata. It is most easily seen in young patients, and is separated from the posterior surface by an optically empty

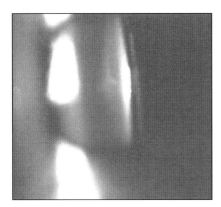

Figure 5.35
Berger's space

space of variable depth, known as Berger's space (*Figure 5.35*). This space is present over the central area to a diameter of 8–9mm, being enclosed by Weiger's ligament, a zone of attachment between the vitreous face and the lens capsule.[44]

In PDS, pigment may collect at this attachment, giving rise to a ring deposit, which may be complete or partial. This is termed the Scheie line or stripe and has only been described in PDS.[22]

The vitreous gel is believed to consist of a 'framework' of collagen fibrils separated by hyaluronic acid molecules. In older eyes, and in myopic or aphakic eyes at a younger age, the vitreous appears less homogeneous. The collagen fibrils aggregate into coarser bundles, visible as irregular tortuous fibres. These are separated by dark, fluid-filled spaces. Eventually, the vitreous may shrink and detach from the retina. The degeneration of the gel may cause calcium soaps to coalesce on the vitreous fibrils. They form white or yellow globules, about 0.5mm in diameter, which move with the gel on eye movement, but always return to their original position, as the framework of

the vitreous is intact. This is termed asteroid hyalosis, and is a benign condition not associated with any systemic condition. It is present in about 0.5 per cent of eyes, more commonly in males and usually unilateral.[45] Some older textbooks call the same condition synchysis scintillans, which is a term now used to describe vitreous opacification secondary to chronic vitreous haemorrhage. The refractile bodies here are flat, golden brown and freely mobile. They always settle at the lowest point of the vitreous when eye movement stops, since the framework of the vitreous is destroyed. The opacities contain cholesterol crystals, and free haemoglobin spherules have also been reported.

A third form of vitreous opacification is associated with amyloidosis, a rare inherited systemic condition. Opacification initially begins near the retina, but later progresses to the anterior vitreous. The early appearance is granular, with wispy fringes, but later the vitreous takes on the appearance of glass wool. No cellular invasion accompanies it. Cells in any number are not a feature of the normal central and retrolenticular vitreous, and their presence indicates either inflammation haemorrhage or neoplastic spread.

Red blood cells *en masse* appear red, but individually they may be yellow, glistening dots that later become a dull white.[46] When they are red, they may be distinguished from pigment cells with the red-free filter, which renders the red blood cells black. The distinction may be difficult, but this is not enormously important since the presence of either is a strong indication of a retinal break.[47] When they are lighter in colour, they may look similar to white blood cells.

White blood cells may appear, along with proteinaceous flare in the anterior vitreous, as a consequence of intermedi-

ate or posterior uveitis. Unpigmented cells may also represent 'seed cells' of neoplastic origin. While these are rare, in a patient over 50 years of age they may signal a large cell lymphoma,[48] if signs of uveitis are absent. The presence of pigmented cells ('tobacco dust') in Berger's space and the anterior vitreous of a phakic eye is a very important sign of a retinal break, even in an asymptomatic patient.[49] The cells arise in Bruch's membrane and they become dispersed throughout the vitreous cavity. The pigment reaches the anterior vitreous within hours of the retinal break.

When posterior vitreous detachment (PVD) occurs, there is a significant risk of a retinal break, though estimates vary widely as to what percentage of patients are affected. Figures of 8–46 per cent have been reported and a recent study found an incidence of 12.5 per cent.[50] It was also concluded that symptoms are a very unreliable indication of a retinal break. Shafer's sign was found to be present in 96 per cent of patients with a retinal break, and none without. The appearance of red blood cells is also significant, as they may arise from damage to small capillaries associated with a retinal break. All patients who have signs or symptoms that suggest either retinal detachment or PVD should have slit-lamp biomicroscopy to detect these signs, and their presence indicates rapid referral. Where no Shafer's sign is present, less urgent referral is indicated in cases of acute PVD, as the occasional patient does show it despite the presence of a retinal break.

Acknowledgements

Figures 5.5, 5.7, 5.8 and *5.9* courtesy of Bausch & Lomb. *Figures 5.21, 5.23–5.25* and *5.28–5.32* courtesy of J Kanski, *Clinical Ophthalmology*, 4th edition, Butterworth–Heinemann.

REFERENCES

1 Henson D (1996). Slit lamps. In *Optometric Instrumentation*, Vol. 1, p. 138–161, Ed Henson D (London, Butterworth–Heinmann).

2 US Department of Health and Human Services, Food and Drug Administration (1998). *Slit Lamp Guidance*, Centre for Devices and Radiological Health, General Services Devices Branch, Division of Ophthalmic Devices, Office of Device Evaluation. http:/www.fda.gov/cdrh/ode/68.html [Accessed 2 June 2001].

3 North RV (1993). *Work and the Eye* (Oxford; Oxford University Press) p. 87–89.

4 Kohnen S (2000). Light-induced damage of the retina through slit-lamp photography. *Graefe's Arch Clin Exp Ophthalmol*. **238**, 956–959.

5 Calkins JL, Hochheimer BF and D'anna SA (1980). Potential hazards from specific ophthalmic devices. *Vis Res*. **20**, 1039–1053.

6 Goldberg JB (1970). *Biomicroscopy for Contact Lens Practice*. (Chicago; The Professional Press Inc.).

7 Kanski J (1994). *Clinical Ophthalmology: A Systemic Approach*, Third Edition. (Oxford: Butterworth–Heinemann) p. 72–97.

8 Woods R (1989). Quantitative slit lamp observations in contact lens practice. *J Br Contact Lens Assoc*. **12** (scientific meetings), 42–45.

9 Sankaridurg PR, Skotnisky C, Pearce D, Sweeney DR and Holden BA (2001). Contact lens papillary conjunctivitis – A review. *Optom Pract*. **1**, 19–27.

10 Osbourne G, Zantos S, *et al.* (1989). Evaluation of tear meniscus heights on marginal dry eye soft lens wearers. *Invest Ophthalmol Vis Sci*, **30** (supplement), 501.

11 Kanski J (1994). *Clinical Ophthalmology: A Systemic Approach*, Third Edition. (Oxford: Butterworth–Heinemann) p. 62.

12 Elliott DB (1997). *Clinical Procedures in Primary Eye Care*. (Oxford: Butterworth–Heinemann) p. 177–180.

13 Morris J and Hirji N (1998). *The Slit Lamp Microscope in Optometric Practice*, Second Edition (Fleet: Association of Optometrists/Optometry Today) p. 7.

14 Mengher LS, Bron AJ, Tonge SR and Gilbert DJ (1985). Effect of fluorescein sodium installation on the pre-corneal tear film stability. *Curr Eye Res.* **4**, 9–12.

15 Gasson A and Morris J (1998). *The Contact Lens Manual*, Second Edition. (Oxford: Butterworth–Heinemann) p. 63.

16 Guillon J-P (1998). Non-invasive Tearscope plus routine for contact lens fitting. *Contact Lens Anterior Eye* **21** (Supplement): S31–S40.

17 Guillon J-P (1997). The Keeler Tearscope – an improved device for assessing the tear film. *Optician* **213** (5594), 66–72.

18 Doughty MJ (1999). *Drugs, Medications and the Eye*, Third Edition. (Helensburgh: Smawcastellane Information Services) p. 4:6–4:9.

19 Lee J, Courtney R and Thorson JC (1980). Contact lens application of Kodak Wratten filter systems for enhanced detection of fluorescein staining. *Contact Lens J.* **9**, 33–34.

20 Hopkins G and Pearson R (1998). Stains. In *Ophthalmic Drugs*, p. 133–138, Ed. Hopkins GA, (Oxford: Butterworth–Heinemann).

21 Doughty MJ (1999). *Drugs, Medications and the Eye*, Third Edition. (Helensburgh: Smawcastellane Information Services) p. 4:7.

22 Collicott T (1998). Pigment-dispersion syndrome, and pigmentary glaucoma. *Optician* **216** (5674), 16–19.

23 Ritch R, Steinberger D and Leibmann JM (1993). Prevalence of pigment dispersion syndrome in a population undergoing glaucoma screening. *Am J Ophthalmol.* **115**, 707–710.

24 Kanski J (1994). *Clinical Ophthalmology: A Systemic Approach*, Third Edition. (Oxford: Butterworth–Heinemann) p. 259.

25 Scheie HG and Cameron JD (1981). Pigment dispersion syndrome: a clinical study. *Br J Ophthalmol.* **65**, 264–269.

26 Hoh HB and Easty DL (1995). *Clinical Cases in Ophthalmology.* (Oxford: Butterworth–Heinemann) p. 53–54.

27 Catania LJ (1988). *Primary Care of the Anterior Segment*, Second Edition (Norwalk: Appleton & Lange) p. 362–363.

28 Cullen A and Jones L (2000). Flare, cells and KP. *Optician* **220** (5759), 28–31.

29 Tomlinson A (1992). *Complications of Contact Lens Wear.* (St Louis, Mosby–Year Book) p. 51.

30 Kanski J (1994). *Clinical Ophthalmology: A Systemic Approach*, Third Edition. (Oxford: Butterworth–Heinemann) p. 153.

31 Muchnick GB. The diagnosis and management of anterior uveitis. *Optometry Today*, **37**(8), 34–37.

32 Catania LJ (1988). *Primary Care of the Anterior Segment*, Second Edition (Norwalk: Appleton & Lange) p. 390.

33 An Y-K and Henkind P (1981). Pain elicited by consensual pupillary reflex: A diagnostic test for acute iritis. *Lancet* **ii** 1254.

34 Kanski J (1994). *Clinical Ophthalmology: A Systemic Approach*, Third Edition. (Oxford: Butterworth–Heinemann) p. 485.

35 Kanski J (1994). *Clinical Ophthalmology: A Systemic Approach*, Third Edition. (Oxford: Butterworth–Heinemann) p. 207–209.

36 Kanski J (1994). *Clinical Ophthalmology: A Systemic Approach*, Third Edition. (Oxford: Butterworth–Heinemann) p. 257.

37 Phelps-Brown NA (1984). The lens. In: *Atlas of Clinical Ophthalmology*, Second Edition, p. 8.20, Eds Spalton DJ, Hitchings RA and Hunter PA (London: Mosby–Year Book Europe Limited).

38 Martonyi CL, Bahn CF and Meyer RF (1985). *Clinical Slit Lamp Biomicroscopy and Photo Slit Lamp Biomicrography*, Second Edition (Michigan: Time One Ink Ltd) p. 42.

39 Phelps-Brown N (1998). Non-opaque human lens defects. *Optician* **216** (5662), 13–17.

40 Franklin NJ, personal communication.

41 Obazawa H, Fujiwara T and Kawara T (1983). The maturing process of the senile 7cataractous lens. N *Acta XXIV International Congress of Ophthalmology*, Ed. Henkind P, American Academy of Ophthalmology. (Philadelphia: JB Lipincott).

42 Sebag J (1992). The vitreous. In: *Adlers Physiology of the Eye*, Ninth Edition, p. 269, Ed. Hart WM (St Louis, Mosby–Year Book Inc.).

43 Hruby K and Posner A (1967). *Slitlamp Examination of Vitreous and Retina* (Baltimore: The Williams and Wilkins Company) p. 37.

44 MacLeod D (1984). Vitreous and vitro-retinal disorders. In: *Atlas of Clinical Ophthalmology*, Second Edition, p. 12.2, Eds Spalton DJ, Hitchings RA and Hunter PA (London: Mosby–Year Book Europe Limited).

45 Sebag J (1992). The vitreous. In: *Adlers Physiology of the Eye*, Ninth Edition, p. 309, Ed. Hart WM (St Louis, Mosby–Year Book Inc.).

46 Hruby K and Posner A (1967). *Slitlamp Examination of Vitreous and Retina* (Baltimore: The Williams and Wilkins Company) p. 45.

47 Novak MA and Welch RB (1984). Complications of acute symptomatic posterior vitreous detachment. *Am J Ophthalmol.* **97**, 308–314.

48 Korolkiewicz M (2000). The management of patients with flashes and/or floaters. *Optician* **219** (5737), 36.

49 Boldrey EE (1997). Risk of retinal tears in patients with vitreous floaters. *Am J Ophthalmol.* **123**, 263–264.

50 Chignell AH, Harle D, Tanner V and Williamson TH (2000). Acute posterior vitreous detachment. *Optom Pract.* **1**, 97–102.

6

Examination of the anterior chamber angle and depth

Frank Eperjesi and Bill Harvey

Gonioscopy is a technique that allows practitioners to examine an area of the eye otherwise hidden from view. The anterior chamber wall cannot be directly observed externally because of the limbal overhang, so as the observer moves parallel to the iris surface, the light rays from the chamber angle undergo internal reflection, which prevents the light from leaving the eye. The word gonioscopy, derived from Greek, means to view the angle. This procedure allows evaluation of the width of the anterior chamber angle, detailed inspection of the structures within the anterior segment of the eye prior to dilation and the investigation of ocular signs or symptoms. Some authorities describe it as an integral part of any complete ophthalmic evaluation. However, gonioscopy can initially seem difficult. This chapter describes the gonio-anatomy and provides a 'how-to' guide to enable those interested in this procedure to develop their skills and use this technique with ease and confidence. It then discusses methods of assessing the depth of the anterior chamber based on the slit-lamp.

Critical angle

A critical angle occurs when light from an object passes from a medium of higher refractive index to another of lower refractive index. The angle of refraction in the lower refractive index medium increases more rapidly than the angle of incidence. At certain angles of incidence, the angle of refraction is 90° and the refracted light runs parallel along the surface. This angle is known as the critical angle. Light that hits the surface at an angle greater than the critical angle does not enter the second medium and is reflected at the surface. In the eye, the light rays from the anterior chamber strike the anterior corneal surface at an angle greater than the critical angle, estimated at 46–49°, and as such are totally internally reflected (*Figure 6.1*).

When a goniolens is placed on the eye, the air interface with the anterior cornea is replaced by the lens surface, which has an index of refraction similar to the index of refraction of the corneal tissue. The critical angle is eliminated because the light is refracted by the steep curved outer surface of the goniolens. Light from the anterior chamber can then be reflected by a mirror into the examiner's eyes. This is the basic concept by which indirect goniolenses, used in conjunction with a slit lamp, allow visualisation of the anterior chamber angle (*Figure 6.2*). The image produced is indirect, virtual and unmagnified, and not laterally reversed about the vertical.

Anterior chamber gonio-anatomy

The purpose of gonioscopy is to permit visualisation of the irido-corneal angle, better known as the anterior chamber angle, and referred to as the angle in this chapter. This is the area in which the trabecular meshwork lies, and is therefore responsible for aqueous outflow.

Before examination of the angle is discussed, it is important to review the anatomy and function of its structures.

The appearance of the anterior chamber angle varies according to congenital individual differences and with acquired changes through age, injury or disease.

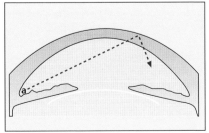

Figure 6.1
Light from the anterior chamber angle 'a' undergoes total internal reflection at the tear–air interface and is not visible to the examiner

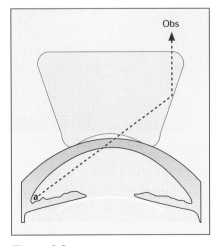

Figure 6.2
Indirect goniolenses use mirrors to reflect the light from the anterior chamber angle 'a' so that it leaves the eye perpendicular to the face of the lens

From anterior to posterior the gonio-anatomy consists of 10 normally visible structures:

- cornea;
- Schwalbe's line;
- Schlemm's canal;
- trabecular meshwork;
- scleral spur;
- ciliary body;
- iris processes (not always present);
- iris root;
- iris surface; and
- pupil border.

The most important are described in detail below (also see *Figures 6.3* and *6.4*).

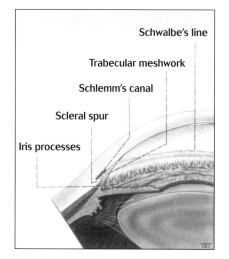

Figure 6.3
Important structures of the anterior chamber angle

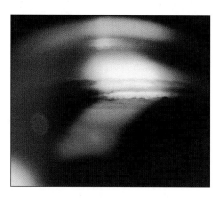

Figure 6.4
View of a normal angle through a goniolens. From posterior to anterior, the pupil margin is just visible in the lower left-hand corner. The larger brown area is the iris, followed by a fine grey line adjacent to the iris, the cilary body, above which is the pale scleral spur, then a brown-pigmented posterior portion of the trabecular, and a less-pigmented anterior portion, with a faint suggestion of Schwalbe's lines, and finally the opaque cornea

Schwalbe's line

Schwalbe's line is a condensation of connective tissue fibres. It forms the termination of Descemet's membrane and marks the transition from the transparent cornea to the opaque scleral tissue. It also forms the anterior boundary of the trabecular meshwork. It is a difficult structure to find and may be barely distinguishable. It appears as a thin white glistening line of variable thickness. Its position can be identified using an optic section, which creates focal lines that represent the anterior and posterior cornea. These focal lines merge at the end of the internal cornea and both denote the internal limbus, as well as mark the location of Schwalbe's line.

Trabecular meshwork

The trabecular meshwork runs from Schwalbe's line to the anterior limit of the cornea, where it inserts into the scleral spur posteriorly. In cross-section, the trabeculum forms an obtuse angle, with the base in contact with the scleral spur, the anterior face of the ciliary body and the iris root. The apex terminates at the corneoscleral boundary – Schwalbe's line.

The trabecular meshwork can be arbitrarily divided into anterior and posterior portions. The former runs from Descemet's membrane to the area anterior to Schlemm's canal. This is considered to be the non-filtering portion of the meshwork because it has no contact with Schlemm's canal. The posterior portion is involved in filtering and overlies Schlemm's canal. The filtering portion has a grey, translucent appearance. In older or in heavily pigmented eyes, the filtering portion of the trabecular meshwork is often pigmented and darker than the remainder of the meshwork. This helps to identify the portion of the meshwork involved in filtration and in localisation of the canal of Schlemm, which lies internal to the meshwork at this point. In eyes without pigmentation, the filtering portion can be identified by its known location from the scleral spur and Schwalbe's line, as well as by its grey, granular appearance in comparison to the white scleral spur.

Schlemm's canal

Schlemm's canal lies within the trabecular meshwork and is approximately 0.2mm to 0.3mm wide. It cannot be detected by gonioscopy unless it is filled with blood, which may appear as a pinkish band anterior to the scleral spur. Normally there is no visible blood in the canal because the pressure within the canal is lower than the pressure in the anterior chamber. The canal of Schlemm connects with the venous system of collector channels that anastomose to form a deep scleral venous plexus. This plexus drains the aqueous into the episcleral veins and anterior ciliary veins.

Scleral spur

The scleral spur is a fibrous ring that is attached anteriorly to the trabecular meshwork and posteriorly to the sclera and longitudinal portion of the ciliary muscle. It is paler than any of the other structures in the angle, and so is the most easily recognised landmark. Its identification and visualisation confirm that the filtering meshwork is not obstructed in the area of observation.

Ciliary body

The ciliary body lies posterior to the scleral spur and varies in colour from grey–white in light eyes to darker grey in pigmented eyes. It may also appear reddish brown, chocolate brown or reddish-grey. Its many functions include:

- manufacture of aqueous humor;
- regulation of aqueous outflow;
- control of accommodation;
- secretion of hyaluronate into the vitreous; and
- maintenance of a portion of the blood–aqueous barrier.

Although most outflow of aqueous occurs through the trabecular meshwork, approximately 10 to 30 per cent is by a non-conventional route, primarily through the ciliary body face into the suprachoroidal space. Uveoscleral outflow is pressure independent, unlike the trabecular outflow. As it is pressure independent, it appears to have more significance with a lower intraocular pressure, probably because the trabecular system can autoregulate and reduce flow-dependent intraocular pressure (IOP).

Iris processes

Iris processes can appear as:

- thin, fine lacy fibres;
- structures like tree branches;
- a coarse dense interlacing network; or
- a membrane attaching the iris to the trabecular meshwork.

The reason for their occurrence is unclear, but they are known to be physiological. Sometimes iris processes can be confused with peripheral anterior synechiae, which are forward adhesions of the iris tissue to the angle wall, and tend to be full-thickness attachments of actual iris tissue that rarely bridge the angle. Compression gonioscopy can be useful to differentiate between the two: a synechia will continue to hold against the wall, whereas the network of iris processes will become lacier in appearance, exposing the wall behind them.

Synechiae result from the iris being placed abnormally against the angle wall. There may be pigment scattering when there is evidence of synechiae. This is characteristic in cases of post-inflammatory conditions such as uveitis or acute angle-closure glaucoma. According to some specialists, synechiae are never found in primary open-angle glaucoma or pure exfoliative or pure pigmentary glaucoma. Their presence is indicative of another abnormality. Peripheral anterior synechia can be an attachment to the ciliary body, or it can be as high as Schwalbe's line or any structure between the two. The low, broad-based attachments may be difficult to recognise, but are critical for identifying early chronic angle-closure glaucoma. Synechiae interfere with aqueous outflow, whereas iris processes do not.

Iris

The iris generally inserts at a variable level into the face of the ciliary body, posterior to the scleral spur. Less commonly, the iris inserts on or anterior to the scleral spur. The iris thins at the periphery near its insertion.

Types of lenses

Gonioscopy is carried out using goniolenses, of which there are two main types – direct and indirect. Indirect mirrored lenses are more commonly used, so the rest of this chapter focuses on this type. Indirect mirrored goniolenses are plastic cone-shaped contact lenses that are available in various sizes and designs and contain one, two, three or four mirrors plus a plano-concave lens in the centre of the cone apex, which effectively eliminates the cornea as a refracting surface (*Figure 6.5*). Lenses may be obtained with or without a flange (lip). Some authorities claim that flanged lenses are easier to insert and keep in the eye. I am not, however, hindered when using flangeless lenses. For some indirect lenses the small difference in curvature between the lens and the cornea is minimised by interposing a viscous coupling gel between the two surfaces (for example, Viscotears® by Novartis Ophthalmics, proprietary artificial tears such as methylcellulose, or a contact lens wetting solution). This solution needs to be optically homogeneous and have a refractive index similar to that of the cornea. From personal practical experience, Viscotears® has the best consistency for this procedure and, as yet, has not resulted in any long-term adverse ocular reaction. There may, however, be a transient superficial punctate corneal epithelial stain, which resolves spontaneously after 30 to 60 minutes,

probably because of a combination effect of the preservative in the gel and pressure from the lens being held on the cornea.

The single-mirror goniolens is useful for teaching purposes and for those new to the procedure. The multi-mirrors of the two-, three- and four-mirror versions can prove confusing for the novice. The single-mirror lens is considered a good choice for children, and adults with small palpebral apertures. In its three-mirror form, the indirect goniolens (often known as the Goldmann 3-mirror) permits angle examination using the smallest arc-shaped

internal mirror. A good view of the mid- and far-periphery of the fundus using the additional mirrors can be obtained through a dilated pupil. As both the single- and Goldmann three-mirror lenses only have one mirror positioned to view the angle, rotation through 270° with an appropriate adjustment to the illumination is required. The slit beam should always be approximately perpendicular to the base of the arc-shaped mirror.

The Thorpe four-mirror goniolens is designed to provide a view of the angle in each mirror. The mirrors are angled at 62°

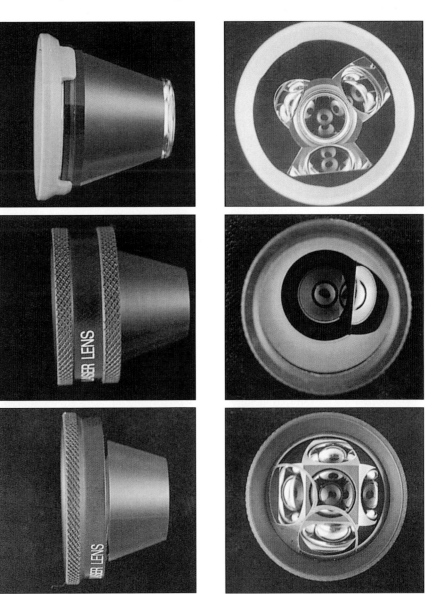

Figure 6.5

(a, b) Goldmann three-mirror lens. The shortest mirror is for examining the angle. The other two mirrors are for examining the peripheral retina. Like all indirect lenses, the central area can be used to examine the fundus. Courtesy of Haag–Streit

(c, d) Goldmann-style one-mirror lens. Courtesy of Ocular Instruments

(e, f) Ritch trabeculoplasty laser lens. Two 59° mirrors are designed to view the inferior angle and two 54° mirrors are designed for the superior angle. A convex button in front of one 59° mirror and one 54° mirror provides extra magnification for examination and laser treatment. Courtesy of Ocular Instruments

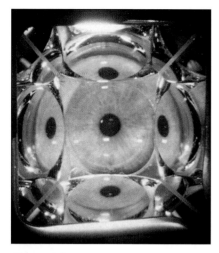

Figure 6.6
View through a four-mirror goniolens

and show the anterior chamber angle in normal size (*Figure 6.6*). This is useful as the lens only has to be rotated slightly for the complete angle to be observed. This lens is the preferred choice of many practitioners for assessing the integrity of the angle. The mirrors are housed in a large cone, which is easier to manipulate for people with large fingers and hands who might find the smaller lens types difficult to control once on the eye. It does, however, require an optical coupling gel.

Sussmann and Volk four-mirror lenses have a small contact surface, so a coupling gel is not required: the lens is coupled to the eye by the tear film. I have found this type of lens difficult to keep on the eye, especially with patients who are eye squeezers. All goniolenses enable examination of the posterior pole through a dilated pupil using the centrally mounted plano-concave lens.

Clinical procedure

As with all invasive ocular surface procedures, corneal health should be assessed with fluorescein before examination. The procedure should not be carried out on a compromised cornea or on an eye that has suffered recent trauma, especially if the globe has been perforated. Tonometry should be performed before gonioscopy, as excessive pressure on the eye can artificially lower IOP.

Two psychological barriers need to be overcome before good results can be obtained with the goniolens. With practice the practitioner will appreciate that the technique is not as difficult as first perceived, that the lens will not damage the

eye and that the patient will not feel any discomfort when it is on the eye.

It is good practice before commencing gonioscopy to explain to the patient what is going to happen and why the procedure is necessary, since the size of the lens can be disconcerting. The patient should be advised that the lens may feel strange, but will not be uncomfortable. This will usually reduce patient anxiety and improve co-operation.

The cornea should be anaesthetised with one drop of topical anaesthetic [for example, oxybuprocaine (Benoxinate®) 0.4 per cent or proxymetacaine 0.5 per cent]. If gonioscopy is performed immediately after contact tonometry, then no further anaesthetic is required. Some patients, usually over 50 years of age, are allergic to the Benoxinate®, and a transient localised or diffuse corneal epithelial desquamation, with fluorescein staining, may occur. Other allergy signs include conjunctival hyperaemia, excessive tearing, pain and photosensitivity. The reaction may develop five to 30 minutes after instillation and lasts for around one hour, but the corneal epithelium regenerates spontaneously. Recovery can be aided with artificial tears and the patient should be reassured of the transient nature of the reaction. A more severe form of reaction can present as a diffuse necrotising epithelial keratitis in approximately one in every 1000 patients.

Examination may take up to five minutes per eye and therefore both examiner and patient comfort are paramount. The patient should be positioned comfortably at the slit lamp, with the lateral canthus of the patient's eye aligned with the marker on the slit lamp. This allows sufficient vertical excursion of the slit lamp to enable the superior and inferior mirrors of a multi-mirrored lens to be viewed. The magnification should be set at approximately ×10–15 and the illuminating slit beam to 2mm width and 2–4 mm in length, with the rheostat at a medium setting. If an excess of light enters the pupil, pupillary constriction may make the angle appear more open than it is under general lighting conditions. The position of the microscope needs to be straight ahead and the light source directly in front of the microscope, so that neither eye is occluded.

Bubble-free coupling gel should be placed into the concavity of the goniolens – any bubbles will adversely affect the view obtained. With the patient looking up, the lower lid can be retracted with the forefinger, then the lower lip of the lens inserted into the lower fornix, the lens brought into contact with conjunctiva at an angle of

approximately 45° and then pushed down along the curve of the globe. This widens the palpebral aperture and allows the practitioner to remove the hand from the lower lid and use it to control the upper lid. The upper lid can be lifted over the upper lip of the lens as the patient is instructed to look forward and the lens quickly pivoted onto the cornea and the upper lid released. This hand can now be used to control the slit lamp. The examiner needs to move smoothly but firmly and with a minimum of drama.

A seal is formed and capillary attraction between the lens, coupling solution and the cornea helps to keep the lens in place. The appearance of folds in Descemet's membrane is an indication that too much pressure is being applied.

When using the single- and Goldmann-type three-mirror lenses, it is advisable to locate the smallest arc-shaped mirror superiorly for orientation purposes, prior to insertion. This enables easier navigation with the slit lamp once the lens is on the eye. In this position, the inferior portion of the angle is available for inspection. The Thorpe- and Sussmann-type four-mirror lenses (each mirror is angled for the anterior chamber viewing) should be inserted with the mirrors initially in the 12, 3, 6 and 9 o'clock positions.

The left hand should be used to hold the lens when viewing the right eye. The hand may be supported and held steady by the forehead strap or by resting the elbow on the slit-lamp table. The angle can now be viewed by moving the slit lamp forwards to focus on the reflected mirror image of the angle and by rotating the lens between forefinger and thumb gently through 270° for single-mirror lenses. The Thorpe- and Sussman-type four-mirror goniolenses need to be rotated only 45° to allow observation of the complete angle. The slit beam will still need to be moved to view each mirror.

The angle is observed by reflected light and the mirror is placed opposite the section being observed. When the mirror is superior, the angle being observed is the inferior angle. The angle under observation is inverted, but not reversed laterally. In the case of narrow angles, the angle recess can be observed easily by tilting the lens to the angle of observation and having the patient rotate the eye towards the gonioscopy mirror.

To avoid or reduce glare from the front surface of the lens, room lights should be dimmed, the illumination arm moved slightly to one side by 5–10° or the lens tilted along the axis of base of mirror. For example, when the mirror is superior, the lens is tilted to the left or right, and when the mirror is temporal, it is tilted up or down.

Deliberate compression (dynamic gonioscopy) gives the observer a certain amount of control over the iris configuration. In an eye with a relatively narrow angle, deeper structures can be visualised by flattening the periphery of the iris gonioscopically. The lens can be shifted or slightly rocked on the corneal surface in any direction for a millimetre or so. Manipulation of the lens in this way allows the practitioner to distinguish between true peripheral anterior synechiae and simple apposition of the iris to the cornea.

The goniolens can be removed by parting the lids so that they clear the lip of the lens. In most cases the lens falls from the eye. If the lens remains attached to the cornea by capillary attraction, the lateral sclera adjacent to the rim of the lens should be pressed firmly with the tip of one finger to break the capillary attraction that holds the lens in place.

Cleaning and disinfection

As soon as the lens is removed from the patient's eye, it should be thoroughly rinsed in cool or tepid water and cleaned by hand using a contact lens surfactant. The lens should then be rinsed with saline and dried with a non-linting tissue. Household bleach can be used to disinfect the lens. The lens is soaked for a minimum of 20 minutes in a mixture of one part bleach to nine parts cool-to-tepid water, rinsed thoroughly with cool or tepid water, dried and placed in a dry storage case. These lenses should never be steam autoclaved or boiled. Acetone, alcohol and hydrogen peroxide all damage the lens.

Indications for gonioscopy

Some optometrists are hesitant to dilate pupils for fear of precipitating an attack of closed-angle glaucoma. Van Herick's slit lamp technique (see below) allows an approximation of the openness of the angle, but the use of a goniolens provides a more accurate evaluation of angle width, as well as an assessment of the structures for anatomic anomalies, disease or the effects of trauma (discussed above). If the angle appears narrow with the van Herick procedure (typically grade 2), gonioscopy is recommended. If only half or less than half of the trabeculum is visible in all quadrants with the goniolens, the eye should be considered at risk for closure during dilation. By taking these precautions the risk of angle closure by pupillary dilation is very low.

Diabetic retinopathy, a particularly severe background, early or established pro-liferation in which the retina is in a state of hypoxia are particularly prone to neovascularisation of the angle (rubeosis irides). As with new vessels on the retina, those in the angle tend to be fragile. They may rupture, and the resultant haemorrhaging and consequential formation of fibrotic tissue close the angle. A similar scenario may occur with branch or central vein occlusion. Neovascularisation at the angle may follow approximately three months after vein closure and hence the possibility of '90-day glaucoma'. Gonioscopic evaluation of these cases enables the optometrist to make a referral at the appropriate level of urgency.

Gonioscopy can give useful information in those cases for which there is historical evidence of angle closure. This includes symptoms of intermittent blur, frontal pain or headaches, haloes around lights, history of a previous attack of angle closure, documented increased IOP from a previous base or IOP greater than 21mmHg.

The differential diagnosis between primary open-angle and chronic closed-angle glaucoma can only be made by gonioscopic evaluation of the anterior chamber angle.

Slit-lamp examination may show evidence of active or past inflammation in the anterior chamber, keratic precipitates, flare or cells in the aqueous, synechiae attachments of the iris to the lens or cornea, ciliary flush, and irregular or poorly responsive pupil. These anomalies can all be investigated further with a goniolens.

The plano-convex contact lens mounted in the centre of most goniolenses is considered by many to be the gold standard for examining the posterior pole, as the clarity of view and degree of stereopsis are unsurpassed. The image is very steady because of the damping effect of the contact lens on ocular movement as well as the prevention of lid closure. However, corneal anaesthesia and the application of contact gel make it more time consuming than other methods and, in addition, the contact gel may interfere with the clarity of view.

Clinical classification

Several grading systems depend on visibility of anatomical landmarks. The most widely used classification is that of Kolker and Hetherington, in which the widest angles are designated grade 4, through narrow angles to the occluded angle, which is graded as zero.

It may be more practical in the clinical setting to describe in words the extent of the visibility of the structures seen, as with the Becker–Shaffer grading system. When the angle is 35–45° it can be described as wide open, incapable of closure and the ciliary body easily visible (grade 4). At 30° the angle is incapable of closure and the scleral spur is identified easily (grade 3). A 20° angle is described as moderately narrow and the trabeculum is the deepest structure that can be identified (grade 2). Angle closure is possible, but unlikely. At 10°, the angle is so narrow that only Schwalbe's line, and perhaps the anterior aspect of the trabeculum, can be identified (grade 1). The risk of angle closure is high. If the angle is zero, with the iris in contact with the chamber wall, occluding the angle, it is described as closed (grade 0). The van Herick technique of angle assessment using a slit-lamp optic section corresponds well with this classification.

Spaeth's classification is more accurate, but also more complicated. Three characteristics need to be noted:
- location of the iris along the angle wall;
- configuration or slope of the peripheral iris; and
- angular approach to the iris recess or the width of the recess.

Although this is considered to be the best system, it is not widely used. It seems too cumbersome for most practitioners.

Gonioscopy and variant Creutzfeldt–Jacob disease

Optical and government agencies have advised against the use of procedures that involve direct contact with the cornea when the optical equipment involved has already been in contact with the cornea of another person, unless clinically required, because of a perceived risk of transmitting the variant Creutzfeldt–Jacob disease (vCJD) prion. No evidenced-based research substantiates these concerns.

In 1999, the Spongiform Encephalopathy Advisory Committee (SEAC) advised the Department of Health (DoH) of a potential theoretical risk of the transmission of prions responsible for variant vCJD by the re-use of lenses and devices that come into contact with the eye. It is important to remember that no such case of vCJD transmission has ever been detected. The College of Optometrists and the Association of British Dispensing Opticians have recommended guidelines about sterilisation procedures in response to the DoH warning. Note, however, that the recommended decontamination (one hour soaking in 2 per cent sodium hypochlorite solution followed by rinsing with sterile saline solution) is only

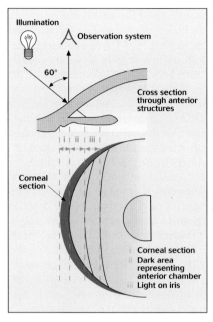

Figure 6.7
Representation of van Herick's method, the ratio of (i) to (ii) is considered for grading

stated as effective for rigid contact lenses and contact tonometry prisms. The efficacy of this procedure in the sterilisation of other instruments, such as gonioscopy lenses, is currently under research.

The use of a goniolens in practice can be justified as a clinical requirement, but the legality of its use for training purposes is less clear. Anecdotal evidence indicates that many teaching ophthalmology departments ignore these guidelines.

Assessment of the anterior chamber depth

Practitioners consistently dilate pupils in everyday practice and need to take some precaution before undertaking this procedure. As well as a measure of IOP, some assessment of the calibre of the anterior chamber is needed to predict the rare occurrence of angle shutdown upon dilation.

Direct viewing of the anterior chamber angle itself, because of the refraction of light by the cornea, requires the use of a contact gonioscopy lens. With the current concerns regarding repeatable-use contact lenses for clinical assessment, many practitioners who work outside hospital departments prefer to use other methods of anterior chamber assessment. Perhaps the most widely used and best-known technique is that first described by van Herick, a brief revision of which is outlined here.

Table 6.1 Van Herick's grading system

Cornea:gap ratio	Grade	Angle
1:1 or greater	4	Open
1:0.5–1.0	3	Open
1:0.25–0.5	2	Narrow, angle closure possible
1:less than 0.25	2	Narrower angle, closure likely
Closed	0	Angle-closure glaucoma

The ease with which van Herick's method may be carried out as part of a routine slit-lamp evaluation has led to its almost universal use. This has, to some extent, overshadowed various other ways to assess anterior chamber depth, some descriptions of which are given here.

Van Herick's technique

It is important to remember that van Herick's method is qualitative in that it does not directly measure anterior chamber depth, but gives a grading of the depth, and so allows some prediction of the risk of angle closure. A typical procedure is as follows:

- The slit-lamp magnification should be set at 10× to 16× to allow an adequate depth of focus.
- With the patient positioned comfortably and staring straight ahead towards the microscope, the illumination system is set at 60° temporal to the patient's eye. The angle is chosen so that the illuminating beam is approximately perpendicular to the limbus and, as the angle is constant whenever the technique is used, this enables consistency of interpretation every time the patient is assessed
- A section of the cornea as close to the limbus as possible is viewed.
  A comparison is made between the thickness of the cornea and the gap between the back of the cornea and the front of the iris where the beam first touches (*Figure 6.7*).
- The ratio of these two measurements may be graded and interpreted, as outlined in *Table 6.1*.
- Many authorities (for example, Elliott[1]) recommend a measure at the nasal limbus also, and that if a large variation is found the narrower angle be considered. When the nasal measurement is carried out on many patients, to avoid the patient's nose with the light beam is problematic. Thus, it is often useful to lock the angle between microscope and illumination system at 60°, swing the whole slit lamp temporally and ask the patient to maintain fixation on the microscope.

Pen-torch shadow or eclipse technique

A very simple, though gross technique, involves shining a pen torch temporal to the patient's eye and interpreting the light and shadow across the iris front surface. This may be done as follows:
- The patient should be asked to stare straightforward in mesopic conditions.
- A pen torch is held at 100° temporal to the eye viewed and brought around to 90°, at which point light is seen reflecting from the temporal side of the iris.
- The amount of iris that remains in shadow may then be interpreted as an indication of the depth of chamber. With a very narrow angle, the forward-bulging iris leaves much of the nasal iris in shadow, whereas a deep chamber with a wide angle allows reflection of light from most of the iris (*Figure 6.8*).

As a very rough guide for use in any situation this technique is claimed by experienced practitioners to be useful.

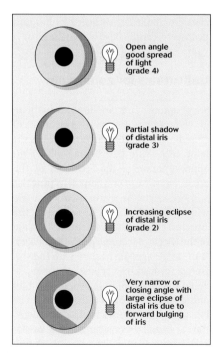

Figure 6.8
Representation of the pen-torch assessment of the anterior angle

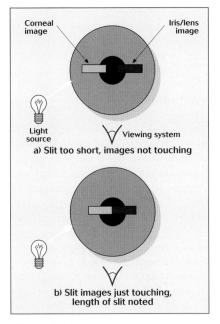

Figure 6.9
Smith's method

Smith's method

First described by Smith in 1979,[2] this technique has been somewhat overlooked, but differs from van Herick's in being quantitative, and so provides the practitioner with an actual measurement (in millimetres) of the anterior chamber depth. The procedure is carried out as follows:

- The microscope is placed in the straight-ahead position in front of the patient, with the illumination placed at 60° temporally. To examine the patient's right eye, the practitioner views through the right eyepiece, and for the left eye through the left eyepiece.

Table 6.2 Conversion of slit length to anterior chamber depth by Smith's method

Slit length (mm)	Anterior chamber depth (mm)
1.5	2.01
2.0	2.68
2.5	3.35
3.0	4.02
3.5	4.69

- A beam of moderate thickness (1–2mm) is orientated horizontally and focused on the cornea. In this position, two horizontal streaks of light are seen, one on the anterior corneal surface and the other on the front surface of the crystalline lens.
- Altering the slit-height adjustment on the instrument is seen as a lengthening or shortening of the two horizontal reflexes.
- Beginning with a short slit, the length is slowly increased to a point at which the ends of the corneal and lenticular reflections appear to meet (*Figure 6.9*).
- The slit length at this point is then measured (it is assumed that the slit lamp is calibrated for slit length).
- This length may be multiplied by a constant to yield a figure for the anterior chamber depth (*Table 6.2*).

Figure 6.10 shows how, for an angle of incidence of 60°, simple geometry shows the depth of the anterior chamber can be calculated by the formula:

$$AC = AC/\sin 60°$$

Note that the diagram does not include the change in the incident beam through corneal refraction, and corneal curvature does introduce a variable into the calcula-

tion. Studies that compared the anterior chamber depth measured by the pachometer (see below) with that by the slit-length method showed a constant ratio of 1.4, which approximates well with the reciprocal of sin 60°.

A more recent study[3] found that when Smith's method is compared with pachometry the constant is around 1.31, a little different, but still predicting an accuracy of ±0.33mm in 95 per cent of the samples assessed. Ultrasonography measurements predicted an accuracy of ±0.42mm in 95 per cent of cases. The constant given by the results using ultrasound, and hence considered to be the more accurate, is that used to calculate the values given in *Table 6.2*. From a clinical point of view, a chamber depth of 2mm should be treated with caution when considering pupil dilation.

Adapted Smith's method

An adapted version of the above method has been proposed[4] for use in those situations in which variable slit height is not possible. In this case, the slit length is noted prior to measurement at a point where it corresponds to 2mm. The instrument is then set up exactly as in the Smith method, but with the initial angle of incidence at 80°. By gradually closing the angle, the two reflected images on the cornea and lens appear to move closer and the angle at which they first touch is noted. A corresponding value for the chamber depth for differing angles is then calculated as given in *Table 6.3*.

Verification of the accuracy of this result with pachometry results showed a good correlation between the methods.

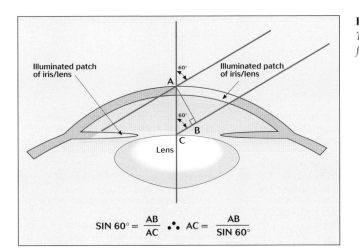

Figure 6.10
Theoretical basis for Smith's method

$$SIN\ 60° = \frac{AB}{AC} \quad \therefore \quad AC = \frac{AB}{SIN\ 60°}$$

Table 6.3 Conversion of slit-to-viewing system angle to anterior chamber depth using an adapted Smith's method

Angle between slit beam and viewing system (°)	Anterior chamber depth (mm)
35	4.22
40	3.87
45	3.52
50	3.17
55	2.83
60	2.48

Ultrasonography

None of the above-mentioned techniques require anything more complex than a slit lamp or pen torch. However, several other methods of anterior chamber assessment are in common usage, albeit more often in a hospital environment, that require more specialised equipment.

Ultrasound allows high-frequency sound echoes to be interpreted and provides a very useful method of measuring distances between structures. An A-scan interprets echoes from a single axial beam through the eye, and so gives peak reflections from the intervening structures. A typical A-scan shows four peaks that correspond to the anterior cornea, anterior lens, posterior lens and retina (*Figure 6.11*). A measurement of the distance between these surfaces is therefore possible, knowing the speed of the beam and the time taken for the echo.

As with ophthalmic lasers, the resolution of image and the penetration within the ocular structure of the ultrasound is a function of its frequency and wavelength. Very low frequency, large wavelength ultrasound scans penetrate well, but the definition of the image gained is less than precise. Very high frequency and short wavelength ultrasound scans have very poor penetration, but the resolution is extremely good. To examine the anterior chamber structure, a poor penetration is of less significance and the image quality is often as good as that gained with light microscopy. Use of a two-dimension (B type) scan of this nature has been described as ultrasound biomicroscopy,[5] and commercially available instruments have been produced. More detailed descriptions of ultrasonography techniques may be found elsewhere.[6,7]

Slit-image photography

By directing a slit beam into the eye along the axis and taking a photographic image from an angle to the axis, the depth of anterior chamber may be visualised. By tilting the objective lens or the film plane, it is possible to keep the slit beam in focus as it passes through the anterior chamber (Scheimpflug's principle). More advanced computerised image-capture systems that interpret images from Scheimpflug video systems are becoming increasingly available and should allow storage of accurate information about the integrity of the anterior chamber over a period of time.

Pachometry

The pachometer slit-lamp attachment is most widely known as a method of measuring corneal thickness, but easily may be used to give a measurement of anterior chamber depth. The pachometer splits the image of a slit beam seen through one eyepiece of a slit-lamp. By moving a calibrated wheel the images move relative to one another, such that is possible to place the back of the corneal section in one image up against the front of the crystalline lens in the other image. Knowledge of the corneal curvature then allows the anterior chamber depth to be calculated.

Conclusion

The use of a goniolens permits visualisation of the structures of the anterior chamber angle that is not afforded by any other procedure. This can be useful in the investigation, diagnosis and management of ocular disease. The technique may be of interest to those optometrists who are keen to develop their skills in this area.

Van Herick's method is a useful qualitative method for assessing anterior chamber depth. However, an actual quantitative measurement need not require expensive or specialised equipment, such as used for pachometry, ultrasound and photography. Smith's method as outlined above is a useful, if often forgotten, technique that yields information about the anterior chamber depth.

Acknowledgments
Figure 6.3 courtesy of J Kanski, *Clinical Ophthalmology*, 4th edition, Butterworth–Heinemann.

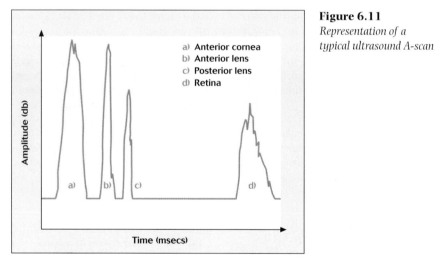

Figure 6.11
Representation of a typical ultrasound A-scan

Amplitude (db)

a) Anterior cornea
b) Anterior lens
c) Posterior lens
d) Retina

a) b) c) d)

Time (msecs)

References
1 Elliott DB (1997). *Clinical Procedures in Primary Eye Care* (Oxford: Butterworth–Heinnemann).
2 Smith RJH (1979). A new method of estimating the depth of the anterior chamber. *Br J Ophthalmol.* **63**, 215–220.
3 Barrett BT, McGraw PV, Murray LA and Murgatroyd P (1997). Anterior chamber depth measurement in clinical practice. *Optom Vision Sci.* **73**, 482–486.
4 Douthwaite WA and Spence D (1986). Slit lamp measurement of the anterior chamber depth. *Br J Ophthalmol.* **70**, 205–208.
5 Pavlin CJ, Harasiewicz P, Sherar MD and Foster FS (1991). Clinical use of ultrasound biomicroscopy. *Ophthalmology* **98**, 287–295.
6 Tromans C (1999). The use of ultrasound in ophthalmology. *CE Optom.* **2**, 66–70.
7 Storey J (1988). Ultrasonography of the eye. In: *Optometry*, pp 342–352, Eds Edwards K and Llewellyn R (Oxford: Butterworth–Heinemann).

Further Reading
Alward WLM (1994). *Colour Atlas of Gonioscopy* (London: Wolfe Publishing).
Carlson NB, Kurtz D, Heath DA and Hines C (1996). *Clinical Procedures for Ocular Examination*, Second Edition. (Stamford: Appleton and Lange) p. 256–263.
Fingeret M, Casser L and Woodcome HT (1990). *Atlas of Primary Eyecare Procedures* (Norwalk: Appleton and Lange) p. 72–84.
Fisch BM (1993). *Gonioscopy and the Glaucomas* (Stoneham: Butterworth–Heinemann).

7

Examination of intraocular pressure

Bill Harvey

Introduction

The measurement of intraocular pressure (IOP) is an important part of the full eye examination. As well as providing useful baseline data for the future examination of a patient's eye, the measurement of IOP has important implications in screening for eye disease.

There is a well-established association between IOP and primary open-angle glaucoma. The insidious nature of the onset of this disease requires that an optometrist, with regular access to examine routinely a patient's apparently healthy eyes, employs a variety of clinical techniques to assess ocular health. The measurement of IOP is one such technique and, as is often the case with a commonly used method, there are many ways to carry it out. In this chapter some of the more widely used methods of IOP measurement are outlined.

Physiology of intraocular pressure

The pressure within the eyeball is related to the secretion and drainage of aqueous fluid. The regulation of aqueous production and its drainage allow control of IOP, which is important for maintaining the structural integrity of the globe and keeping the refractive elements of the eye in the appropriate relative position.

The aqueous is secreted from the epithelial layer of the processes of the ciliary body at a rate of around 2µl per minute, which enables complete aqueous renewal every 100 minutes, though this is subject to variation as outlined later.

The method of secretion has been explained as a combination of passive diffusion from the capillaries in the ciliary body, hydrostatic filtration from the blood to the anterior chamber and an active transport mechanism. Most recent research favours the last of these theories. Passive diffusion appears only to allow movement of lipid-soluble molecules, and the pressure gradient from the capillaries to anterior chamber appears too low for a filtration mechanism.[1]

Aqueous passes through the narrow passage between the anterior crystalline lens surface and iris into the anterior chamber, and drains away via one of two routes. The flow of aqueous towards the drainage routes appears to follow a distinct pattern as illustrated by the way in which pigment is laid down on the corneal endothelial surface in pigment dispersion syndrome (Krukenberg spindle).

About 80–90 per cent of aqueous drains via the so-called trabecular or conventional route. The fluid passes via the trabecular meshwork into the canal of Schlemm, to leave the eye through the aqueous veins into the general venous drainage.

The remaining 10–20 per cent (or higher in non-primate mammals) passes into the suprachoroidal space from the iris root and anterior ciliary muscle, to drain into the scleral vascular system; the so-called uveoscleral or unconventional route. This is summarised in *Figure 7.1*.

Range of intraocular pressure in the population

Most population studies among patients over 40 years of age indicate that IOPs measured with a Goldmann tonometer (see later) are distributed in a manner similar to a normal distribution with a mean pressure reading of approximately 16mmHg. However, the normal distribution curve is slightly distorted, since IOPs over two standard deviations above the mean (that is greater than 21mmHg) account for 5–6 per cent of the patients rather than the 2.5 per cent predicted by a normal distribution.[2]

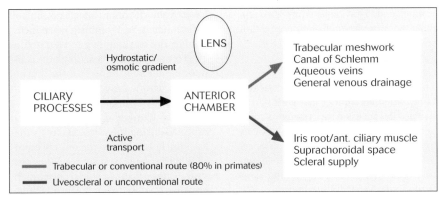

Figure 7.1
Production, secretion and drainage of the aqueous humour

A patient with an IOP greater than 21mmHg on a consistent basis is said to be ocular hypertensive. The vast majority of ocular hypertensives are detected by optometrists.

For patients under 40 years of age, IOP distribution tends towards lower values. The aqueous drainage structures become less efficient with age, and so the tendency is to higher values throughout life, though this is somewhat counteracted by a reduction in aqueous production in older patients.

This dependence of IOP upon the physiological processes outlined below results in a wide variation of inter- and intrapersonal IOPs.

Physiological variables of intraocular pressure

A great many factors affect IOP measurement and have some bearing on the interpretation of any result gained when measuring IOP. The following factors affect IOP.

Accommodation

Accommodation has been found to cause a transient initial increase, possibly because of the increase in curvature of the crystalline lens surface, followed by a small sustained decrease (4–5mmHg over 4 minutes measured for a +4.00D change). This drop may also be linked to an associated miosis linked with accommodation. The initial increase may also be enhanced by the convergence action of the extraocular muscles (see below).

Age

As already stated, IOP is found to increase with age, possibly by as little as 1–2mmHg.[3]

Gender

Females are found to have a very slightly higher IOP (1mmHg), even when allowing for the age factor in a population; women tend to live longer so are often represented more frequently in population studies relating to glaucoma and IOP.

Genetic factors

Though environmental factors are also to be remembered, the clear variation in IOP profiles between races suggests some genetic influence. Far Eastern races appear to have less of a gender difference, and in Japan IOP has even been shown to decrease with age. Many studies confirm an increased increment in IOP with age among Afro-Caribbeans and a somewhat higher baseline level than Caucasians.

Blinking

It is not surprising that any pressure directly applied to the globe may cause a change in IOP. This is one factor to be considered during many of the methods of tonometry. Lifting a lid inappropriately, or applying a tonometer probe for too long, may affect IOP values. A blink may cause a rise of up to 10mmHg in IOP, and a forced blink one even higher than this.

Extraocular muscle action

An increase in IOP occurs upon horizontal and downward gaze, as the extraocular muscles obviously exert varying pressure upon the outside of the globe. Convergence may cause an increase in IOP of up to 4mmHg.

Respiration

IOP increases on expiration, and decreases on inspiration. The fluctuation may vary, but it is occasionally as high as 2–3mmHg during the breathing cycle.

Ocular pulse

The IOP varies with the cardiac cycle, often by as much as 3–5mmHg between systole and diastole, and corresponds to arterial pulse and choroidal filling. This may result from the influence of a hydrostatic secretory mechanism, a direct effect of vessel influence upon the anterior chamber or (most likely) an effect upon the drainage of aqueous fluid. This pulse is the main reason for the need to repeat readings taken with a non-contact tonometer. A contact tonometer, with the probe held on the eye for a finite period, may allow a measurement of the IOP fluctuation and some researchers have used measurements of differing ocular pulses between the eyes as evidence of more profound systemic vascular disease.

Diurnal variation

IOP varies in a sinusoidal fashion over a 24-hour period, and generally seems to peak in the early morning and reach its lowest value 12 hours later. This diurnal variation may be 3–6mmHg when measured in the working day to as much as 10–16mmHg when measured over a 24-hour period. It is found that the diurnal range is significantly higher in a patient with primary open-angle glaucoma and a measured change of greater than that expected during the working day (usually 5mmHg is taken as the cut-off point) should be treated as suspicious. A recent study[4] suggests that a borderline or high-pressure reading taken in the afternoon should be checked the following morning, when a second high reading could confirm the possibility of ocular hypertension.

Monitoring IOP over a period of time, so-called phasing, is a useful technique used in hospital clinics to verify the reliability of a suspect hypertensive referral.

If the pattern of variation between individuals was repeatable, then comparison would be simplified by screening everyone at a chosen time in the morning to coincide with the peak reading. Unfortunately, such repeatability is not found, probably because of the variety of factors thought to contribute to diurnal fluctuation. Sleep itself could influence IOP in many ways (dilated pupils, relaxed accommodation, closed lids, supine position, slower heart and respiration rates, absence of external agent intake and so on).

There also appears to be a link with our metabolic body clock and the diurnal cycles of hormones, regulated in part by secretions of adrenocorticotrophic hormone (ACTH). This has been shown to influence the secretion of melatonin from the pineal gland, which itself has been demonstrated to have an effect upon IOP. The activity of the pineal gland is maximal during rapid eye movement sleep, usually towards the end of a sleep phase, which is reflected in an IOP rise some 30 minutes later. In most lifestyles this corresponds with an IOP rise in the early to mid-morning.

This diurnal fluctuation necessitates the times at which readings of IOP are taken, and variations of greater than 5mmHg over a diurnal cycle should be treated as suspicious and possibly indicative of a less than 'flexible' system..

Seasonal variation

IOP is on average 1mmHg lower in the summer and the individual variation may be as much as 5mmHg.

Food and drugs

Though more pharmacological than physiological, it is important to remember the influence of food and drugs on IOP. Water intake increases IOP, as does excessive caffeine. Reports suggest a transient increase with smoking tobacco, but smoking marijuana or heroin may induce a reduction in IOP. Many legal drugs have an effect on IOP, such as the well-known link with systemic steroids (increase IOP) or beta-blockers (decrease IOP), but a full list is beyond the scope of this chapter (a pharmacological text should be consulted for more detail).

IOP and ocular disease

The measurement of IOP is useful in the investigation of several ocular diseases.

Glaucoma

Glaucoma describes a wide range of ocular diseases in which there is progressive damage to the optic nerve that leads to a loss of visual function and, frequently, a rise in IOP. With many of the secondary glaucomas and with primary angle-closure glaucoma the rise is very dramatic and produces symptoms such as corneal oedema. With primary open-angle glaucoma, perhaps the disease which optometrists are most likely to be the first to detect, the association with IOP is not so clear-cut.

Though the very many population studies in this area show some significant variation, overall they indicate that around 50 per cent of patients who develop glaucoma have an IOP greater than 21mmHg and that only 10 per cent of ocular hypertensives go on to sustain glaucomatous damage.[5]

However, before dismissing tonometry completely, it should be remembered that the higher the IOP, the greater the risk of glaucoma. Furthermore, the risk of glaucoma starts to rise above unity at 16mmHg (not the usually quoted 21mmHg). Clear evidence for the importance of IOP in the development of glaucoma is seen in eyes with asymmetric pressures, of which the eye with the higher pressure is usually the one to deteriorate first.

So IOP is a significant risk factor for primary open-angle glaucoma.

Other ocular disorders

As a diagnostic tool for conditions other than the glaucomas, tonometry may often be considered of limited use. However, a high IOP is often a causative factor in central retinal vein occlusion.

Low IOP may indicate that intraocular fluid is being lost. It is commonplace for IOP to be reduced subsequent to intraocular surgery, so the stabilisation of IOP after surgery is often sought. A choroidal detachment after filtration surgery may result in an unusually low IOP reading.

In eyes with no history of surgery or traumatic penetration, a very low IOP reading can sometimes indicate a rhegmatogenous retinal detachment, and this measurement may be particularly useful to an optometrist when the tear is in the extreme periphery and difficult to visualise directly. A drop in IOP accompanying 'tobacco dust' in the anterior vitreous should warrant urgent action.

Furthermore, a measurable difference between the two eyes of the transient fluctuation in IOP that relates to the ocular pulse may give some indication of a general systemic vascular perfusion problem.

The role of ocular blood flow is discussed more fully in Chapter 8.

Tonometry in the routine eye examination

There are many indications for tonometry to be carried out. Most practitioners, aware of the link with open-angle glaucoma, the major risk factor for which is age, measure IOP routinely on all patients over a certain age. 40 years of age is a cut off point at which epidemiological studies suggest the incidence of glaucoma becomes significant. 1–2.1 per cent of Caucasians and 4.7–8.8 per cent of Afro-Caribbeans over the age of 40 years suffer the disease.[6] The incidence increases dramatically to 3.5 per cent of Caucasians and 12 per cent of Afro-Caribbeans over the age of 70 years.

These figures, and the great variability of the disease, are both reflected in the occurrence of open-angle glaucoma in those under 40 years of age, so I measure IOP on all patients over 30 years of age.

It is also often useful to have a baseline measurement of IOP on all patients to help interpret any future readings taken.

IOP is also routinely measured prior and subsequent to dilation. A rise of more than 5mmHg that fails to stabilise may indicate an induced angle closure requiring medical attention. Remember also that cycloplegic drugs may interfere with aqueous flow, so IOP measurement, even in the very young, may need to be considered.

Finally, younger patients may present with signs that could indicate a risk of secondary open-angle or primary and secondary closed-angle glaucoma, for example a very narrow angle or the presence of material on the corneal endothelium or in the anterior chamber. An IOP measurement is useful in these instances.

Techniques for measuring intraocular pressure

Many methods have been used to measure IOP, some more successfully than others; those that are likely to be used or have been used widely in the past are described here.

Before discussing some of the available mechanical methods, some mention is required of digital palpation. Despite this method being largely discounted as inaccurate by many authorities, the palpation of the superior sclera with the forefingers of both hands on the closed eyes is still used, often by practitioners who claim great accuracy. Certainly, a large difference between the eyes should be detectable to

an experienced practitioner and there may well be situations, in an emergency, for example, in which it is the only available technique.

Tonometry relies upon the application of an external force to cause a deformation of the cornea (or the sclera in eyes where this is not possible, such as when anaesthesia cannot be used and the cornea is grossly scarred) and relating the deformation to the eye's internal pressure. Tonometers may thus be classified according to the deformation produced.

Indentation or impression tonometry

These tonometers rely upon a plunger of variable weight to deform the cornea by a shape that resembles a truncated cone. The level of indentation with differing weights is related to the IOP. The prototype, and most famous indentation tonometer, is the Schiotz (*Figure 7.2*).

While the instrument is held on the cornea, successive weights are added to the plunger and the measurements of indentation are plotted on a graph (a Freidenwald nomogram). This allows extrapolation of a line through the points for each reading to the *y*-axis, which

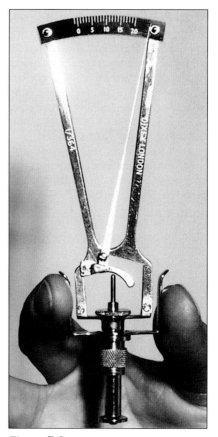

Figure 7.2
Schiotz tonometer

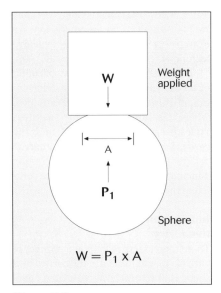

Figure 7.3
Imbert–Fick principle

denotes IOP. There is also a curve outlining a coefficient of rigidity that attempts to quantify the scleral rigidity. A soft eye distends more than a hard eye, which affects the pressure readings.

The patient needs to be supine for the technique, which itself affects the reading. There is also the risk of corneal compromise, though some practitioners still quote this as the preferred technique in nystagmus patients. Perhaps the greatest disadvantage is the inaccuracies that result from the instrument and plunger promoting aqueous outflow. This so-called ocular massaging results in a gradual decrease in IOP. Despite this, newer variations of the Schiotz are currently under trial as a rapid screening test to assess indentation through the closed lid of a patient.

Ocular massaging itself has had some application in studying the efficiency of an eye's aqueous outflow and adapted Schiotz tonometers have been used to measure the gradual decrease in IOP over a period of time under a constant applied force. This technique is called tonography.

Applanation tonometry

As suggested by the name, this technique relies upon the tonometer flattening or applanating an area of cornea. The weight applied may be related to the pressure within and the area applanated by the application of the Imbert–Fick Law (also originally known as the Maklakov–Fick Law).

This law states that an external force (W) against a sphere equals the pressure in the sphere (P_1) times the area applanated or flattened by the external force (A), as shown in *Figure 7.3*.

This physical law assumes that the sphere is perfectly spherical, dry, perfectly flexible and infinitely thin. The cornea fails to satisfy any of these criteria. It is aspheric, wet and neither perfectly flexible nor infinitely thin. The tear film creates a surface tension (S) that has the effect of drawing the applied weight onto the eye, while the lack of flexibility requires an extra force to deform the cornea. Furthermore, as the cornea has a central thickness of around 0.55mm, the area applanated is larger on the external surface (A) than the internal surface (A_1).

To overcome this, the Imbert–Fick law may be modified to:

$$W + S = P_1 A_1 + B$$

Here B represents the force needed to bend the cornea. When A_1 is 7.35mm^2, then S balances out B and therefore:

$$W = P_1$$

An area of 7.35mm^2 has a diameter of 3.06mm and the above cancelling out holds true for areas of diameter between 3 and 4mm. 3.06mm is useful because if that diameter is chosen then an applied force of 1 gram corresponds to an internal pressure of 10mmHg, so making calibration of any applanation instrument easier. Furthermore, the volume displacement for this applanation is approximately 0.50mm^3, such that ocular rigidity does not significantly affect the reading. Ocular massaging plays no part in applanation either.

The very first applanation tonometers employed a fixed weight applied to cause a variable area of applanation, such as the Maklakoff, Tonomat and Glaucotest instruments. These instruments are now rarely used as, with a lower IOP, a particular force can applanate a larger area and so promote aqueous displacement.

Much more widely used and usually taken as the standard technique is that of Goldmann, which uses a variable weight and a fixed (7.35mm^2) area.

Goldmann contact tonometer

The Goldmann contact tonometer is widely used and is generally accepted as the international standard by which other instruments are compared and with which the vast majority of research in IOP measurement is carried out.

The applanation is caused by the probe, which consists of a cone with a flat end containing two prisms mounted with their apices together. On contact with the cornea, the tear film forms a meniscus around the area of contact and the ring so formed is seen by the practitioner through the probe. The split prism allows the ring to be seen as two semicircles that may be moved in position relative to one another by varying the weight of the probe applied to the cornea (*Figure 7.4*).

This use of a vernier reading method adds to the accuracy of the instrument, and when the inner edges of the semicircles just touch, the diameter of the applanated area is 3.06mm.

The basic instrument itself, into which the cone is inserted, is basically a lever weight system with an adjustable scale, with the scale calibrated in grams to allow a varying force to be applied to the cornea by the probe when the wheel is turned.

Procedure

The basic procedure for Goldmann tonometer use should always involve a thorough cleaning of the probe head. As well as the common infective agents found in the tear film, cases have been reported of hepatitis B and human immunodeficiency virus (HIV) isolated in the tears. The recent fuss with regards to the Creutzfeldt–Jacob disease (CJD) prion and trial contact lenses should also be borne in mind, though at the moment of writing no action relating to this regarding the use of contact tonometer probes has been taken beyond the advice to sterilise as usual. Most recently single-use disposable tonometer probes have been made available for all Goldmann and Perkins (see below) instruments. Initial reports on these Tonosafe probes are encouraging, though the price may be a little discouraging.

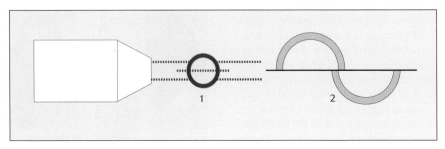

Figure 7.4
(1) Tear meniscus without prismatic effect. (2) Tear meniscus seen through the prism when the weight applied is at the correct level for IOP measurement.

Adequate sterilisation may be carried out with a weak solution of sodium hypochlorite or swabs impregnated with 70 per cent isopropyl alcohol. Though it is tempting to air dry the probe, dry residue of the cleaning agent has been found to aggravate the cornea occasionally, so a rinse with saline is advised.

The probe should be inserted so that the white marking on the head aligns with that on the instrument to ensure that the split between the rings is horizontal. For astigmatic corneas (of greater than 3.00DC), it has been shown that the probe should be aligned such that the interprism face is set at 43° to the meridian of the lowest power, and then the area applanated is still correct. A little red marker on the probe head allows this adjustment.

The cornea is anaesthetised (I prefer 0.5 per cent proxymetacaine, which seems to cause less stinging and reactive tearing) and fluorescein instilled. Though difficult to quote an exact amount that is meaningful in practice, too much fluorescein and therefore too wide a ring width tends to give a high reading. If too little is instilled it is difficult to visualise the rings and vernier adjustment is less easy. Some experienced clinicians carry out the procedure without any stain at all.

The instrument is set on the plate on the slit lamp before the eye to be examined, which usually allows the probe to be directed slightly from the nasal aspect to allow the incidence to be on axis despite any slight convergence by the patient. To minimise the contact time with the cornea it is useful to set the instrument to a weight setting of 1g (10mmHg), or a previous reading if known. On low-to-medium magnification, the probe is viewed through the microscope with the cobalt-blue light incident on the probe head, and the lamp set at 60° temporally.

The probe is moved onto the cornea and the rings visualised and adjusted as described. If the semicircles are not of equal size, then small vertical adjustments may be needed. If the semicircles are not equal, the reading will be too high.

The probe should be removed from the cornea, the weight reading on the scale noted (in grams or ×10 for mmHg), and the cornea checked for staining. If staining is induced, most epithelial stain will disappear within a matter of several hours, but caution by the optometrist should be exercised; if worried, monitor and consider prophylactic antibiotic drops.

Prolonged contact should be avoided to minimise corneal compromise, but it does allow the practitioner to visualise the ocular pulse, seen as small oscillations of the semicircles relative to each other. Prolonged contact also has the effect of reducing IOP by an ocular massaging process. A reduction in this effect or a marked difference between the ocular pulse in each eye may indicate vascular occlusive disease.

The thickness of the cornea may also cause some error, as a very thin cornea produces low IOP readings. A very irregular cornea may make visualisation of the rings difficult, but a contact method is probably more accurate in such cases than a non-contact method. In cases of extreme corneal vulnerability or for which anaesthesia is not advisable, the contact methods may not be the first-choice method.

As with any accurate measuring instrument, regular calibration is necessary and is easily carried out by the practitioner.

Perkins contact tonometer

This instrument was developed as a hand-held, and therefore portable, version of the Goldmann. Having its own light source and viewing lens negates the need for the slit lamp (*Figure 7.5*). The probe is held on a counterbalanced mounting with a coiled spring, which allows the instrument to be used accurately in either the horizontal or vertical position, and so is useful for the supine patient in a domiciliary visit. This mechanism originally required a probe weighted slightly differently to maintain accuracy, denoted by a red ring marking as opposed to the black ring marking on Goldmann probes. The advent of newer designs for both instrument and probe has done away with this discrepancy.

The instrument has a headrest attachment that may be extended and held in position on the patient's forehead to minimise instrument shake, possibly one of the main problems with this instrument. The Mark 2 version now available has two light sources for ease of viewing and may be fitted with a magnifying device (the Perkins Examination Telescope), which allows the rings to be viewed at arm's length.

As already stated, Tonosafe probes may be used with this instrument. Its operation is as with the Goldmann. Calibration should be carried out regularly and may be done by the practitioner. Not surprisingly, the results gained are comparable to those of the Goldmann.

Tonopen XL mentor

The Tonopen XL mentor is a small portable electronic contact tonometer that has a stainless steel probe which, on contact with the cornea, measures IOP by an electronic signal from a solid-state strain gauge held within. The short contact time requires several readings to be taken and averaged, but this, combined with its small appearance, appears to make it patient friendly (*Figure 7.6*). Its re-use requires a sterile rubber sheath to be placed over the probe for each applanation.

Results appear to be reliable in comparison with the Goldmann tonometer, albeit with some greater spread, as may be expected in any instrument that is used to take a series of instant readings compared with one prolonged reading.

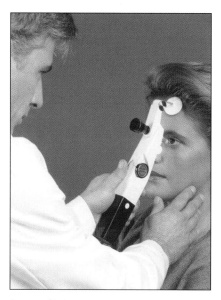

Figure 7.5
Perkins tonometer fitted with examination telescopes

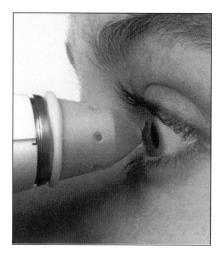

Figure 7.6
The Tonopen XL

Non-contact tonometers

The non-contact tonometer (NCT) was first introduced in 1972 and has the obvious advantage of not requiring contact with the cornea. This minimises the potential for corneal compromise, negates the need for anaesthesia and in many cases is preferred by the patient. Automation of the mechanism means that the instruments are often used by non-professional staff as a screening instrument.

A wide variety of instruments are on the market, and rarely a year goes by without some new upgrade of an instrument. The basic operation relies upon the applanation of an area of cornea by a jet of air, which is usually switched on and off at a point dictated by the quality of image of reflected light from a source on the tonometer. Either the time taken to flatten the cornea or the pressure of air needed is converted electronically into a reading of IOP by the instrument.

As all the NCTs take an instantaneous reading of IOP, there is some variation between readings. If the reading is taken at the peak of the ocular pulse or respiratory cycle, or immediately after a blink, then a disproportionately high reading may be found. It is standard practice, therefore, to take 3 or 4 consistent readings with the NCT before arriving at a useful value.

The overall perception that NCTs give higher readings is likely to be based on practitioners using an inappropriate average or not taking enough readings. In fact, any significant studies suggest that if there is any difference it is that the NCT method gives lower readings than the contact method.[7]

A substantial body of literature compares results taken from the various NCTs with the Goldmann standard, certainly within the non-hypertensive population. At higher readings, certainly above 30mmHg, the correlation breaks down and NCT readings seem less consistent, even though most incorporate adjustments to deal with higher values. It is for this reason, which is becoming increasingly debatable, that many ophthalmologists recommend referral of consistently measured high IOPs taken with a contact method, or that high NCT readings be confirmed with a contact method before referral.

Many NCTs are available, a full description of each being outside the scope of this chapter. Most incorporate a calibration mechanism and a demonstration setting that enables the patient to know what to expect from the 'puff of air'. This action usually also serves to clear any dust particles from the air chamber, which could otherwise be transferred to the patient's cornea.

Some well-known models and their basic features described next

Pulsair EasyEye

The Pulsair (*Figure 7.7*) was the first hand-held NCT and has proved very reliable and popular. It measures pressure in the range 4–59mmHg, with an adjustment for IOPs over 30mmHg, and fires automatically upon alignment of a projected image on the cornea. It converts the flow of air into a pressure reading and has been found to compare favourably with the Goldmann tonometer. The latest model is yet more portable and has an image of the eye in the viewer to aid centration and alignment.

Nidek NT-3000, Topcon CT-60, Xpert NCT Plus

Other examples of NCTs are the Nidek NT-3000, Topcon CT-60 (*Figure 7.8*) and Xpert NCT Plus (*Figure 7.9*), which are widely used, and all employ a video image of the cornea to make them very user friendly. They are automatic, but have a manual override. For individual details the operator manuals should be consulted

As all NCTs rely on some interpretation of a reflected image from the corneal surface, irregular corneas reduce the accuracy of the technique. Similarly, poor fixation, such as in a nystagmus patient, makes accuracy difficult. Most NCTs give some indication that a reading may not be as accurate as might be wished. Most recently on the market, Reichert have introduced a very small hand-held NCT and the quest for improved portability of NCTs is likely to continue.

Ocular blood flow tonometry

It has already been suggested that there is a close correlation between IOP and the ocular blood flow. Over recent years a contact tonometer has been developed, the Ocular Blood Flow Tonometer, which measures IOP and the ocular pulse in terms of pulse amplitude, pulse volume and pulsatile blood flow. This is discussed in full in Chapter 8.

Analysis of results

It would be a very easy, if possibly boring, world if it were possible to have a list of situations that would warrant referral, including a cut-off IOP measurement. It should now be clear that IOP alone as a predictor of eye disease is not reliable and that referral in the absence of any other risk factor is only agreed to be necessary at consistently very high values.

A safe policy is for the optometrist to find out what local hospital policy is regarding referral on IOP alone. In the practices I work in, local ophthalmologists are happy to see patients with repeatable IOP readings over 25mmHg, and consider treatment if verified to be over 30mmHg. It is not unheard of for the patients in the 25–30mmHg group to be checked and discharged with advice

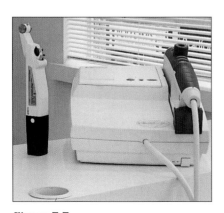

Figure 7.7
The Pulsair EasyEye and a Mark II Perkins Tonometer

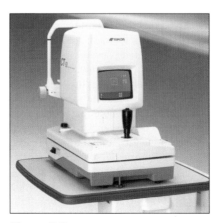

Figure 7.8
Topcon CT 60

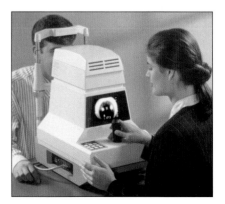

Figure 7.9
Xpert NCT Plus is the latest generation of NCTs, which project a video image of the eye

to attend regularly at the optometric practice for IOP monitoring. A very high IOP reading in an asymptomatic eye may occasionally occur in chronic secondary glaucoma conditions, such as Posner–Schlossman syndrome, in which the history of inflammatory activity may be vague and the IOP rise only transient.

It is also a significant finding if there is a significant and repeatable difference between the IOPs of each eye (5mmHg or more) if this finding cannot be related to previous history, such as intraocular surgery.

As already stated, an unusually low IOP (less than 8mmHg, for example) may be clinically significant.

Conclusion

The aim of this chapter is to give an overview of the theory behind IOP measurement and the techniques used in carrying it out. Further details, particularly with regard to specific points of design and operation of the individual instruments mentioned, are widely available from the manufacturers.

Acknowledgments
Figure 7.2 courtesy of J Kanski, *Clinical Ophthalmology*, 4th edition, Butterworth–Heinemann.

References

1 Lawrenson J (1997). Anatomy and physiology of aqueous production and drainage. In *Continuing Professional Development – Glaucoma*, Ch 1 (Fleet: Association of Optometrists/Optometry Today).
2 McAllister JA and Wilson RP (1986). *Glaucoma*. (Oxford: Butterworths).
3 Ruskill G (1997). Intraocular pressure variations in glaucoma. In *Continuing Professional Development – Glaucoma*, Ch 9 (Fleet: Association of Optometrists/Optometry Today).
4 Pointer JS (1997). The diurnal variation of intraocular pressure in non-glaucomatous subjects: relevance in a clinical context. *Ophthalmic Physiol Opt.* **17**, 456–465.
5 Flanagan JG (1998). Glaucoma update: epidemiology and new approaches to medical management. *Ophthalmic Physiol Opt.* **18**, 126–138.
6 Tielsch JM (1991). A population-based evaluation of glaucoma screening: the Baltimore Eye Survey. *Am J Epidemiol.* **134**, 1102–1110.
7 O'Kelly H and Macnaughton J (1997). Examination of the glaucomatous eye. In *Continuing Professional Development – Glaucoma*, Ch 5 (Fleet: Association of Optometrists/Optometry Today).

8

Measurement of ocular blood flow in optometric practice

Andrew Morgan and Sarah Hosking

In recent years a new instrument, the Ocular Blood Flow Analyzer (OBFA; Paradigm Medical Industries, Utah, USA), has entered the domain of the optometrist. This instrument records a measure known as pulsatile ocular blood flow (POBF) and allows optometrists an insight into the vascular status of their patients.

This chapter reviews the importance of blood flow to the eye and those diseases in which it appears to be defective. In addition, the various methods available for measuring ocular blood flow (OBF) are discussed, with particular attention to POBF and its place in the optometric examination.

Vascular anatomy

Blood supply to the eye

Like most tissues in the body, the eye requires blood to perform its various haematic functions: delivery of oxygen and nutrients; removal of waste products; and, of particular relevance to the irradiated retina, control of tissue temperature. In fact, the choroid has one of the fastest tissue blood flows in the body in order to prevent thermal damage to the retina.[1] How blood is delivered and extracted from the eye is therefore of great importance.

Freshly oxygenated blood, destined for the eye, first starts at the left side of the heart. It courses briefly along the aorta, before entering the common carotid artery, which divides into right and left carotid arteries. Each carotid artery rises with the spine and, before reaching the base of the skull, divides further into the external carotid, responsible for the arteries to the face, and the internal carotid, which enters the skull. Soon after entering the cerebral cavity the ophthalmic artery branches off from the internal carotid.

The ophthalmic artery is an end-artery responsible for blood flow to the orbit and some of the surrounding scalp. The significance of being an end-artery is that it is the sole artery to that region and if blocked, for example by an embolus, there is no alternative arterial back up. The eye receives its blood supply from two sources of the ophthalmic artery: the ciliary arteries and the central retinal artery (CRA; *Figure 8.1*).

The ciliary supply accounts for over 95 per cent of total ocular blood flow. It is responsible for supplying all the uveal tissue, from the choroid at the back of the eye to the iris at the front. The uveal supply enters the eye posteriorly (via the lateral and medial posterior ciliary arteries) and anteriorly (via each muscle insertion) as anterior ciliary arteries. The entry points of the anterior ciliary arteries can often be discerned on ophthalmoscopy as small light-coloured streaks anterior to the equator. The posterior ciliary supply divides into numerous smaller arteries, known as the short posterior ciliary arteries.

The short posterior ciliary arteries, 10 to 20 in number, pierce the sclera as a corona that surrounds the optic nerve. Two offshoots from these ciliary arteries continue slightly further forwards on either side of the globe and are known as the long posterior ciliary arteries. These long posterior ciliary arteries are often also seen, particularly in fair-skinned patients, on ophthalmoscopy. They appear as white horizontal lines at the 3 and 9 o'clock positions at the retinal equator. The white colouring is, in fact, from the nerve associated with the artery, the long posterior ciliary nerve, and their positions serve as useful anatomical landmarks.

The more familiar CRA enters the optic nerve about 10mm behind the globe and travels at its core before appearing at the surface of the disc. There it branches to form four retinal arterioles, one for each quadrant of the retina. Occasionally, the retinal blood supply is supplemented by an offshoot, from the choroid, at the temporal disc margin: a cilioretinal artery.

Once its function has been performed in the capillary beds of the eye, blood drains from the uveal tissue into the vortex veins and from the retinal tissue into the central retinal vein. Vortex veins are often easily seen on ophthalmoscopy. They

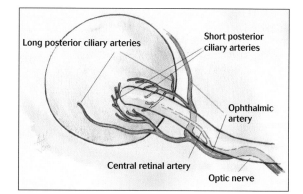

Figure 8.1
Posterior arterial supply to the eye

Long posterior ciliary arteries

Short posterior ciliary arteries

Ophthalmic artery

Central retinal artery

Optic nerve

appear as dark spider-like shapes near the equator, usually one in each quadrant.

Blood supply to the optic nerve

Its possible importance in glaucoma means the vascular anatomy of the optic nerve head has been studied in detail.[2] *Figure 8.2* illustrates the anterior portion of the optic nerve and its vascular supply.

The intraorbital portion of the nerve, between the CRA entry to the nerve and the globe, is supplied by pial arteries that surround the nerve (centripetal branches) and by the CRA at its core (centrifugal arteries). The vascular distribution of the intraocular portion of the nerve is more complex and can vary considerably in individuals. It can be divided into three portions, the laminar, the prelaminar and the surface nerve fibre layer:

- The laminar portion is supplied by recurrent branches from the choroid and centripetal branches from an extensive meshwork of arterioles that originates from the short posterior ciliary arteries. This anastomosis of arterioles often forms a complete elliptical arterial ring around the nerve: the circle of Zinn and Haller.
- The prelaminar portion, between the laminar cribrosa and the surface nerve fibre layer, is primarily supplied by the short posterior ciliary arteries. Angiographic studies indicate a strict sectorial blood supply in this layer. An occlusion to an arteriole here would therefore result in nerve infarction.
- The surface nerve fibre portion is mostly supplied by arterioles from the CRA.

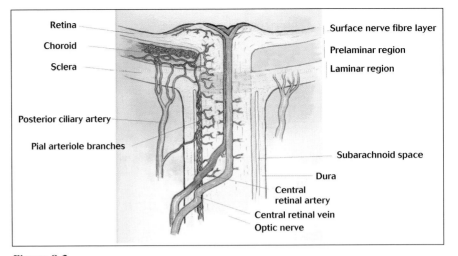

Figure 8.2
Cross-section of the optic nerve

Methods of assessing ocular blood flow

Until quite recently, measurement of OBF was limited to such subjective techniques as quantifying the entoptic phenomenon of white corpuscles against a blue screen, or the relatively invasive use of fluorescein angiography to measure circulation time. In the past decade or so a number of new non-invasive objective methods to quantify OBF have become available. A summary of these is given in *Table 8.1*.

Pulsatile ocular blood flow

Of all these methods, POBF most commonly extends into clinical practice and for that reason it is discussed fully here.

POBF is derived from the natural variation found in intraocular pressure (IOP), which varies slightly in phase with the heart and respiratory cycles. This variation is noticed clinically as the movement of the fluorescein rings during applanation tonometry. It was Perkins *et al.*[3] who devised a pneumatic tonometer that allowed the continuous recording of a subject's IOP. Langham[4] took this further by arguing that if the IOP change, associated with the heart rate, is caused by a bolus of blood entering the eye then it is possible to back-calculate the volume change needed to cause a defined pressure change.

The calculation of POBF from the original IOP recording can be broken into four stages:[5]

Table 8.1 Methods of assessing ocular blood flow					
Technique	*Measurement location*	*Basis of measurement*	*Haemodynamic outcome*	*Reproducibility*	*Application*
Blue field entoscopy	Macular region	Subjective match to leukocyte velocity	Leukocyte velocity and density	Poor	Research
Velocimetry	Retinal arteries and veins	Laser Doppler frequency shift	Velocity	Fair	Research
Flowmetry	Retinal and optic nerve head capillary beds	Laser Doppler frequency shifts/volume	Flow (rate and number of moving corpuscles), volume, and velocity	Fair/good	Research Clinically for qualitative retinal blood flow mapping
Scanning laser angiography	Retinal arteries, veins and capillaries; choroid	Dye intensity; visualisation of capillary transit time	Velocity and flow mapping	Good	Clinical ophthalmology
Ocular pulsatility	All pulsatile inflow; predominantly choroidal flow	IOP variation during cardiac cycle	Pulsatile blood flow volume	Fair/good	Research Clinical practice
Colour Doppler imaging	Larger retrobulbar vessels (ophthalmic) artery, central retinal artery/vein	Ultrasound Doppler frequency shifts	Velocity; colour coded for direction to or from probe	Good	Ophthalmology research

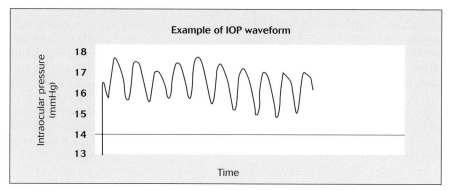

Example of IOP waveform

Figure 8.3
Example of intraocular pressure waveform

1 A continuous IOP measurement of sufficient quality is required. The OBF tonometer records the IOP at a frequency of 200Hz and an example of a 10 second recording is shown in *Figure 8.3*.

2 The pressure profile is then transformed into a volume profile by using Friedenwald's formula for ocular rigidity (*Figure 8.4*) and data on the pressure–volume relationship from living and cadaver eyes.

3 The volume profile is then differentiated to produce a rate of volume change against time (*Figure 8.5*).

4 The rate of volume change calculated in stage 3 can only give information about pulsatile flow and not the steady 'background' blood flow. Any point on the graph can be thought of as a mixture of increasing and decreasing blood flow. For example, the ascending portion of the profile contains a larger proportion of inflow than outflow and thus there is

a net rise in inflow. The crucial point on the profile is the lowest part of the graph, which represents maximum net outflow. Since the net inflow must balance net outflow (otherwise the eye would expand or shrink), the lowest point on the graph represents the negative of the net pulsatile inflow. This value, averaged over time, is used to calculate POBF.

The ocular blood flow tonometer

A number of refinements since the original Langham POBF system have culminated in the presently available instrument: Ocular Blood Flow Analyzer (OBFA; Paradigm Medical Industries, Utah, USA). This instrument consists of a probe and a base unit connected via plastic piping (*Figures 8.6* and *8.7*).

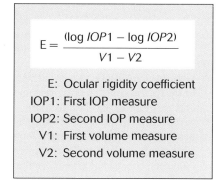

$$E = \frac{(\log IOP1 - \log IOP2)}{V1 - V2}$$

E: Ocular rigidity coefficient
IOP1: First IOP measure
IOP2: Second IOP measure
V1: First volume measure
V2: Second volume measure

Figure 8.4
Friedenwald's formula for ocular rigidity

The disposable probe tip is of a similar design to the original Perkins' pneumatonometer and has a central channel along which pressurised air, produced from the base unit, flows. The tip of the probe is capped, but not sealed, with a thin viscoelastic membrane.

The cornea is applanated and the opposing corneal pressure under the centre of the probe is balanced against the pressurised air produced by the base unit. If the pressurised air exceeds the corneal pressure, the seal between probe and membrane is broken and excess air escapes into the probe's side channels. A transducer in the base unit calculates the IOP continuously from the air pressure in the probe.

Taking a measure of POBF

The probe, either mounted on a slit lamp or hand held (*Figures 8.8* and *8.9*), is placed against an anaesthetised cornea (*Figure 8.10*). The recording of the measurement lasts between 5 and 20 seconds. The instrument searches for five similar and satisfactory pulse waveforms; if these are not found within 20 seconds an error message occurs.

The capture time is long, but a number of practical steps can be taken to improve the chance of a successful measurement:

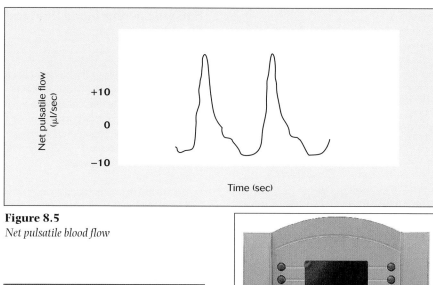

Figure 8.5
Net pulsatile blood flow

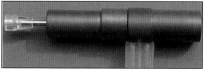

Figure 8.6
OBF system tonometer

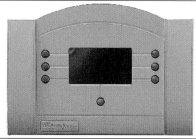

Figure 8.7
OBF system base unit

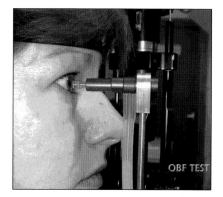

Figure 8.8
OBF tonometer mounted on slit lamp

- The patient's steadiness and position of fixation is crucial. It is useful to have a selection of detailed fixation points for the patient to look at.
- Make sure the patient is relaxed; this helps to steady the systemic pulse rate and improve the reliability of the measure.
- In some cases saline artificial tears may help to prevent drying from the long period without blinking. This improves tonometer contact and sustains epithelial integrity.
- Particularly with the hand-held instrument, a steady hand is essential; with practice, the technique is quick and reliable and often preferred by patients who feel more relaxed.

As well as producing a measure of POBF, the standard output also provides average IOP, pulse amplitude, pulse volume and pulse rate.

Reference values

Mean (SD given in brackets) POBF values for normal subjects have been reported as 669µl/min (233µl/min) for males and 842µl/min (255µl/min) for females.[6] The greater value in females may be attributed, at least in part, to their higher pulse rate. The distribution of normal values, as can be seen from the standard deviation, is large and they are positively skewed: that is, the distribution stretches further towards higher values than towards lower ones.

Reproducibility and limitations

Although the OBF instrument has been shown to be reliable[6–8] and the theory that POBF is based on is sound,[9] there are a number of points to bear in mind when dealing with this measure:[10]

- The theory depends on a continuous non-pulsatile outflow of blood.[9] The calculation of POBF would be erroneous if venous outflow had a significant pulsatile quantity.
- The measure of POBF cannot quantify how much non-pulsatile blood enters the eye. Colour Doppler ultrasound studies indicate that the steady flow is significant and, perhaps more importantly, the proportion of pulsatile to non-pulsatile flow varies under different physiological conditions.[11] Factors that affect the proportion of pulsatile flow are: the compliance or distensibility of blood vessels; the heart rate;[12] and the IOP and systemic blood pressure.
- The conversion from pressure to volume is dependent on scleral rigidity and ocular volume. Indeed, it has been shown that POBF is negatively correlated with increasing axial length.[13] That is, as the level of myopia and therefore ocular volume increases, the measure of POBF falls.
- Given the proportions of uveal and retinal vasculature to total blood inflow, POBF is best described as a measure of choroidal circulation.

OBF tonometry – a measure of IOP

Obviously, the OBF system can be used in its more humble role as a tonometer. As one would hope, it shows good agreement with the gold standard of Goldmann tonometry.[8] Furthermore, although pneumotonometry is just as affected by corneal thickness as Goldmann tonometry[14] in normal corneas, it may have a role in measuring IOP after photorefractive surgery when the ablation zone is small (5 mm or less). Abbasoglu et al.[15] found that pneumotonometry measured the IOP reliably after photorefractive keratectomy, which produces a thinner cornea, whereas central Goldmann tonometry underestimated the IOP by 2.40 ± 1.23mmHg.

Pulsatile ocular blood flow and eye disease

Glaucoma

A blood flow abnormality has long been suspected as part of the cause of glaucoma, particularly its normal tension variant (NTG).[16] The precise vascular defect in glaucoma is not known, but a number of factors are suspected.[17] These include:

- cardiovascular deficiencies;
- vasospasm;
- nocturnal hypotensive episodes;
- blood coagulation abnormalities.

Broadway et al.[18] have defined four types of glaucomatous disc, each believed to result from a relatively isolated causative factor. These glaucomatous disc types are summarised in *Table 8.2*. Two types are specifically associated with vascular defects.

Findings from studies with POBF support the contribution of vascular disturbance to the aetiology of glaucoma. Both NTG and primary open-angle glaucoma patients have lower mean POBF compared

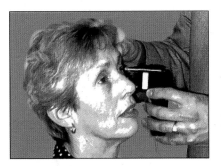

Figure 8.9
Hand-held OBF tonometer

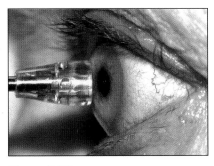

Figure 8.10
Close up of OBF tonometer against the cornea

Table 8.2 Types of glaucomatous disc[18]

Type of glaucomatous disc	Classic disc appearance	Characteristics associated with disc type	Classic field defect appearance
Focal ischaemic	Notch type loss at the neuroretinal rim Disc haemorrhages relatively common	Female to male ratio of 65:35 High vasospasm score (e.g., Raynaud's disease) Normal or raised IOP	Dense field defect, frequently threatening fixation
Myopic glaucomatous	Large disc and often tilted	Younger patients Higher ratio of males High myopia Normal or raised IOP	Dense field defect
Senile sclerotic	Relatively low cup:disc ratios	Higher incidence of cardiovascular disease Older patients Even male:female ratio Normal or raised IOP	Relative scotomas with diffuse loss
Generalised cup enlargement	Cup:disc ratio high	High IOP	Diffuse field loss

to normals and ocular hypertensives respectively.[19–22] An elegant study by Fontana *et al.*[23] compared NTG patients with unilateral field loss to normal subjects' eyes. They found POBF was reduced in both eyes of the NTG group and, furthermore, the eye with the field loss had the worst POBF. Such studies raise the possibility of using POBF as an indicator of early glaucoma and therefore early intervention.

Certain glaucoma treatments have been shown to affect POBF. POBF increases significantly after trabeculectomy[24] and with certain eye drops thought to increase perfusion, such as latanoprost.[25] Other drops, such as the staple beta-blocker timolol, decrease POBF,[26] a finding that may, in part, result from reduced pulse rate.

Diabetes

Compared with glaucoma, POBF results in diabetic patients are more confusing: some investigators[27] found that POBF decreases with progression of retinopathy, while others found it increases.[28] This variability in outcome may result from differences in the degree of control of diabetes between the study groups. The consensus that fits best with other blood-flow investigations is that, as the duration of diabetes increases, there is a transition from negative to positive retinal blood-flow progression.[29]

Carotid artery disease

Considering that reduced pulse amplitude has been a diagnostic sign of carotid artery stenosis for some time,[30] it is surprising to find that POBF is unaltered in these cases.[31]

POBF and eye disease: summary

To conclude, mean values of POBF have been found to be abnormal for a number of different ocular diseases. However two points must be borne in mind:

• First, because of the large spread of normal values for POBF (212μl/min to 1126μl/min for males; 342μl/min to 1340μl/min for females), it is difficult to predict the onset of disease in individual suspects or patients, unless the values are profoundly reduced. As such, the data are only of value in clinical case-findings when considered as part of a battery of information.

• Although findings from case-control studies highlight departures from normality in various vascular diseases, whether this is a cause or a consequence of the disease remains uncertain.

POBF in optometric practice

So, where does this leave the optometrist who has an OBF tonometer?

We suggest that the OBF measure of IOP provides an enhanced method for IOP measurement. Pneumotonometry may have a role in measuring IOP in post-photorefractive surgery patients as it appears to be less influenced by small ablation zones than does Goldmann tonometry. *When would it provide useful information to influence the clinical management of a patient?*

Perhaps the OBF instrument should be considered not as a tonometer solely, but also has an instrument that provides a measure of ocular blood flow, in which case its clinical application becomes more obvious. To optometrists, the apparatus is of greatest value in screening for glaucoma of all types.

The OBF system thus measures two indications for glaucoma in patients:
• those with high IOP;
• those whose glaucoma is likely to be vascular in origin.

In addition to an elevated IOP measurement, the finding of an abnormally low or asymmetric POBF measurement provides the practitioner with an additional risk factor to weigh up in the management of the glaucoma suspect.

OBF tonometry has yet to reach the domain of the general ophthalmologist, although its role has become more widely recognised by glaucoma specialists. Referrals in which OBF data are included should indicate whether the flow readings are considered low, moderate or high and the importance of this finding in relation to other data, such as the level of IOP, disc appearance or visual field status.

Is the OBF tonometer of use in other diseases?

The OBF tonometer may provide useful additional information in those patients who complain of transient washing out or loss of vision (amaurosis fugax) or when retinal emboli are seen on ophthalmoscopy. However, it appears pulse amplitude and pulse volume are better diagnostic indicators than POBF.[31,32]

Conclusion

Optometrists now have, we believe, an enhanced method for IOP measurement coupled with a means of taking a measure of ocular blood flow. This allows them to investigate a further parameter in a patient's ocular and systemic health.

References

1 Alm A (1992). Ocular circulation. In: *Adler's Physiology of the Eye*, Ninth Edition, p. 198–227, Ed. Hart WM (St Louis, Mosby–Year Book Inc.).

2 Bill A (1993). Vascular physiology of the optic nerve. In: *The Optic Nerve in Glaucoma*, p. 37–50, Eds Varma R, Spaeth GL and Parker KW (Baltimore: Lippincott, Williams and Wilkins).

3 Perkins ES, Edwards J and Saxena RC (1977). A new recording tonometer. *Trans Ophthalmol Soc UK* **97**, 679–682.

4 Langham ME and To'mey KF (1978). A clinical procedure for the measurements of the ocular pulse–pressure relationship and the ophthalmic arterial pressure. *Exp Eye Res*. **27**, 17–25.

5 Silver DM and Farrell RA (1994). Validity of pulsatile ocular blood flow measurements. *Surv Ophthalmol*. **38**, S72–S80.

6 Yang YC, Hulbert MFG, Batterbury M and Clearkin LG (1997). Pulsatile ocular blood flow measurements in healthy eyes: Reproducibility and reference values. *J Glaucoma* **6**, 175–179.

7 Butt Z and O'Brien C (1995). Reproducibility of pulsatile ocular blood flow measurements. *J Glaucoma* **4**, 214–218.

8 Spraul C, Lang GE, Ronzani M, Hogel J and Lang GK (1998). Reproducibility of measurements with a new slit lamp-mounted ocular blood flow tonograph. *Graefe's Arch Clin Exp Ophthalmol*. **236**, 274–279.

9 Krakau CET (1995). A model for pulsatile and steady ocular blood flow. *Graefe's Arch Clin Exp Ophthalmol*. **233**, 112–118.

10 James CB (1998). Pulsatile ocular blood flow – Editorial. *Br J Ophthalmol*. **82**, 720–721.

11 Canning CR and Restori M (1988). Doppler ultrasound studies of the ophthalmic artery. *Eye* **2**, 92–95.

12 Trew DR, James CB, Thomas HLS, Sutton R and Smith S (1991). Factors influencing the ocular pulse – the heart rate. *Graefe's Arch Clin Exp Ophthalmol*. **229**, 553–556.

13 James CB, Trew DR, Clark K and Smith SE (1991). Factors influencing the ocular pulse – axial length. *Graefe's Arch Clin Exp Ophthalmol*. **229**, 341–344.

14 Doughty MJ and Zaman ML (2000). Human corneal thickness and its impact on intraocular pressure measures: A review and meta-analysis approach. *Surv Ophthalmol*. **44**, 367–408.

15 Abbasoglu OE, Bowman RW, Cavanagh H D and McCulley JP (1998). Reliability of intraocular pressure measurements after myopic excimer photorefractive keratectomy. *Ophthalmology* **105**, 2193–2196.

16 Jay JL (1992). The vascular factor in low tension glaucoma: alchemist's gold? *Br J Ophthalmol*. **76**, 1.

17 Chung HS, Harris A, Evans DW, Kagemann L, Garzozi HJ and Martin B (1999).Vascular aspects in the pathophysiology of glaucomatous optic neuropathy. *Surv Ophthalmol*. **43**, S43–S50.

18 Broadway DC, Nicolela MT and Drance SM (1999). Optic disk appearances in primary open-angle glaucoma. *Surv Ophthalmol*. **43**, S223–S243.

19 Ravalico G, Pastori G, Toffoli G and Croce M (1994). Visual and blood flow responses in low-tension glaucoma. *Surv Ophthalmol*. **38** (Suppl.), S173–S176.

20 James CB and Smith SE (1991). Pulsatile ocular blood flow in patients with low tension glaucoma. *Br J Ophthalmol*. **75**, 466–470.

21 Kerr J, Nelson P and O'Brien C (1998). A comparison of ocular blood flow in untreated primary open-angle glaucoma and ocular hypertension. *Am J Ophthalmol*. **126**, 42–51.

22 Trew DR and Smith SE (1991). Postural studies in pulsatile ocular blood flow II. Chronic open-angle glaucoma. *Br J Ophthalmol*. **75**, 71–75.

23 Fontana L, Poinoosawmy D, Bunce CV, O'Brien C and Hitchings R (1998). Pulsatile ocular blood flow investigation in asymmetric normal tension glaucoma and normal subjects. *Br J Ophthalmol*. **82**, 731–736.

24 James CB (1994). Effect of trabeculectomy on pulsatile ocular blood flow. *Br J Ophthalmol*. **78**, 818–822.

25 McKibbin M and Menage MJ (1999). The effect of once-daily latanoprost on intraocular pressure and pulsatile ocular blood flow in normal tension glaucoma. *Eye* **13**, 31–34.

26 Kitaya N, Yoshida A, Ishiko S, Mori F, Abiko T, Ogasawara H, Kato Y and Nagaoka T (1997). Effect of timolol and UF-021 (a prostaglandin-related compound) on pulsatile ocular blood flow in normal volunteers. *Ophthalmic Res*. **29**, 139–144.

27 Langham ME, Grebe R, Hopkins S, Marcus S and Sebag M (1991). Choroidal blood flow in diabetic retinopathy. *Exp Eye Res*. **52**, 167–173.

28 MacKinnon JR, O'Brien C, Swa K, Aspinall P, Butt Z and Cameron D (1997). Pulsatile ocular blood flow in untreated diabetic retinopathy. *Acta Ophthalmol Scand*. **75**, 661–664.

29 Konno S, Feke GT, Yoshida A, Fujio N, Goger DG and Buzney SM (1996). Retinal blood flow changes in Type I diabetes: A long-term, follow-up study. *Invest Ophthalmol Vis Sci*. **37**, 1140–1148.

30 Best M and Rogers R (1974). Techniques of ocular pulse analysis in carotid stenosis. *Arch Ophthalmol*. **92**, 54–58.

31 McKibbin M and Verma D (1999). Recurrent amaurosis fugax without haemodynamically significant ipsilateral carotid stenosis. *Acta Ophthalmol Scand*. **77**, 224–226.

32 Kerty E and Horven I (1995). Ocular haemodynamic changes in patients with high-grade carotid occlusive disease and development of chronic ocular ischaemia. I. Doppler and dynamic tonometry findings. *Acta Ophthalmol Scand*. **73**, 66–71.

9
Assessment of the fundus

Frank Eperjesi and David Ruston

There can be little doubt that a thorough examination of at least the central fundus should form part of even the most rudimentary eye examination. When any of the patient's age, symptoms, medication, family history or signs indicate, a complete fundus examination should always be undertaken.

In view of the variety of different examination techniques, this chapter is split into two sections:
- Examination of the central region of the fundus;
- Visualisation of the periphery and vitreous.

The full extent of the fundus is shown in *Figure 9.1*. The larger of the circles indicates the region described as the central retina. The smaller circle indicates the typical field of view with a direct ophthalmoscope.

Should the patient be dilated?

It is for the practitioner to decide when dilation is required. Certainly when a full central and peripheral examination is indicated, it is mandatory in the vast majority of cases. However, in routine cases and patients with large pupils, particularly when the direct ophthalmoscope is employed, it is unnecessary. Prior to dilation the remote possibility of triggering an acute attack of closed-angle glaucoma needs to be considered. Normal symptom and history taking should have identified those patients who have already experienced prodromal attacks or those who have a genetic predisposition to angle closure. The anterior chamber depth should be assessed using the Van Herick technique,[1] as discussed in Chapter 6. Approximately 6 per cent of normals have narrow angles and it is thought that less than 10 per cent of these are at risk of closure.

If gonioscopy is a technique that the practitioner is not familiar with, then dilation should take place in the morning and the IOP checked 30 minutes post-dilation. In addition, the practitioner should ensure that there is an eye casualty department within reasonable proximity to refer the patient should there be a significant rise in IOP post-dilation. It is a generally held view that, provided medical aid is at hand, the practitioner who dilates a symptomatic patient and discovers a predisposition to angle closure has done that patient a favour.

Aside from patients who have extremely narrow angles, only the following patients should not be dilated:
- Those with iris clip intraocular lenses (very rare).
- Patients who have to drive immediately on leaving. It should be remembered that, with sunglasses, the visual acuity on a bright day is not greatly impaired following dilation and that if one suspects a serious retinal pathology, the examination is more important than the patient driving home.
- History of recent penetrating injury – these patients should be referred unexamined.

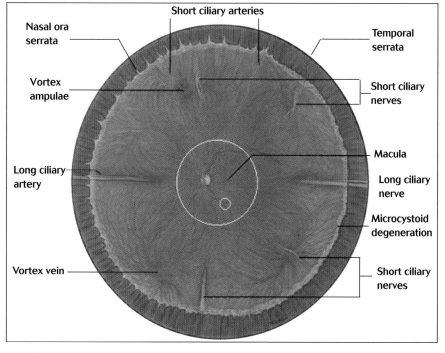

Figure 9.1
View of entire fundus. The larger circle indicates the central area, while the smaller circle is the field of view through a direct ophthalmoscope. Localising features are shown.

What should be used for dilation?

- One drop of 2.5 per cent phenylephrine, then one drop of 0.5 per cent tropicamide. This produces maximal dilation and improves patient comfort, as there is less attempted constriction on examination.
- Or two drops of 0.5 per cent tropicamide separated by one minute.
- Or an anaesthetic may be used first to facilitate movement of the mydriatic drug through the cornea.

Examination of the central retina

The typical instruments used for examining the central 45° are:

- direct ophthalmoscope;
- hand-held indirect lens [slit-lamp binocular indirect ophthalmoscopy (BIO)];
- Hruby lens (slit-lamp direct);
- fundus contact lenses;
- modified (monocular) indirect ophthalmoscopy;
- head-borne indirect ophthalmoscopy (headset BIO).

In addition, some practitioners are now using a non-mydriatic fundus camera linked to digital imaging software to screen the central area of the fundus. Without doubt this new technology offers some advantages over any of the other techniques described below and is discussed in Chapter 10. Most importantly, the entire image is seen at once on the computer monitor. This makes rapid and comprehensive screening of the central fundus much easier than any of the techniques in which scanning the fundus is necessary to build up a mental image of the whole area. The permanent image, stored as a digital file, makes systematic evaluation of a lesion or structure much easier than if a drawing is made. It can also be stored in a variety of ways, printed out or e-mailed to another practitioner. There is a considerable disparity in quality between the different systems; an excellent review of the technology is provided by Meyler and Hodd.[2]

Direct ophthalmoscopy

In routine optometric practice, the mainstay of examination is still the direct ophthalmoscope. Although regarded as being an inferior instrument by some practitioners, it has several favourable attributes, which (along with its failings) are set out in *Table 9.1*. In view of the familiarity of the optometric profession with this instrument, it tends to be forgotten how difficult it was to develop proficiency in its use during the period of training. This should be borne in mind when attempting to learn a new technique like slit-lamp indirect ophthalmoscopy. As indicated in *Table 9.1*, direct ophthalmoscopy is particularly useful for examination through a small pupil for specific fine features, for example neovascularisation of the disc and microaneurysms. It is least useful when a stereoscopic view is required, such as in macular oedema or in the assessment of depth of cupping in potentially glaucomatous discs. It is also of little value when an overall view of the posterior pole is required, as is the case in diabetic retinopathy. No further discussion of this technique is given here in view of its universal usage.

Slit-lamp binocular indirect ophthalmoscopy

Hand-held indirect lenses are now becoming widely used by the profession, particularly when a thorough binocular scan of the central area is required. Assuming that there is a slit lamp to hand, all that is required is a suitable lens. The features of those most readily available are set out in *Table 9.2*. (NB different manufacturers quote different figures for the magnifications and field of view of similarly powered lenses. Therefore, these figures are indicative only.) As a general principle, the higher the lens dioptric power, the lower the magnification and closer the lens must be held to the eye, but the higher the field of view. Lenses are available with detachable yellow filters (which reduce the blue-light hazard in prolonged examination), lid adapters (which help separate the lids and set the correct working distance), graticules to record the size of features, and mounts which steady the lens at the slit lamp.

A stereoscopic low-magnification wide-field view of the fundus is obtained.

Table 9.1 Features of direct ophthalmoscopy compared to indirect ophthalmoscopy

Advantages	*Disadvantages*
High magnification view (15×)	Magnification varies with patient's refractive error: higher in myopes
Relatively good imaging through a small pupil	Very small field of view (10° in an emmetrope): difficult to scan fundus
Readily portable: good for domiciliary use	Monocular view
Relatively inexpensive	Difficult to use on small children
View of fundus is correct way up and non-reversed	Image degrades significantly with media opacities
	Poor at showing colour and elevational changes
	Close proximity to patient essential

Table 9.2 Basic features of some hand-held slit lamp indirect lenses[3]

Power	*Magnification*	*Field of view (degrees)*	*Working distance from cornea*	*General usage*
60D	1.15×	76	11.0	Disc and macula
78D	0.93×	84	8.0	General screening
90D	0.75×	94	6.0	General screening, smaller pupils
SuperField	0.76×	95	7.0	Wider field than 78/90
Variable zoom	0.77 to 0.94×	78 to 100	5.0	General screening with zoom feature
132D SP	0.45×	99	4.0	Small pupils, wide field

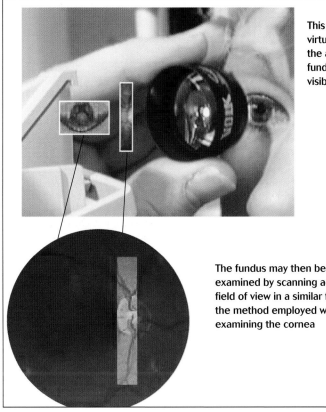

This figure shows the virtual inverted images of the anterior eye and fundus, not normally visible from a side angle

The fundus may then be examined by scanning across the field of view in a similar fashion to the method employed when examining the cornea

Figure 9.2
Use of the hand-held slit lamp BIO lens showing the image formation and fundus view.
Courtesy of Andrew Field

Unfortunately, this is laterally reversed and upside down, which makes disc analysis and spatial localisation a little more difficult. *Figure 9.2* shows how this virtual image is formed by the lens.

Technique
- Instil a mydriatic as necessary. For the general routine examination of a young patient, a mydriatic is not essential, especially for the higher-powered lenses with shorter working distances. However, for older patients and for all instances in which a thorough binocular examination of the central fundus or foveal area is required, a mydriatic should be used.
- Position the patient comfortably at the slit-lamp microscope (SLM). Ensure the lens is spotlessly clean and that the magnification is set to low.
- Select a beam height approximately equal to the patient's pupil diameter and a width of about 3mm.
- Pull the SLM back towards the practitioner and laterally align the slit beam so that the blurred slit-beam illuminates the centre of the patient's pupil.
- Interpose the BIO lens centrally and at about 2cm from the eye. It is generally not important which way round the BIO lens is held. The surfaces must be clean.

- The SLM should then be moved forwards towards the patient and focused on the aerial image of the patient's inverted pupil. Then continue moving forwards to focus through the pupil onto the retina. This image is between the BIO lens and the aerial image of the pupil/iris.

- The BIO lens should then be moved forwards towards the patient to enlarge the pupil image and, by doing so, increase the field of view.
- The practitioner should then scan over the fundus using the same approach adopted when scanning the cornea.
- The patient should be instructed to look in the different directions of gaze (eight positions) and the lens repositioned each time to optimise the view, tilting where necessary to avoid reflections.
- The magnification can be increased where necessary. The amount of magnification is limited by the particular slit lamp used.
- Finally, the patient is asked to look towards the practitioner's ear (right ear for right eye, left ear for left eye), which enables visualisation of the disc.
- If the vitreous is to be examined, the microscope must be pulled back and the focus shifted onto the floater or hyaloid membrane. Visualisation of the vitreous is difficult and the practitioner is recommended to begin with patients who have widely dilated pupils and who have suffered posterior vitreous detachment.
- If necessary the field of view can be increased by moving the lens either vertically or horizontally in the frontal plane. The lens is moved in the same direction to the region that requires investigation. For example, if more of the superior fundus needs to be imaged, then the patient is instructed to look up as far as possible and the lens is moved upwards.

The technique has advantages and disadvantages (*Table 9.3*). As is highlighted, slit-lamp BIO is particularly useful for

Table 9.3 Features of hand-held slit-lamp indirect ophthalmoscopy compared to direct ophthalmoscopy

Advantages	*Disadvantages*
Wide field of view, relatively easy to scan fundus	View of fundus is upside down and laterally reversed
Image degrades significantly less than direct image with media opacities	Magnification limited by quality of slit-lamp optics
Good at showing colour and elevational changes	Very difficult to use with a small pupil
Relatively inexpensive if slit lamp available	Difficult to use on small children
Magnification does not vary with patient's refractive error	Unsuitable for domiciliary use
Comfortable distance from patient maintained	Takes some practice to become comfortable with technique
	Less pleasant for patient
	Reflections are a problem
	Scanning of fundus required to build up general picture

stereoscopic examination of the disc and macula, principally to assess the depth of cupping in glaucoma and to detect subtle macular oedema in diabetics. With further experience, the vitreous can be inspected and the hyaloid membrane visualised. It is certainly not an easy technique to become comfortable with and requires practice.

Hruby lens slit-lamp direct ophthalmoscopy

Slit-lamp direct ophthalmoscopy can be performed with the non-contact Hruby lens (−58.6D). The high minus power of this lens produces an upright virtual image that is not laterally reversed. Direct ophthalmoscopy using a slit lamp and negative auxiliary lenses can provide a very high level of magnification, even greater than that of the monocular hand-held direct ophthalmoscope. The actual level of magnification depends on that available through the slit lamp. Stereopsis is provided to a greater degree than in all the other examination techniques, except for contact lenses designed for fundal viewing. The Hruby lens produces a very detailed image.

The main disadvantage of this technique is the field of view. It is smaller than all the other examination methods, with the exception of direct monocular ophthalmoscopy (less than two disc diameters for an emmetropic patient). More dilation is required than in other binocular techniques. The quality of the image is easily degraded by media opacities; increasing the slit-lamp illumination can reduce this problem.

As the magnification is so high, small movements of the practitioner, lens or patient have an immediately noticeable negative effect on image quality. Patient co-operation is extremely important and can be enhanced with the use of a fixation device (present on most slit lamps). The non-contact Hruby lens is generally incorporated into the slit-lamp design. This allows a stable relationship between the patient's eye and the lens to be maintained. As the lens is mounted on the slit lamp, the practitioner's hands are free to manipulate the slit lamp and the fixation device.

Technique
- Ensure pupils are maximally dilated.
- Patient co-operation is extremely important and can be enhanced by attention to comfort beforehand.
- Set the magnification to the lowest setting, usually 6–10×.
- Set a slit height of about 5mm and width of 2mm and place the illumination system midway between the oculars.
- Place the fixation device in the centre of the patient's field in front of the contralateral eye.
- Image slit in patient's pupil.
- Introduce the lens in front of the patient's eye as close as possible, without touching the cornea or lashes. The concave side should face the eye.
- Position the slit beam in the centre of the lens and then view the red reflex through eyepieces.
- Move the slit lamp towards the patient; any opacities in the crystalline lens or vitreous become apparent.
- Once the retina comes into focus, moving the patient's fixation with the fixation device on the slit lamp can control the area of the fundus examined. Adjustments in the vertical and horizontal positions of the slit lamp are necessary to keep the practitioner's view in the pupil. It is helpful to use major retinal vessels for orientation. These can be followed back to the optic nerve head.
- Adjust the magnification and increase the width of beam to enhance the view.

The view produced by slit-lamp direct ophthalmoscopy is upright and requires no translation, which the view in the condensing lens does require. As the magnification and stereopsis obtainable are significantly greater with this technique, subtle thickening of the retina may be apparent, even though it may not have been observed with other procedures.

Indications for the use of slit-lamp direct ophthalmoscopy are:
- The suspected presence of diabetic retinopathy, especially if the macula may be involved.
- Symptoms of macular disease not previously explained, unexplained reduction in visual acuity and metamorphopsia.
- High stereopsis visualisation of the optic disc.
- If a high stereopsis view is required, but a fundus contact lens is not available.

Fundus contact lenses

Various manufacturers make this type of lens. Apart from the lens, the only other requirement is a coupling solution to provide an optically smooth interface between the lens and the eye, the slit lamp and an anaesthetic. Perhaps the best-known lens of this type is the Goldmann three-mirror (*Figure 9.3*). However, there is a plethora of different lenses, some of which are summarised in *Table 9.4*.

Some of these lenses are available with or without flanges, which help hold the lids apart. In addition, versions are designed to function without a coupling fluid. While having the advantage of not blurring the vision, these can be more difficult to use. The view obtained with Goldmann three-mirror (*Figure 9.3*) has the following properties:

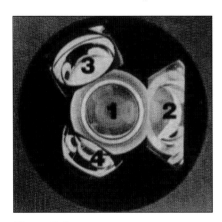

Figure 9.3
The Goldmann three-mirror contact lens

Table 9.4 Résumé of some of the wide range of contact lenses designed for fundal viewing

Name	Magnification	Field of view	Recommended usage
3-Mirror 'Goldmann'	0.93×	36	High stereoscopic evaluation of disc and macula
Area centralis	1.06×	70	General inspection of posterior pole
Super macula 2.2	1.50×	60	High magnification view of disc and macula
Quadraspheric	0.51×	120	General wide-field and small pupils
Equator plus	0.44×	114	Wide-field view and/or small pupils
Mainster ultra field PRP	0.53×	140	As above
Superquad 160	0.50×	160	Widest field possible

- The central part of the lens contains a negative powered region, which provides a 30° view of the posterior pole. The image is not reversed nor inverted, and is therefore like that of direct ophthalmoscopy, but it is brighter and possesses a very high degree of stereopsis. It is ideal for examination of the macula and disc, particularly when checking for macular oedema and papilloedema, or if an accurate assessment of disc size is required
- The equatorial mirror (largest and oblong shaped) enables visualisation from 30° to the equator.
- The peripheral mirror (intermediate in size and square shaped) enables the practitioner to see from the equator as far as the ora serrata.
- The gonioscopic mirror (smallest and dome shaped) is normally to visualise the angle, but can also be used to see the extreme retinal periphery and pars plana.
- The view obtained through each of the mirrors is upside down, but not laterally reversed. Therefore, to see the superior retina, the mirror is placed at 6 o'clock.

The view obtained with other non-mirrored lenses has properties with some variation to those of the Goldmann three-mirror. The rest of the fundus contact lenses described in *Table 9.4* produce a wide-field, laterally reversed upside-down view of the fundus in a similar way to the hand-held lenses described in the section on slit-lamp BIO above. However, the contact with the globe, via the coupling solution, produces a vastly superior view. The image is brighter, clearer, suffers from far fewer reflections and possesses a higher degree of stereopsis than that with the hand-held lenses. Scanning the image is easier and the lens can still be moved slightly to extend the field of view. These advantages are the reason why these lenses are used so extensively by ophthalmologists to examine diabetic patients and for laser treatment of the posterior segment.

Technique

This procedure involves placing a hand-held high-precision lens against the anaesthetised eye and viewing the image through the slit lamp. It is easier than is commonly believed, although scanning the fundus with a mirror lens does take practice as the lens has to be rotated. It is contraindicated in those situations in which the minimal trauma associated with the technique would be harmful to the patient, such as:

- The period immediately following an eye operation.
- If there is any active corneal disease.
- The presence of a penetrating or perforating injury.
- Before other ocular procedures that depend on corneal clarity (e.g., fundus photography).

The presence of any of these requires the contact-lens examination to be deferred, unless absolutely necessary.

As a topical anaesthetic oxybuprocaine (Benoxinate®) 0.4 per cent is typically used, although other types of anaesthetic, such as proxymetacaine 0.5 per cent, amethocaine 0.5 per cent and lignocaine, are acceptable. The patient should be asked about drug allergies before any drug is applied. One to two drops should be instilled into the lower conjunctival sac of each eye one or two minutes before the examination is to take place.

Many diagnostic contact lenses have a curvature that is steeper than that of the cornea and most need to be coupled to the cornea by a material with an index of refraction that is close to that of the cornea. Recommended solutions are:

- Viscotears® eye lubricant (Novartis Ophthalmics);
- GelTears® (Chauvin);
- Proprietary gonioscopic solutions such as Gonak (Cerium Visual Technologies). These tend to be rather viscous and are expensive.

Dilation is highly desirable for the full benefits of this series of lenses to be enjoyed. To insert the lens, patient co-operation is extremely important and can be enhanced by an explanation of the procedure and attention to comfort beforehand:

- Set up the slit lamp as normal and set the magnification to low, about 6–10×, with medium light output and a square slit of about 4mm width.
- The height of the patient is adjusted with the chin rest so that the fixation device is in the centre of the patient's field in front of the contralateral eye.
- Scan the anterior segment of the patient's eye with the microscope to rule out conditions that contraindicate use of this procedure.
- Instil topical anaesthetic.
- Ensure the lens is disinfected correctly.
- Half-fill the lens concavity with the coupling solution. Avoid introducing bubbles into the solution.
- Place the illumination in the straight-ahead position between the oculars.
- The slit lamp should be moved in front of the contralateral eye to provide easier access to the eye that is to be examined first.
- While seated, lift the lens with the first finger and thumb of the dominant hand in such a way that the lens can be tilted up easily to contact the patient's eye; take care not to spill the coupling solution.
- The patient is directed to look down while the practitioner grasps and retracts the upper eyelid with the thumb of the opposite hand.
- The patient then looks up while the examiner places the lower rim of the contact lens into the patient's lower conjunctival sac (*Figure 9.4*).

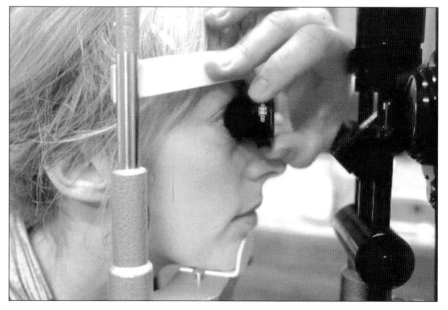

Figure 9.4
Three-mirror contact lens in situ with slit-lamp viewing. (NB The lens is usually held with the left hand for the right eye)

- The lens is quickly tilted up to contact the cornea, and the tension on the upper lid is slowly released while light pressure against the patient's eye is maintained. This last step needs to be done quickly and in one movement.
- Light but positive pressure against the eye is necessary to keep the patient from blinking the lens out of the eye.
- It may be necessary to remind the patient not to back away from the instrument or the pressure will be lost. A failed attempt at lens insertion is frustrating for both the examiner and the patient.
- It is better to be firm and succeed at the first attempt rather than to be overly concerned with the patient's reaction and fail several times.
- Firmly support the hand that holds the contact lens by resting your elbow on the slit-lamp table. If the length of your forearm is too short to reach the slit lamp table, an inverted tissue box may be placed under the elbow.

Examination technique

View the fundus through the lens, scanning across it using the slit-lamp beam. When a mirror lens is used, move onto the oblong mirror to view up to the equator. To visualise the entire central fundus using the mirror, the lens is rotated starting at 6 o'clock (superior fundus) and working clockwise in approximately 20° steps. To maintain the optimum view, the following rules apply:
- For vertical meridians the illumination column can be left or right of centre.
- For horizontal meridians keep the column centrally placed.
- For 2 and 8 o'clock keep the column to the right.
- For 11 and 5 o'clock keep the column to the left.
- Rotate the beam axis so that it is always at right-angles to the mirror.

Removal of the lens

Once the examination has been completed the contact lens is removed from the patient's eye. The suction that helps to hold the lens in place must be broken before the lens can be removed. The globe may be slightly distorted by digital pressure through the lower lid, while the lens is gently pulled from the eye, or the patient may look up and blink. Any remaining coupling solution can be irrigated from the patient's eye using ophthalmic sterile saline.

Disinfection and cleaning of all fundus contact lenses should be carried out using the same guidelines described for gonioscopy lenses in Chapter 6. After use, clean off any residual coupling solution with rising-mains tap water. Clean the contact surface with a few drops of mild soap on a moistened cotton ball, employing a circular motion, and dry on a soft tissue. If necessary, clean the lens surface with proprietary cleaner and/or cloth suitable for anti-reflection coated lenses. Disinfection of the contact surface is achieved by filling the cup with a 1:10 dilution of sodium hypochlorite (household bleach) in fresh tap water. The lens should then be rinsed thoroughly in running rising-mains tap water and dried carefully with a soft tissue. It is then stored in a dry storage case.

Complications

It is very common for mild, transient, superficial, punctate keratitis to be induced following diagnostic contact-lens fundoscopy. Usually, reassurance to the patient that a transient foreign-body sensation may develop, as the anaesthetic wears off, is all that is necessary, although artificial tears may be advised for 12–24 hours. As with all techniques that involve pressure to the globe, the patient may experience vasovagal syncope and pass out from a rapid decrease in blood pressure. Should this occur, basic first-aid measures should be taken to revive the patient.

Since the coupling fluid will mar the view of the fundus for a while, direct and indirect ophthalmoscopy should be carried out before examinations with the mirror or wide-field contact lenses.

Modified (monocular) indirect ophthalmoscopy

Examination of very young children can be difficult, especially when a detailed view of the macula and optic nerve is required. The magnification and patient co-operation required with head-mounted BIO using a 20D lens or slit-lamp biomicroscopy using a 90D or other similar lens means that fundus examination is usually difficult or impossible on young children. Also, the magnification may be inadequate to allow an accurate evaluation of the posterior pole details. The direct ophthalmoscope is often the best available instrument for a detailed retinal examination in young patients. However, children often become frightened as the examiner approaches closely, as is necessary with the direct ophthalmoscope, and co-operation is lost. Additionally, children often fixate the ophthalmoscope light and track it as it is moved by the examiner, which allows examination of the macula but not of the disc. The field of view is small and the magnification is more than that usually required. This prevents the examiner from seeing the overall picture.

To avoid these difficulties the direct ophthalmoscope can be used in conjunction with a condensing lens, the type used with head-mounted binocular indirect ophthalmoscopes.[4] This combination provides a moderately magnified, and wider angle, view of the posterior pole. It avoids the close proximity between the patient and examiner required when using a direct ophthalmoscope alone. The technique is called modified (monocular) indirect ophthalmoscopy and has been noted for its ability to provide a good view of the retina through a small pupil.

Examination technique
- Visualise a red reflex through the direct ophthalmoscope held approximately 18cm from the patient's eye.
- Place a 20D, 28D or ×2.2 panretinal lens 3–5cm in front of the patient's eye in the path of the ophthalmoscope light beam (*Figure 9.5*).
- Move slightly towards or away from the patient until a clear image of the retina is observed.

An inverted, laterally reversed aerial image of the retina is produced, located between the observer and the lens. The apparent magnification gradually increases as the examiner moves closer to this image (i.e., closer to the patient), which enables a more detailed examination. A magnification of 4–5× is obtained by moving closer to the image. As the examiner moves closer, additional lenses in the ophthalmoscope are needed to keep the image clear, depending on the accommodative needs of the examiner. Experience has shown that a viewing distance of approximately 18cm from the patient is optimal, as it provides suitable magnification and a wide field of view.

A disadvantage of the technique, as with conventional direct ophthalmoscopy, is the lack of a true stereoscopic view. However, lateral movement and rotation of the direct ophthalmoscope during the examination gives good parallactic clues to depth.

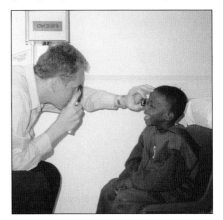

Figure 9.5
Modified (monocular) indirect ophthalmoscopy

Head-borne indirect ophthalmoscopy (headset BIO)

This technique, which is described in greater detail later and by Austin,[5] is not generally used to examine the central fundus because of the low magnification (about 3×, see *Table 9.5*), but it is particularly useful for young children, like the modified monocular indirect technique described above. The child should be dilated, so usually this technique is performed after a cylcoplegic refraction. An ideal lens to use for screening children is the 40D, since it gives a very wide field of view and reduced working distance. It is, however, portable, and could be used in conjunction with the direct ophthalmoscope in domiciliary visits. Dilation is generally essential for this technique. Like all indirect methods, the view through hazy media is better than that of the direct methods.

Examination of the peripheral retina and vitreous

It could be argued that an examination of the peripheral retina and vitreous is desirable in every eye examination for every patient, particularly myopes. However, a careful and extensive examination is mandatory in the following circumstances:

- Recent-onset floaters or increase in number of floaters.
- Any floater that appears to reduce best-corrected acuity.
- Flashes, particularly if unaccompanied by headache and of an arcuate form arising with change of posture.
- Symptoms of peripheral visual loss.
- Any suggestion of vitreal haze during normal fundoscopy or of tobacco dust in the retrolental space.

- History of blunt ocular trauma.
- High myopia or family history of detachment.
- Patients with lattice degeneration or retinal holes seen on normal fundoscopy.
- Patients with a recent history of posterior vitreal detachment (PVD).
- Any patients for whom a wide-field view and stereoscopic imaging will enhance observation of a lesion (examples are peripheral tumours, retinoschisis, diabetic retinopathy).
- All diabetic patients with any evidence of retinopathy.
- Any patient taking tamoxifen, because of the possibility of secondary tumour in the eye.

How should an optometrist examine the peripheral retina?

It is a pointless exercise to attempt a full peripheral retinal examination without maximally dilating the pupil. From a medico-legal point of view, it is also a foolish omission, since there is no way in which pathology could be satisfactorily excluded without a clear view. It is not considered good practice to examine a patient with a suspected peripheral retinal anomaly with the direct ophthalmoscope. It is extremely difficult to view and systematically scan the peripheral retina to locate a lesion, particularly in high myopes. In addition, it is very difficult to detect subtle colour and elevational changes in any part of the fundus, particularly the periphery.

Three main methods are used to examine the peripheral retina and vitreous:

- Headset BIO with or without scleral indentation.
- Goldmann-type three- or four-mirror contact lens and slit lamp.
- Wide-field indirect ophthalmoscopy with contact lens and slit lamp.

The advantages, disadvantages and techniques associated with each method are dealt with below.

Head-borne binocular indirect ophthalmoscopy (headset BIO)

The head-borne illumination and binocular observation system is used in conjunction with a hand-held condensing lens in patients with dilated pupils. A scleral depressor is required if scleral indentation is attempted.

The condensing lens captures the emergent light from the patient's eye and presents this for binocular viewing (*Figure 9.6*). The larger the lens and the bigger the pupil, the wider the field of view obtainable. The lower the condensing lens' power, the greater the magnification and the smaller the field, as shown in *Table 9.5*. Higher-power lenses are held closer to the patient. The view is a bright wide field (about 10× wider than that of direct ophthalmoscopy). There is reasonable stereopsis and negligible alteration in magnification with the refractive error of the patient or examiner. An addition of +2.00D or +2.50D is incorporated in the viewing system, so that presbyopic examiners can view the aerial image comfortably. The image is upside down and laterally reversed. The most peripheral part of the image seen is in the opposite direction to the patient's gaze, so that on looking up the superior periphery is seen at the bottom of the image (*Figure 9.6*).

For a peripheral retinal examination, a wide field of view is preferable. However, too little magnification leads to small lesions being missed. A good compromise is afforded by the Pan Retinal 2.2® (Volk), which delivers a 56° field and a magnification of 2.68×.

Technique

The first time an instrument is used by a practitioner adjustment of the headband is required. This is done as follows:

- Slacken the head size and height adjustment knobs and place the headband on the head like a hat.
- Tighten the height adjustment control until the headband sits level on the head and is located about 2cm above the eyebrow. Tighten the head size adjustment knob to comfortably lock the unit into position. It should not feel excessively tight, but be stable.
- Slacken the browbar knob and the hinge adjustment control to locate the eyepieces level with the eyes and as close as possible to them. Tighten the knobs to maintain this position.

Table 9.5 Properties of condensing lenses used for headset BIO

Lens power, size	Working distance from corneal apex (mm)	Magnification obtainable	Typical field of view (degrees)
15D, 52mm	72	4.11×	36
15D, 45mm	72	4.10×	31
20D, 50mm	50	3.13×	46
20D, 35nn	51	3.08×	34
Pan retinal 2.2, 52mm	40	2.68×	56
25D, 45mm	38	2.54×	52
25D, 33m	39	2.48×	39
28D, 41mm	33	2.27×	53
30D, 43mm	30	2.15×	58
30D, 31mm	31	2.09×	44
40D, 40mm	20	1.67×	69
40D, 31mm	21	1.61×	57

- Provided that the unit is used by the same practitioner, the above should not need to be reset each time it is used.

The oculars of the observation system then need to be set accurately for the examiner:

- Look through the eyepieces at an object about 40cm away (e.g., one's thumb).
- Slide the two knobs for PD adjustment laterally while looking monocularly through each eyepiece, so that the view of the object is centred exactly in front of the eye.
- Move the illumination beam so that it overlaps an object in the centre of the field of view through the eyepieces.
- Select the appropriate beam size. Generally, the largest beam is the most suitable for peripheral examination. Smaller diameters are better for undilated pupils or high-power lenses. Put the diffuser (if available) into the system as it improves the peripheral view.
- A filter can be selected if appropriate, although for peripheral assessment white light is generally used.

The observational technique requires practice and requires several weeks of experience before the practitioner becomes confident. The procedure is as follows:

- Instruct patients that their eyes are going to be examined using a bright light, but that it will not be at all harmful. Both eyes should remain open throughout the examination.
- Lie patients down in a darkened room so that they are at waist height and their head is in front of the examiner.
- Start by examining the superior periphery. This will entail the patient looking up and the examiner standing 180° in the opposite direction (i.e., towards the patient's feet).
- Once the red reflex is seen, insert the lens with the steeper curvature of the bi-aspheric lens facing the examiner. The side facing the patient has a silver or white band at the edge.

- Hold the lens parallel to the patient's iris plane and a short distance from the cornea with the fingers steadied on the patient's forehead or cheek.
- If necessary, hold the lids apart with the fingers of the other hand.
- The anterior segment of the eye should be seen through the lens with a red reflex in the pupil.
- Move the lens away from the eye until the fundus image fills the lens, but not so far that an inverted minified image of the anterior segment is seen.
- Adjust the illumination, if necessary, to the minimum that permits clear visualisation of the fundal details.
- Progressively cover all peripheral quadrants by asking the patient to adjust the direction of gaze and moving to a position opposite to the gaze direction. The lens needs to be re-aligned each time. Tilting the lens can improve the image dramatically by moving the lens' surface reflections out of the examiner's way.
- Finally, examine the posterior pole, limiting exposure time to reduce dazzle.
- Release the lids before each re-fixation to allow the patient to blink and separate as necessary to improve your view.

Scleral indentation

This is usually essential should the examiner wish to examine to the extreme periphery. The compression of the sclera caused by pressure from a scleral indentor places the ora serrata within the field of view of the headset BIO (*Figure 9.7*). In addition, it permits a kinetic evaluation of the peripheral retina to be made. Any break in the retina located beyond the equator will move or be more easily seen on indentation. However, it is not easy and should not be attempted until the art of this type of BIO has been mastered. While scleral indentation does not make retinal lesions worse or cause a detachment, it should not be attempted in any eye that has had

intraocular surgery in the previous 8–10 weeks, because the large increase in IOP it temporarily produces could cause damage. It should not take place if the eye has had a penetrating or orbital injury.

The technique is as follows:

- A thimble-type scleral indentor is placed on the first finger of the dominant hand.
- The indentor should always be tangential to the eye and wherever possible the force should be applied through the lids, beyond the tarsal plates.
- The patient looks initially in the opposite direction to the region to be viewed. The superior temporal region is easiest to examine.
- Therefore, start with the patient looking down. Press the indentor on the upper lid behind the tarsal plate. Remember the ora begins at least 7mm behind the limbus.
- With the indentor gently pressed against the eye, ask the patient to look up. At the same time, advance the indentor parallel to the globe back into the anterior orbit.
- While looking through the headset the indentor is pressed into the eye, applying force tangentially. The mound produced in the superior retinal periphery is seen like a mouse under a carpet and appears darker than surrounding tissue.
- The indentor should be removed and the procedure repeated at each clock hour while working clockwise over the eye. The motion of the mound (or mouse) is observed, while keeping the examiner's eyes, the condensing lens, the fundus image and the indentor all in a straight line.
- At the 3 and 9 o'clock positions indentation can be done by dragging the lids from the 10 or 2 o'clock position. If this is not possible, gentle pressure on the conjunctiva itself may be required, with or without anaesthesia.

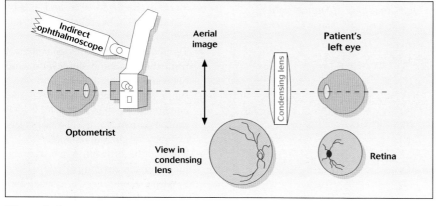

Figure 9.6
Headset BIO schematic showing magnified, reversed, inverted image. Courtesy of David Austen

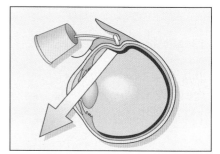

Figure 9.7
Manipulation of globe to view the ora serrata using a sceral indentor. Courtesy of David Austen

Goldmann-type three- or four-mirror contact lens

As described in the section on fundus contact lenses, the peripheral mirror (intermediate in size and square shaped) enables the practitioner to see from the equator as far as the ora serrata. The gonioscopic mirror (smallest and dome shaped) is normally used to visualise the angle, but can also be used to see the extreme retinal periphery and pars plana. The procedure is exactly as described in the section on fundus contact lenses, except that the peripheral mirrors are used. Where general screening of the peripheral retina is required, it is normal practice to start with the appropriate mirror placed inferiorly (viewing the superior periphery) and to rotate the lens clockwise in approximately 20° steps. As above, to maintain the optimum view, the following rules apply:

- For vertical meridians the illumination column can be left or right of centre.
- For horizontal meridians keep the column central.
- For 2 and 8 o'clock keep the column to the right.
- For 11 and 5 o'clock keep the column to the left.
- Rotate the beam axis so that it is always at right angles to the mirror.

It is possible to see the ora serrata through the gonioscopy mirror by displacing the lens on the globe, so that indentation is not required to see to the far periphery provided the pupil is fully dilated. As for the central retina, the magnification can be increased when required by altering the slit-lamp settings. As with the indirect techniques, the vitreous can be inspected (where it is not optically empty) by focusing more anteriorly. However, with all contact systems a disadvantage is that the patient cannot flick the eye laterally to enhance visibility of a liquefied vitreous.

Wide-field indirect ophthalmoscopy with contact lens and slit lamp

Apart from the lens, the only other requirement is a coupling solution to provide an optically smooth interface between the lens and the eye, the slit lamp and an anaesthetic. Lenses are made by a variety of manufacturers. Typical examples are the Volk SuperQuad 160 and Mainster Ultra Field PRP lenses.

The lens contains a positive-powered aspheric lens system, which provides up to a 160° view of the posterior pole. The image is laterally reversed and inverted, just as with the headset BIO or other slit-lamp indirect lenses. The extremely wide-field view is magnificent and free of some of the bothersome reflections inherent in other techniques. The technique is not excessively difficult and scanning of the image is relatively easy. However, it is not possible to see to the ora serrata without displacing the lens and/or employing scleral depression. This is more challenging and is better done with headset BIO. The view obtained is upside down and laterally reversed. The field of view is so large that the lens can be used in the centred position to observe up to the equator.

The technique is very similar to that for the mirror lenses described above, except the lens does not have to be rotated and it is easier to locate the image. Contra-indications are as per the mirror lenses. Topical anaesthetic, insertion, optical coupling solution and dilation are all governed by the same rules already mentioned.

Examination technique

- Fewer reflections will occur if the illumination column is tilted at all times.
- Place the slit-lamp beam in the middle of the lens and a few centimetres away so that the red reflex is seen.
- Push forwards until the fundal image comes into focus.
- Widen the beam and begin to scan the fundal image, starting superiorly and moving horizontally. This can be done more rapidly than with the mirror lenses.

- To examine further into the periphery requires that the lens be moved in the opposite direction to the quadrant to be examined, with the patient looking in the expected direction. For example, to examine the superior periphery, the patient looks up, the lens is moved down and the examiner scans the inferior part of the image.
- To examine as far as the ora serrata, scleral indentation needs to be used, just as with headset BIO. This is difficult and requires an assistant.

Removal and complications are as per the mirror lenses.

Which peripheral examination technique should be used?

Headset indirect is the instrument conventionally used to screen the peripheral retina for holes or tears following symptomatology characteristic of PVD. This is supplemented by mirror examination for a more detailed view of suspicious areas. Scleral indentation is used when the ora serrata needs to be visualised. This might arise when there is very high suspicion of a retinal break or following blunt trauma. Contact indirect techniques are finding favour with the new generation of ophthalmologists for screening in cases of flashes and floaters, sometimes combined with scleral indentation. For the patient with diabetic retinopathy and suspected neovascularisation of the peripheral fundus, these offer a magnificent view to the practitioner.

In general, for optimum examination (and better immunity from medico-legal action) the practitioner is advised to use two out of the three techniques described.

Acknowledgement
Figure 9.1 courtesy of J. Kanski. *Clinical Ophthalmology Photo CD Volume 5: Retinal Disorders*, Butterworth–Heinemann.

References

1 Van Herick W, Schaffer RN and Schwartz A (1969). Estimation of width of angle of anterior chamber. *Am J Ophthalmol.* **68**, 626–629.
2 Meyler J and Hodd NB (1988). The use of digital image capture in contact lens practice. *Contact Lens Ant Eye* **21**(Suppl), 3–11.
3 Ocular Instruments *Ocular Instruments Optometry Catalogue*. (Washington: Ocular Instruments Inc).
4 Eperjesi F (1997). Paediatric ocular evaluation. *Optician* **214**(5618), 31.
5 Austin DP (1993). Binocular indirect ophthalmoscopy. *Optom Today* **March 22**, 13–19.

Further Reading

Fingeret M, Casser L and Woodcome HT (1990). *Atlas of Primary Eyecare Procedures*. p. 72–84 (Norwalk: Appleton and Lange).
Johnston RL and Cakanac CJ (1995). *Retina, Vitreous and Choroid. Clinical Procedures*, p. 89–99 (Newton: Butterworth–Heinemann).
Kanski JJ (1994). *Clinical Ophthalmology*, Third Edition, p. 318–322 (London: Butterworth–Heinemann).

10

Laser imaging techniques for assessment of the ocular fundus

Anita Lightstone

Optometric examination of the fundus has consisted chiefly of examination by either direct or indirect ophthalmoscopy with or without dilation. Binocular indirect ophthalmoscopy may also be used with optical devices such as the Goldman three-mirror contact lens to improve peripheral viewing of the retina and give better magnification, but the technique requires considerable patient co-operation and gives a smaller field of view.[1]

Scleral depression is another method that can be used to give an increased view of the periphery. This involves indenting the patient's sclera, either through the lids or on the bulbar conjunctiva using an instrument designed for the purpose. All these methods of fundus investigation mainly use drawings by the practitioner to record all findings, although photography can be used in conjunction with some of these techniques.

The drawings show what the practitioner noted during the course of the examination. They do not give a complete record of the fundus at the time of examination. The drawings do not give the practitioner the facility to re-inspect the fundus on a separate occasion and do not provide a positive defence if he or she is accused of failure to detect pathology after examining an eye. It can be argued that a more definitive record of the fundus can be obtained with a retinal imaging system.

Although fundus cameras have been available for many years, the complexity and the cost of these instruments have prevented them from becoming part of the standard routine of the optometrist. However, with the advances that have taken place in the field of digital imaging and with the increased power of computers to facilitate the processing and manipulation of the image, optometrists can now include imaging of the fundus as part of the routine examination.

More recent advances in the field of imaging include the introduction of the Scanning Laser Ophthalmoscope (SLO) in a form that can be used by optometrists to image the retina and also, in a confocal form, for tomography and analysis of the optic nerve head. This chapter concentrates on the use of digital imaging with both conventional light sources and laser sources, looks briefly at the use of tomography in practice, and also considers the other applications of laser for fundus investigation.

Fundus imaging using conventional light sources

Cameras that use conventional light sources follow two design types – those intended for use when the pupil has been dilated (mydriatic cameras) and those capable of imaging through an undilated pupil (non-mydriatic cameras). However, even the non-mydriatic cameras require a relatively large pupil to allow enough light to enter the pupil for a good image to be obtained. Most non-mydriatic cameras require the pupil size to be at least 4mm, although the Canon CR6 produces an image through a 3.7mm pupil using a special setting, but this gives a reduced field of view. Consequently, it is often necessary, when using a non-mydriatic camera, which is based on a conventional light source, to carry out pupil dilation.

Although mydriatic cameras are used in some optometric practices, they are more often found in a hospital photography department. They are highly sophisticated instruments and allow capture of the image using 35mm film, Polaroid, digital imaging, and video. Some people claim that the resolution and quality of the image obtained by using 35mm film far exceeds that of other techniques. However, with the advances that have taken place over recent years, this claim is now dubious and the quality of the digital images can be regarded as equal to that of 35mm film for most systems. This depends not only on the quality of the camera optics, but also on the resolution capabilities of the computer monitor and on the specification of the software that is used. The mydriatic cameras all incorporate a series of filters within their systems that allow imaging by alternative techniques. Among other functions, the filters are used for imaging during retinal angiography. This technique is a valuable way to investigate the functioning of the retinal and choroidal circulation systems and to assess macular change. During angiography, either fluorescein or indocyanine green is injected into a vein in the patient's arm. Imaging is then carried out at about 1 second intervals, starting about 5 seconds after the injection and continuing for up to 25 seconds. In some cases, images may be taken up to 20–30 minutes after the injection, known as late-stage images. Fluorescein is imaged with blue light and generally used when disruption to the retinal circulation is suspected, while indocyanine green dye is used to investigate choroidal circulation. Ophthalmologists use this method extensively, particularly to investigate diabetic retinopathy, macular degeneration, retinal vein thrombosis and retinal tumours.

The mydriatic cameras are capable of various modifications to the light levels and alteration of focus to give optimum images. Probably the best images are obtained when skilled and specially trained

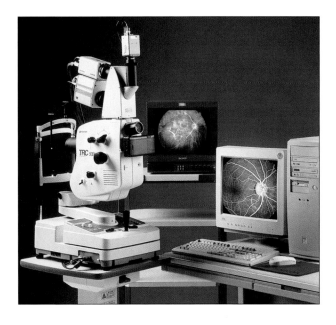

Figure 10.1
Topcon retinal camera

Although the ability to see results immediately was previously the main benefit with the Polaroid system, the film is expensive, which means additional cost for the optometrist if more than one image needs to be taken. In addition, the resolution with Polaroid film is not as high as that obtained with 35mm film and most modern digital systems.

Once a satisfactory image has been obtained digitally, it is possible for this to be printed, if required, although most manufacturers recommend that the screen image should be used for diagnosis. These images may also be sent by email when the patient needs further referral or for a second opinion.

photographers use the cameras. The maximum field of view in a single image with these cameras is 60°, although multiple images can be built into a 'mosaic' picture to increase the size of the field. Topcon has now developed software to facilitate this process automatically when digital images have been taken (*Figure 10.1*). This allows a field of view of the retina of up to 85°. In addition, the cameras can also be set to image smaller field sizes, which is often used when images of higher magnification are required for specific areas, such as the optic nerve head.

Non-mydriatic cameras

Non-mydriatic cameras require a pupil size of 4mm or above to provide a good image. For a pupil size less than this, dilation is advisable to obtain a useful image with minimum reflections and shadows, as well as to be at the optimum level of brightness. The pupil size tends to decrease with age, which means that many older patients need to be dilated. As pathology also tends to increase with age, the optometrist will probably find that a high proportion of patients that he or she wishes to image will need to be dilated.

Non-mydriatic cameras are generally very easy to use with devices that facilitate the automatic setting of the camera for optimum illumination levels and focus. The latest generation of these can be operated by optometric assistants, provided pupil dilation is not required. When this is necessary, mydriasis should be carried out by the optometrist before the patient is handed over to the assistant for imaging.

With the advent of digital imaging, the non-mydriatic camera makes a much

more useful tool for the practising optometrist. Good pictures can be produced from lower light levels when the image is being captured for digital processing and focusing is carried out with an infrared monitor. The infrared monitor helps to keep the levels of light as low as possible, and so keep the pupil size at a maximum before the image is taken. As the light level used to grab the image is also relatively low, it is not necessary to wait before taking further images, as the pupil will not have undergone any marked degree of constriction during imaging.

The maximum field size obtainable with these cameras is 45° and, as with the mydriatic cameras, some of the cameras can produce different field sizes. The software supplied with the Topcon camera also allows a series of 'mosaic' images to be created to give a bigger field, as with the Topcon mydriatic camera. In addition, some of the cameras also have facilities that allow modification of the settings as an override to the camera's automatic settings usually employed. Again, some of the cameras may also be used with 35mm or Polaroid film.

The use of the computer has enabled fundus photography to become a much more feasible task for the optometrist to carry out. It is no longer necessary for a roll of film to be completed before the results of the imaging can be assessed for their usefulness. With rolls of film, if the result is found to be deficient in any manner, the patient has to be recalled for further imaging. This involves further cost for the optometrist, inconvenience for the patient, and a possible delay in the start of treatment or further referral, all avoided if computer images are taken.

The use of laser

Scanning laser ophthalmoscope
Laser is an acronym for light-stimulated emission of radiation and consists of atoms of a medium, such as a rare gas, that has been excited by an appropriate energy source, which leads to the spontaneous emission of photons. When the conditions are such that there are more excited than unexcited atoms, the result can be a build up of emitted photons with the same direction, wavelength and phase. By use of amplification techniques, a highly concentrated and powerful light source of relatively low illumination level is produced.

The principle of SLO is that the laser is focused to form a highly collimated beam that is passed through a series of mirrors, including a rotating polygon mirror, to pivot in the plane of the pupil and form a raster at the patient's retina. Light is then reflected back through the system and passed through signal amplification (and other devices to reduce reflections) to form an image via a computer and specifically designed software or to a video device. The main advantage of this system is that it can be used to carry out retinal investigations in ways that enable the ophthalmologist or optometrist to gain more information about the retina than can be obtained from conventional imaging techniques.

The SLO tends to be superior to standard imaging methods when cataract is present[2] and can be used for both fluorescein and indocyanine green angiography. Research has shown that the image obtained using an SLO with infrared for indocyanine green imaging suffers from fewer scattered-light effects than does conventional imaging.[3] Consequently, a more useful image is produced by this method in terms of the amount of information that can be obtained from it. Most of the images produced by SLO systems are monochromatic and of relatively small dimension. A further function that can be performed by a scanning laser system is that of retinal tomography or three-dimensional imaging to allow quantitative data to be obtained. For these measurements, a confocal system is needed by which the laser beam is focused onto the retina.

Until recently, SLOs had been used only in hospitals. The setting of the instrument to provide maximum information was highly complex and in most cases carried out by ophthalmic photographers. The instruments are also extremely expensive. However, in 2000 two instruments were introduced to the market for use by both optometrists and ophthalmologists. These are the Panoramic 200 and the Heidelberg Retinal Tomograph 11 (HRT11).

The Panoramic 200

The Panoramic 200 was developed by Optos in Dunfermline, Scotland. The instrument is designed to enable an area of up to 200° × 200° internally of the fundus to be produced as one image and without the use of collaging or pupil dilation. The instrument uses two lasers (red, wavelength 633nm, and green, wavelength 532nm). There is also a third laser channel available. In due course, the third channel may be used for a blue laser source, and thus enable fluorescein angiography to be carried out. Another possibility for the development of this channel would be to incorporate an infrared source to allow imaging with indocyanine green. As with other SLOs, a series of mirrors and a high-velocity polygon create the sweep lines that form the raster. However, by using a series of ellipsoidal mirrors and also by causing the light to scan effectively from a virtual focus point at the centre of the pupil, the technology has achieved the remarkable feat of imaging an extensive area of the fundus without mydriasis or invasive techniques (*Figure 10.2*). This technology also means that the process does not cause discomfort to the patient through either the installation of drops or the use of bright lights. The image created consists of 2000 × 2000 pixels × 2 colours. The resolution of the image is smaller than 20μm on the axis and 40μm at the far periphery. The image is captured within 0.25 seconds.

Although the two lasers image simultaneously, the images gathered are separate, which is highly valuable when carrying out a diagnosis of any abnormalities noted on inspection of the image. Images from the red laser relate mainly to

structures from the pigment epithelium and choroidal levels, while images from the green laser relate to the neural layers of the retina. The images captured may be viewed as monochromatic reds and greens, combined colours or as grey tones of red and green. Although the combined colour comes nearest to the colour of the image that is obtained during standard photography, the image does appear different, with some areas of the retina seeming to be green in colour. However, this should not prove to be difficult for the experienced optometrist to learn to interpret and the colour can be modified, using appropriate software, to bear a greater resemblance to the images obtained using conventional light sources.

Since over 80 per cent of the retina can be seen in one image, the optometrist is able to view nearly all areas of the fundus in one view. This often makes it easier to assess the significance of any pathology. In addition, as the usual reference markers to pathology location and size (i.e., optic nerve head) can be seen in the same image as the abnormality, to reference the location and size of the anomaly is simplified. From clinical trials by Baumal and Puliafito,[2] the Panoramic 200 has been shown to match a standard fundus camera for specificity and to exceed it slightly for sensitivity, although this difference did not reach statistical significance. Both cameras showed a specificity (proportion of true negatives that are detected by the camera) of 100 per cent. The Panoramic 200 had a sensitivity (proportion of true positives that were detected by the camera) of 95.8 per cent, while the standard fundus camera had a sensitivity of 91.6 per cent. The gold standard for this study was indirect ophthalmoscopy (method not specified).

As the system can be used without dilation and by auxiliary staff, it is envisaged

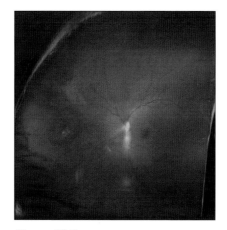

Figure 10.2

An image produced by the Panoramic 200 from Optos

that the instrument could be used to screen for pathology on all patients, and thus reduce the need for patients to be dilated in most cases[4]. From this, it can also be deduced that it is probable that an increase will occur in the amount of ocular pathology that is detected before there is loss of sight. A study by Amer *et al.*[5] suggests that the Panoramic 200 can increase practice efficiency by increasing patient flow and reducing the number of occasions when a second appointment is needed so that mydriasis can be carried out.

Previously, the use of SLOs was inaccessible to optometrists not only because of the complexity of operation, but also through the cost of the equipment. Having overcome the former problem, Optos has also brought the Panoramic 200 within the budget of most optometrists. This has been made feasible by the use of a payment scheme known as 'access technology now'. This means that the optometrist has no capital outlay, but pays each time a patient is imaged successfully. In return, the optometrist has the use of the equipment, including an additional computer for viewing of the images in a separate location, and image storage. The scheme also covers training of staff, maintenance of the Panoramic 200, and any upgrades that may be introduced by the company at a later date. The disadvantage of this method of payment is that to make it financially viable at least 200 patients need to be imaged by the practice each month.

The system is non-invasive, so it can be used for a wide variety of patients from very young children (a few weeks old) to the very elderly. The instrument is designed to be accessible to wheelchair-bound patients and a small feedback camera is installed to assist with patient alignment for those who, for various reasons, have difficulty in correctly positioning themselves. The guidance that the practitioner can obtain from the feedback camera means it should be possible to image people who have very low vision. Currently, the Panoramic 200 is a large instrument and so requires a reasonable amount of space. This is a new and developing technology and it is to be expected that in due course the size of the instrument may decrease and so become even more optometrist friendly.

The HRT and HRT11

The HRT11, which is distributed by Clement Clarke, is also very new to the optometric field. It is based on the Heidelberg Retinal Tomograph (HRT), which has been used by both research

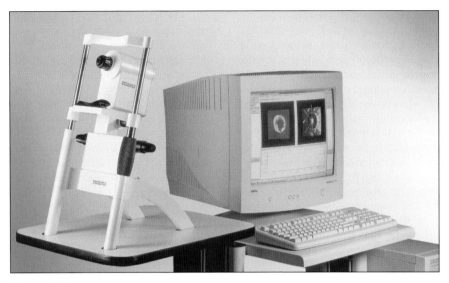

Figure 10.3
The HRT11 from Clement Clarke may come to be regarded as an essential instrument for screening for glaucoma, particularly in shared or managed care schemes

institutions and hospitals for many years. The HRT is a highly sophisticated and complex instrument that can be used for many purposes. It has a confocal laser-scanning system for the acquisition of three-dimensional images of the posterior segment. This involves building up a series of numerous sequential two-dimensional images from which a three-dimensional image can be computed. This image is produced from more than 65,000 local measurements of the retinal surface height. The image is colour-coded to give a map effect, in which dark colours represent the elevated structures, while lighter colours represent the depressed structures. With the HRT it is possible to vary the field size between a $10° \times 10°$ field and a $20° \times 20°$ field. It can be used for analysis and follow-up of pathologies such as macular holes, macular oedema, retinal detachments and tumours. An important application of the instrument, which is supported by sophisticated computer software, is the quantitative analysis of the optic nerve head.

The HRT11 (*Figure 10.3*) has been simplified in use so that its sole function is to carry out analysis of the optic nerve head. This made the instrument much easier to use, less expensive and smaller. It is sufficiently small and light to be regarded as a portable instrument, although it needs computer support. As a result of this re-engineering of the HRT, the HRT11 is an instrument that is applicable in everyday optometric practice. The HRT11 conducts the same scanning process as the HRT, but the field size is $15° \times 15°$. Each frame that is captured has 384×384 pixels, which gives an extremely high resolution of 10μm per pixel. Sixteen images per

milimetre of scan are obtained, with the number of images acquired per eye varying according to the depth of the optic cup. After acquisition, quantitative and graphic analyses are carried out. For this analysis, the optic nerve head is divided into seven areas: global, temporal, temporal/superior, temporal/inferior, nasal, nasal/superior, and nasal/inferior. This method gives data that are very easy for the optometrist to interpret, and is based on research carried out by Wollstein *et al.*[6] at Moorfields Eye Hospital.

This quantitative approach to analysis of the optic disc may eventually become part of the standard routine for patients with either ocular hypertension or suspicious discs in both the hospital setting and the optometric practice. Certainly, it can be expected that the HRT11 will become regarded as an essential part of the screening procedures carried out for glaucoma, particularly in shared or managed care schemes. However, at present, it is not recommended that the optometrist should rely solely on data from this instrument when deciding whether to refer a patient as a suspect glaucoma case, but should follow the current College of Optometrists' guidelines and continue to monitor intraocular pressures and visual fields as well.

Other Heidelberg SLO systems found in the hospital situation are designed to carry out angiography investigation using both fluorescein and indocyanine green, and the Heidelberg Retina Flowmeter is for the two-dimensional mapping of blood flow in the capillary system. This is achieved by using an infrared laser source. The Doppler effect causes light reflected or scattered by moving objects to undergo a frequency

shift, which results in interference happening with light that has been unchanged following reflection from stationary objects. The Heidelberg Retina Flowmeter measures this temporal intensity variation at each point in the two-dimensional scan by multiple scanning. The Doppler frequency shift of the reflected light is computed and these data are used to quantify the local velocity of the moving particles, which gives the information on blood flow.

The Rodenstock SLO
For many years, Rodenstock has produced an SLO designed for hospital use.[7] Using a confocal system, the Rodenstock SLO can use lasers of four different wavelengths (red, HeNe 633nm, blue argon ion, 488nm, green argon ion, 514nm, and infrared diode laser, 780nm). There are also four different imaging fields available, which are 20° and 40°, with an option of 30° and 60°. It can be used not only to obtain stationary retinal images (*Figure 10.4*), but also (via the compatible Rodenstock Videomed system) dynamic processes, such as blood-flow velocity and pulsation of the retinal vessels may be observed. In addition, the system can be used for techniques such as fluorescein angiography and indocyanine green investigation, and these can be viewed in real-time. As with the Panoramic 200, the red laser source images well on the deeper layers of the retinal choroidal structures, while the blue and green argon sources image the more superficial layers and can be used for angiography. The confocal laser beam used in this SLO means that the corneal scattering of light is reduced. Another feature of the Rodenstock SLO is that the modules incorporate specific fixation targets, which may be viewed on the retina and allow the exact location of a scotoma to be found. These targets are available as Snellen E test or Landolt rings and are sized to enable them to be used for a wide variety of acuity levels. This increases the safety of the laser treatment by allowing an exact analysis of the area that is used for fixation by the patient and by plotting areas of the retina that are intact and functioning normally.

Other laser applications

Retinal laser polarimetry
Another interesting advance in retinal assessment is the use of retinal laser polarimetry.[8] This is a non-invasive technique that does not require the pupil to be dilated and the data are collected in less

than 1 second. Commercially, the instrument that can carry out this investigative technique is the GDx Nerve Fiber Analyzer, produced by Laser Diagnostic Technologies in California.

The laser source for this instrument is in the near infrared with a wavelength of 780nm. The beam is passed through a polarisation modulator, which continuously changes the polarisation of the laser output. The focused laser beam of about 35μm is scanned in a vertical and horizontal raster across the retina. The laser beam double-passes through the retinal nerve fibre layer (RNFL), which is birefringent because of the presence of the retinal ganglion cells. The birefringent property of the RNFL causes the beam to be split into two parts, which are plane polarised at right angles to each other. One of these beams continues to obey the laws of refraction (the ordinary beam), while the other (the extraordinary beam) does not. This results in a phase-shift between the two beams. A polarisation detector is used to measure the change in polarisation and Fourier analysis is used to calculate the phase shift or retardation that has occurred. This retardation is proportional to the thickness of the RNFL. It is claimed that the reproducibility of the lateral measurements is 20μm, and for the thickness it is 15μm or better.

The GDx is being used to measure the nerve fibre layer to detect glaucoma early, as there is a loss of nerve fibres before the field loss measurable by standard perimetry methods. The maps produced by these techniques are colour coded, with brighter colours representing the thicker areas of nerve fibre layers and the darker colours indicating the thinner layers. Horizontal and vertical cross-sections are also plotted and displayed, giving useful information.

At present, the results may be difficult to interpret, as there is considerable variation in the RNFL among normal subjects. However, there is obvious value in the longitudinal monitoring of any patients suspected of having the early stages of glaucoma. The technique can also be used to plot and monitor other optic neuropathies. The GDx is an extremely expensive instrument and so this technology is currently limited to hospital use. It is possible that as the technology develops, the cost of these instruments may decrease and reach a level that would be affordable for an optometric practice. If so, then retinal laser polarimetry is likely to become another valuable tool in assessing retinal function.

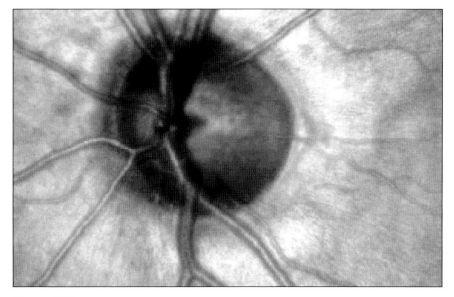

Figure 10.4
Image created by the scanning laser ophthalmoscope from Rodenstock

Laser biomicroscopy[8]

The laser source for this technique is a green helium source with a wavelength of 543nm. A map is generated of the retina using a scanning mirror and fundus-imaging lens. A total of nine scans are involved in producing a retinal map and each scan has 10 optical sections in a 2mm × 2mm area. Laser biomicroscopy is used to give a visualisation of the retinal structures and a measurement of retinal thickness. This can be valuable for early diagnosis and also for monitoring retinal conditions, such as macular oedema, epiretinal membrane and macular holes. The instrument used to carry out this procedure is the Retinal Thickness Analyzer by Talia Technology, a highly specialised instrument that is only used in hospitals.

Future uses of diagnostic laser[8]

Many exciting possibilities are currently still at the development and research stage for the future use of laser as both a qualitative and a quantitative diagnostic tool to investigate the structure and function of ocular tissues. These include the use of fluorescence spectroscopy to detect and monitor diabetes by looking at the fluorescent light and back-scattered Rayleigh radiation. Changes in the ratio of these aspects, after allowing for age-related changes, are proportional to changes in haemoglobin A_{1c} levels. This reflects the mean blood glucose level over the preceding 6–12 weeks.

Another application that is already commercially available is that of holographic interferometry. In this procedure, the laser beam is used as a radiation source that is split into two beams, the reference beam and the object beam. The object beam is reflected off the object of interest and on return interferes with the reference beam in the plane of the film. Using thermoplastic film, a high-resolution holographic interferogram is formed. Interferograms of both the back surface and the front surface of the cornea can be generated. These allow assessment of the outcome of keratorefractive surgery as well as evaluation of corneal wound strength and the effect of postoperative treatment. This instrument is produced in the US as the Kerametrics CLASS 1000 Corneal Analyzer.

Laser interferometry can also be used for clinical application through the production of an interference fringe pattern on the retina. The fringe spacing is determined by the wavelength of the light and the distance between the two beams, while the contrast is determined by the amount of stray light and relative beam intensities. The technique gives a quantitative measurement of macular function and is useful in predicting the possible improvement in visual acuity after treatment, such as for cataracts and corneal opacification, although sometimes the predicted improvement may not happen. This instrument is produced by two companies – Rodenstock as the Retinometer and Haag–Streit as the Lotmar Visometer.

Conclusions

The use of new imaging techniques is providing much more information about the state of the retina and retinal function than has previously been possible. As the use of the laser for investigative examination becomes available to the optometrist, it should be possible to detect eye disease at an earlier stage and before loss of vision has occurred. As these new instruments continue to reach levels of higher resolution and are developed to give stereo images, so the use of more invasive techniques will become redundant. However, until that stage is reached, the new instruments should be regarded as being able to provide the optometrist with additional and valuable information about the patient's eye, rather than as replacing the standard methods of ophthalmoscopy. No doubt within 10 or 20 years the optometrist will only have to place on his or her head a virtual reality headset to have the effect of actually exploring a patient's eye from the inside. This will give the optometrist the advantage of being able to view every aspect of the eye from the ora serrata to the cupping of the optic nerve head. The same approach may also become the standard method used by surgeons to carry out operative treatment. The care of eyes will have entered a new era in which, hopefully, loss of sight will be greatly reduced.

References

1 Jones WL (1998). *Atlas of the Peripheral Ocular Fundus* (Oxford: Butterworth–Heinemann).
2 Baumal CR and Puliafito CA (2000). *Evaluation of the Retina with the Optos Panoramic 200 Non-mydriatic Retinal Imaging System*. Poster, ARVO 2000.
3 Flower RW, Csaky KG and Murphy RP (1998). Disparity between fundus camera and scanning laser ophthalmoscope indocyanine green imaging of retinal pigment epithelium detachments. *Retina* **18**, 260–268.
4 Lightstone A and Harris MB (1999). Preliminary evaluation of an ultra-widefield fundus imaging system. *Optom Vis Sci.* **76**, 118.
5 Amer A, Wilson G, Brundenell L, Lightstone A and Edwards JR (2000). *Evaluation of an Ultra-Widefield Non-Mydriatic Scanning Laser Ophthalmoscope within an Optometric Practice*. Poster, American Academy of Optometry Meeting, Madrid, April 2000.
6 Wollstein G, Garway-Heath DF and Hitchings RA (1998). Identification of early glaucoma cases with the scanning laser ophthalmoscope. *Ophthalmoscopy* **105**(8), 1557–1563.
7 Ellingford A (1994). The Rodenstock scanning laser ophthalmoscope in clinical practice. *J Audiovis Media Med.* **17**(2), 67–70.
8 Wormington CM (1999). *New Diagnostic Uses of Lasers*. Lecture: American Academy of Optometry Meeting, December 1999, Seattle.

Multiple-choice questions, Section 2

There is one correct answer per question. The answers are given at the end of the book.

1 **Which of the following factors does not govern the resolution of the microscope on a slit lamp?**
A   Its numerical aperture.
B   The diameter of the objective lens.
C   The diameter of the eyepiece lenses.
D   The working distance.
E   The wavelength of light.

2 **Which statement on focusing and setting up a slit lamp is false?**
A   Both the illumination system and the microscope have a variable focus.
B   The illumination system has a fixed focus while the microscope has adjustable eyepieces.
C   Ideally, the slit lamp should be focused with a focusing rod.
D   When setting the focus of the instruments the magnification of the microscope should be high.
E   Focusing the microscope on the patients' eyelids is inaccurate.

3 **Which one of these statements about sclerotic scatter is true?**
A   A wide beam should be used.
B   The technique relies on total internal reflection.
C   The slit height should be 8mm.
D   The illumination and observation systems should be set at 90°.
E   Scarred corneal areas do not scatter light and so are difficult to detect.

4 **Which of the following statements about specular reflection is true?**
A   The corneal endothelium cannot be visualised using this technique.
B   This technique is completely independent of Purkinje images
C   The corneal endothelium can be viewed by utilising the second Purkinje image.
D   It is essential that the illuminating system and microscope are placed either side of the centre of the eye.
E   It is not possible to view the anterior surface of the lens (orange peel effect) using the technique.

5 **Which statement on assessment of the anterior chamber depth is false?**
A   Van Herick's method is the technique most commonly used to assess the anterior chamber depth.
B   Van Herick's method is based on forming a section at the limbal/corneal boundary.
C   The ratio between corneal thickness and aqueous space is assessed in van Herick's technique.
D   The ratio between the aqueous space and the corneal thickness is assessed in van Herick's technique.
E   An alternative to the van Herick technique was described by Smith in 1979.

6 **Which of these statements about conic sections is true?**
A   This technique is useful for assessing the presence of inflammatory material in the anterior chamber.
B   The technique should be performed in a brightly illuminated room.
C   The area between the reflex of the cornea and the lens should always appear bright.
D   The slit height should be no less than 8mm for this technique.
E   The microscope should always be decoupled when performing this technique.

7 **The anterior chamber can only be viewed with a goniolens because:**
A   Other instruments cannot focus enough light in this part of the eye.
B   The iris prevents a clear view with any other procedure.
C   The cornea is milky white with other techniques.
D   Scleral limbal overhang and total internal reflection by the cornea prevent a clear view with any other procedure.
E   The critical angle of the cornea is too high.

8 **In gonioscopy the critical angle of the cornea is eliminated by:**
A   The anaesthetic.
B   Slit-lamp magnification.
C   Light refracted by the steep curved outer surface of the contact lens.
D   The small thumbnail mirror.
E   The tear film.

9 **The most important part of the anterior chamber angle is the posterior portion of the trabecular meshwork because:**
A   Behind it lies the canal of Schlemm.
B   It can easily be occluded by the iris.
C   It can often fill with blood.
D   It is involved in uveoscleral outflow.
E   It is a site often involved in neoplastic activity.

10 **The Thorpe four-mirror lens has:**
A   One mirror angled for the anterior chamber and three for the retina.
B   Does not need any viscous coupling gel.
C   Has four mirrors angled for the anterior chamber.
D   Is useful in children and those with small palpebral apertures.
E   Has to be rotated through 270° for the optimum viewing angle.

11 **Optimum initial magnification and slit beam dimensions are:**
A   ×15, 2mm width and 5mm height.
B   ×6, 1mm width and 4mm height.
C   ×10, 3mm width and 5mm height.
D   ×10 to ×15, 3mm width and 5mm height.
E   ×10 to ×15, 2mm width and 2–4mm height.

12 Prior to dilation, for what van Herick's grade is gonioscopy recommended:
A 1
B 2
C 3
D 4
E 0

13 Aqueous is secreted at which of the following rates?
A 2ml per minute.
B 2ml per hour.
C 2μl per minute.
D 2μl per hour.
E 20ml per hour.

14 Which of the following is not associated with a rise in intraocular pressure (IOP)?
A Age.
B Systemic beta-blockers.
C Cardiac systole.
D Blinking.
E Winter time.

15 Which of the following statements regarding an IOP measurement below the normal range within a population is not true?
A It is not of clinical significance.
B It may result from rhegmatogenous retinal detachment.
C It may result from postoperative choroidal detachment.
D It may be associated with a central retinal vein occlusion.
E It may be iatrogenic.

16 Which of the following factors does not influence the application of the Imbert–Fick principle to the eye?
A Corneal thickness.
B Surface tension of the tear.
C The direction of the force applied perpendicular to the sphere.
D Corneal flexibility.
E Area of applanation.

17 The area of applanation of a Goldmann tonometer probe at which a reading of IOP is made is:
A $3.06mm^2$.
B Between 3 and $4mm^2$.
C $7.35mm^2$.
D $0.5mm^2$.
E $10mm^2$.

18 Which of the following statements about non-contact tonometers (NCTs) is true?
A They cannot be calibrated.
B They are never as accurate as contact methods.
C They never cause corneal compromise.
D They cannot be used on scarred corneas.
E They may require many readings to be taken to achieve a consistent result.

19 Which statement is correct?
A The optic nerve head receives its blood supply from the anterior ciliary arteries.
B The optic nerve head receives its blood supply from the posterior cerebral artery.
C The optic nerve head receives its blood supply from the ophthalmic artery.
D The optic nerve head only receives its blood supply from the posterior ciliary arteries.
E The central retinal artery provides the majority of blood flow to the optic nerve head.

20 Which statement is incorrect?
A Pulsatile ocular blood flow (POBF) is the only non-invasive way to measure blood flow in the eye.
B Colour Doppler ultrasound reveals the velocity of retrobulbar arterial blood.
C Digitalised fluorescein angiography can measure retinal blood flow.
D Blue-field entoscopy allows a subjective measure of retinal blood flow.
E Flowmetry uses the Doppler effect to calculate retinal blood flow.

21 Which statement is correct?
A POBF is predominantly a measure of choroidal blood flow.
B POBF measures total uveal blood flow.
C POBF detects pulsatile retinal blood flow.
D POBF is unaffected by gender.
E POBF is a measure of pulsatile flow in the posterior ciliary arteries.

22 Which statement is incorrect?
A Focal ischaemic-type discs commonly have splinter haemorrhages.
B Low blood pressure at night may cause ischaemic damage of the nerve head.
C Raised IOP is not the sole cause of glaucoma.
D Glaucomatous discs have been classified into four distinct types.
E Glaucoma is caused by normal-tension blood pressure.

23 Which statement is correct?
A Systemic medications do not affect POBF.
B A diabetic patient with high POBF definitely has proliferative retinopathy.
C A patient with a low POBF definitely has normal tension glaucoma.
D Other signs of ocular disease should be sought in a patient with a significantly asymmetric POBF.
E Optometrists should refer all patients with low POBF.

24 Which statement is correct?
A POBF can only be measured when used with a slit lamp.
B The ocular blood flow (OBF) system only measures POBF and IOP.
C The IOP measured by the OBF system is equal to the pulse amplitude.
D The OBF system is influenced less by corneal thickness when measuring IOP.
E Fluorescein drops are required to measure the IOP with the OBF system.

25 A 78D slit-lamp indirect fundus lens has:

A Lower magnification and field of view compared to a 125D lens.

B Higher magnification and field of view compared to a 125D lens.

C Lower magnification and greater field of view compared to a 125D lens.

D Higher magnification and smaller field of view compared to a 125D lens.

E The same magnification and field of view if held at the same distance from the eye as a 125D lens.

26 To visualise more of the peripheral fundus using a slit-lamp indirect lens one must:

A Pull the lens further away from the eye.

B Tilt the lens away from the incident light beam.

C Move the lens in the direction one wants to visualise.

E Have the patient look towards the area of interest and move the lens in the opposite direction.

27 Headset BIO is the most appropriate technique for:

A Screening in children under the age of five years.

B Optic nerve assessment.

C Stereoscopic examination of a fundal lesion.

D A diabetic patient.

E Patients who cannot be dilated.

28 The Hruby lens is particularly appropriate for:

A Use when a patient has difficulty maintaining stable fixation.

B Wide-field examination of the posterior pole.

C High-magnification non-inverted stereoscopic examination of the disc and macula through a non-dilated pupil.

D Locating retinal tears in the far periphery.

E High-magnification non-inverted stereoscopic examination of the disc and macula through a fully dilated pupil.

29 The best examination routine on a patient complaining of recent-onset floaters is pupil dilation followed by:

A Headset BIO examination.

B Examination of the anterior vitreous by direct ophthalmoscopy, followed by headset BIO.

C Slit-lamp examination of the anterior vitreous, followed by headset BIO or slit-lamp BIO, followed by mirror contact lens where appropriate.

E Hruby lens examination of the anterior vitreous followed by retinal examination with the central region of a mirror contact lens.

30 The various examination techniques in ascending order of stereopsis are:

A Direct ophthalmoscopy, slit-lamp BIO, headset BIO, Hruby lens, fundus contact lens.

B Slit-lamp BIO, headset BIO, Hruby lens, fundus contact lens, direct ophthalmoscopy.

C Direct ophthalmoscopy, slit-lamp BIO, headset BIO, fundus contact lens, Hruby lens.

D Slit-lamp BIO, direct ophthalmoscopy, headset BIO, Hruby lens, fundus contact lens.

E Direct ophthalmoscopy, headset BIO, slit-lamp BIO, Hruby lens, fundus contact lens.

31 For the majority of conventional, non-mydriatic fundus cameras, the minimum pupil size must be at least:

A 1mm.

B 2mm.

C 3mm.

D 4mm.

E 5mm.

32 Which of the following statements about digital imaging is false?

A Good-quality images are only obtainable when the light levels are high.

B The light level used to grab the image is relatively low.

C Focusing is performed with the aid of an infrared monitor.

D Marked pupil constriction is reduced, which allows rapid, consecutive images to be taken.

E A large field of view of 45° can be obtained with this application.

33 In which pathological condition is the scanning laser ophthalmoscope (SLO) most superior to standard imaging for viewing the fundus?

A Blepharitis.

B Conjunctivitis.

C Iritis.

D Cataract.

E Age-related macular degeneration (ARMD).

34 The Panoramic 200 SLO utilises two lasers. Images from the red laser mainly relate to the:

A Level of the photoreceptors.

B Inner nuclear layer.

C Inner plexiform layer.

D Nerve fibre layer.

E Level of the choroid and retinal pigment epithelium.

35 Which of the following statements about the HRT II is true?

A Its main function is in the analysis of the retinal nerve fibre layer 15° temporal to the macula.

B Its main function is in the analysis of the optic nerve head.

C It can be used in the analysis of macular pathologies such as holes.

D The resolution of this instrument is poor because of the low number of pixels.

E The HRT II does not allow accurate quantitative analysis of the optic nerve head.

36 Retinal laser polarimetry can be used to detect early glaucomatous changes in which retinal area or feature?

A The optic nerve head.

B The lamina cribrosa.

C The retinal nerve fibre layer.

D The small blood vessels at the optic nerve head.

E The circle of Zinn.

Section 3
VISUAL FIELDS

A Glossary of Terms used in Perimetry

Full threshold
Stimuli are presented at a level at which the viewer is just able to perceive them. The stimulus brightness is usually specified in decibel units (dB) or as a log unit. The two are related by a factor of 10, 1 log unit equals 10dB.

Suprathreshold
Stimuli are presented at a brightness level above threshold by a specified amount.

Algorithm
In a generic sense, this term may be applied to any set of rules that outlines a sequence of actions undertaken to solve a problem. The rules are precise and so may be carried out automatically. In field screening, the algorithm normally describes the settings a machine will operate in terms of stimulus brightness and location to establish sensitivity data for specified locations in the visual field.

Up–down staircase thresholding
The method commonly used to establish threshold, whereby perceived stimuli are succeeded at the same location by fainter stimuli, and non-perceived stimuli followed by brighter ones.

Crossing or reversal of threshold
The situation in which a stimulus crosses from seen to unseen or *vice versa*. Typically, a double-crossing technique may be used whereby the stimulus brightness is reduced until no longer seen (first crossing or single reversal) and then increased until seen again (second crossing or double reversal).

A 4-2dB algorithm
A program in which there is a change in stimulus brightness in 4dB steps until the first reversal is achieved and then in 2dB steps until second reversal is reached.

SITA
This stands for the Swedish interactive thresholding algorithm, and is incorporated as an option in Humphrey field analysers, 700 series onwards. It was designed as an attempt to decrease the time taken for a traditional staircase method assessment (a 4-2dB algorithm typically takes 15 minutes) and yet maintain good sensitivity in glaucoma detection. Time is reduced in several ways as the algorithm specifies the appropriate stimulus brightness to be presented at each point, may monitor the time of response to adopt appropriate subsequent presentations and is able to stop once sufficient information has been taken. The presentation of stimuli at levels around that at which 50 per cent are seen greatly reduces the speed of testing. So by better pacing of the test, and the useful interpretation of false positives and false negatives, the SITA appears to correlate well with standard perimetric assessment, but in less time. The reduced timing is likely to help the accuracy of response.

Heijl–Krakau technique
A method of monitoring fixation throughout a field assessment by projecting a stimulus to an assumed location of the blind spot. If fixation is not present, the patient will respond to this stimulus and the machine will note the number of errors. The technique relies on an estimate of the exact location of the optic disc, and is thus open to error.

Gaze-tracking
As opposed to individual blind-spot assessment at specified times during assessment, often primarily at the beginning of the test, gaze tracking allows a continual assessment of fixation throughout by monitoring the relative positions of every stimulus presented.

False negative
Usually used to describe a stimulus presented at a specified increased brightness to a previously seen point that is now not seen. For example, in a FASTPAC screening, a false negative will be recorded when a seen point is then missed when presented at 9dB brighter.

False positive
Typically describes the point at which a patient responds to a stimulus that was not presented. This usually occurs during pauses incorporated into the programme when no stimuli are presented, to allow for some assessment of accuracy of response.

11

Frequency doubling and short-wave perimetry

Robert Cubbidge

New developments

In recent years, visual field testing (perimetry) has become an integral constituent of the eye examination and should be considered as an essential diagnostic tool for the optometrist. In private practice, perimetry is primarily used to screen for glaucoma. Prevalence studies indicate that approximately 50 per cent of the population are unaware that they have chronic primary open-angle glaucoma,[1] which is not surprising considering the asymptomatic nature of the disease. This underlines the importance of the optometrist's role in glaucoma detection as the front line in the prevention of blindness from this disease.

Glaucoma is defined as an optic neuropathy that produces characteristic cupping of the optic nerve head and visual field loss. It is important to note that elevated intraocular pressure has not been included in this definition and should be considered as a risk factor for the development of primary open-angle glaucoma. Indeed, screening for primary open-angle glaucoma using tonometry alone has been reported to produce 12 false positives for every patient with a confirmed diagnosis of glaucoma.[2] Numerous histological studies in both primates and humans have shown that up to 50 per cent of ganglion cells are damaged before a visual field defect becomes manifest.[3] Even after treatment is commenced, damage to the optic nerve often continues, albeit at a slower rate, with the result that the visual field deteriorates (visual field loss progression) and ultimately blindness occurs. Consequently, a number of research groups have been developing novel investigative techniques to detect glaucoma, with

the aim of detecting glaucoma at an earlier stage, so that the numbers of patients who go blind can be reduced. Such developments include structural investigations, imaging the optic nerve using scanning laser technologies and tests of visual function such as perimetry. Moreover, if psychophysical examination of the visual function could identify whether visual function deficits were due to dead ganglion cells or merely damaged ones, neuroprotective drug therapy might offer a significant benefit to glaucoma patients.

Conventional perimetry

Conventional perimetry consists of measuring the subject's sensitivity to white-light stimuli projected against a white background at selected locations in the visual field. Sensitivity may be measured using suprathreshold or full threshold techniques. The full threshold technique is preferable, since it yields more information about the visual field and is particularly suited for statistical analysis and, therefore, for monitoring glaucomatous disease progression. Until recently, however, the full threshold technique was not particularly suited to optometric practice and was confined mainly to the hospital eye service because of the time constraints in a typical optometry clinic. Traditionally, a full threshold visual-field examination would take approximately 50 minutes to complete. In the past few years, sophisticated new threshold algorithms, which are based on knowledge of normal and abnormal visual-field behaviour, have become commercially available (e.g., the SITA algorithms of the Humphrey field analyser or tendency-oriented perimetry with the Octopus perimeters). The substantial

reduction in examination time that these algorithms offer has now made full threshold testing in routine clinical practice a viable and preferable alternative to suprathreshold visual-field examination.

Short wavelength perimetry

Conventional perimetry is thought to be a relatively insensitive detection method for primary open-angle glaucoma because the white stimulus simultaneously stimulates all the visual pathways. The general consensus among histologists and physiologists is that two anatomically and functionally specific pathways segregate and convey visual information from the retina to the lateral geniculate nucleus, namely the parvocellular and magnocellular pathways. The parvocellular, or P-pathway, conveys information on colour, high spatial frequency detection and fine pattern discrimination, whereas the magnocellular, or M-pathway, predominantly contributes to motion, luminance and the detection of coarse patterns.[4,5] There is evidence to support the hypothesis that specific groups of ganglion cells are damaged early in the glaucomatous disease process.[6,7] A stimulus that specifically taps into these pathways should, in theory, permit earlier detection of the disease. This was the original premise behind the development of short-wavelength automated perimetry (SWAP), which specifically investigates the visual pathway sensitive to short-wavelength. The parvocellular pathway responsible for coding blue spectral information contains larger diameter nerve fibres than the parvocellular pathways that mediate red and green chromatic information.[8,9] Two theories attempt to explain this:

- The selective damage theory suggests that the short-wavelength pathway is preferentially damaged early in the glaucomatous disease process because larger nerve fibres are thought to be preferentially damaged.[6,7] Latterly, this hypothesis has been disputed.[10]

- The redundancy theory supports the view that all pathways are equally damaged in the disease process. Visual field losses in SWAP can be explained by the smaller distribution of blue cones in the retina. They constitute between 5 and 10 per cent of the total number of cones.[11] If all cone pathways were equally damaged, the blue response pathway would become adversely affected earlier in the disease process than the other spectral pathways.

SWAP is commercially available on models of the Humphrey visual field analyser (Zeiss Humphrey Systems) and Octopus perimeters (Haag–Streit; *Figure 11.1*), and has demonstrated the ability to detect glaucomatous visual field defects up to 5 years before that found using conventional perimetry.[12]. Visual field progression also precedes that of conventional perimetry by up to 3 years.[13,14] It may also be useful in the investigation of neuro-ophthalmological conditions.[15] SWAP differs from conventional perimetry in that the background is yellow and of higher luminance (to suppress activity in the medium wavelength, long wavelength and rod pathways). The stimulus is larger (Goldmann size V), contains a narrow range of blue wavelengths, and evaluates the short-wavelength pathway sensitivity using a conventional staircase method. The short-wavelength sensitive pathway is only isolated from the other pathways over a range of approximately 15dB,[16] and the low spectral transmission of the stimulus filter gives the procedure a reduced dynamic range in comparison to conventional perimetry, which has a dynamic range approaching 40dB. Consequently, problems may be encountered when evaluating a markedly damaged visual field. In the presence of moderate age-related cataract, absorption of the blue stimulus by the human lens may render examination with SWAP ineffective. The between-subject variability of SWAP is substantially greater than that of conventional perimetry.[17] This results in a wider range of normality for short-wavelength thresholds, which makes statistical separation of normal visual fields from abnormal fields difficult. Research into the development of new statistical procedures to delineate visual field abnormality in SWAP is ongoing. Although SWAP is a

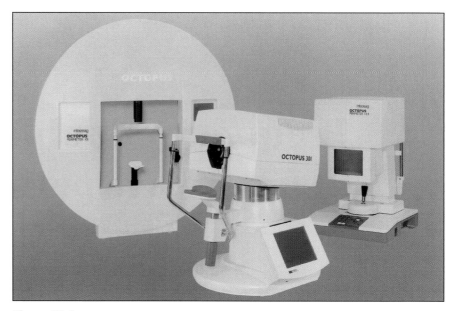

Figure 11.1
The Octopus 301 has an option for blue–yellow screening

useful technique for the evaluation of glaucoma, it still requires further work to make it a viable procedure in the clinical setting.

Frequency doubling technique

More recently, a new instrument has become commercially available, the FDT Visual Field Instrument (Zeiss Humphrey Systems), which purports to detect glaucoma at an earlier stage than conventional perimetry.[18,19] This instrument is based on

the frequency doubling illusion. When a sinusoidal grating that possesses a low spatial frequency (less than 1 cycle per degree) undergoes counterphase flicker at a frequency greater than 15Hz, the spatial frequency of the grating appears to double (i.e., the grating will appear to have twice as many light and dark bars as are physically present. *Figure 11.2* represents the target that the patient sees. This illusion is known as the frequency doubling illusion. The illusion is thought to be mediated by a subset of retinal ganglion cells, called M(y) cells, in the magnocellular pathway. M(y)

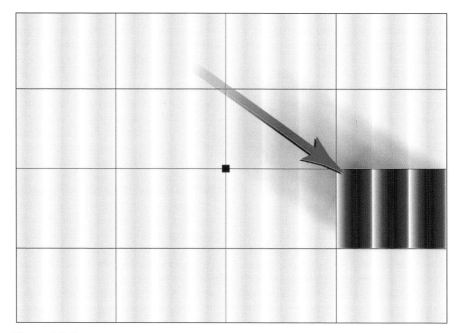

Figure 11.2
Segmental presentation of the frequency doubling sine-wave target

cells constitute between 5 and 25 per cent of the total number of magnocellular nerve fibres,[20] and tend to have the greatest diameter of the retinal ganglion cells. Similarly to SWAP, the ability of the frequency doubling technique (FDT) to detect glaucoma at an earlier stage than conventional perimetry can be explained by both the selective damage and redundancy theories.

The instrument

The instrument has a smaller footprint than a perimeter and principally consists of a backlit liquid-crystal display at the back of the instrument, with a viewing eccentricity of 40°, which is projected to infinity by means of a viewing lens at the front of the instrument. The machine is operated by a simple graphic display located on the front of the instrument (*Figure 11.3*). The frequency doubling stimulus is generated using a sinusoidal grating with a spatial frequency of 0.25 cycles per degree, undergoing a counterphase flicker of 25Hz, presented for a maximum of 720ms.[21]

Testing can be carried out under normal room illumination. An objective lens at the front of the instrument negates the need for a near-refractive correction to be used and the patient can undergo the test with their own single vision-distance correction, or with multifocal spectacles. Since the stimulus is a low spatial frequency sinusoidal grating, it should be relatively insensitive to the influence of optical defocus. The manufacturers suggest that a refractive correction is not necessary up to 7D. However, to date, no clinical studies have investigated the influence of optical defocus on FDT thresholds, which suggests that it is prudent to employ a distance refractive correction wherever it is possible. During the test, patients have to press a response button whenever they detect the presence of flickering dark and light vertical bars in the visual field. The operator display shows a progress indicator, test grid and reliability criteria (fixation losses, false-positive and -negative responses), which enable the examiner to monitor the test effectively (*Figure 11.4a*). Once the test is completed, the results can be printed for each eye (*Figure 11.4b*). A typical 17-stimulus location, full threshold C-20 program takes approximately four and a half minutes to complete, whereas a suprathreshold examination takes approximately a minute. The printout is via a thermal printer incorporated into the machine and can be interpreted in a similar way to full threshold perimetry. The provision of FDT data from the normal population within the machine software enables statistical interpretation of the results to be provided. Global indices for mean deviation (MD) and pattern standard deviation (PSD) give an indication of the magnitude of diffuse and focal loss in the visual field, respectively. Probability analysis provides information on the spatial location of visual field loss. Defects are shown as varying shades of grey to indicate 'mild relative loss', 'moderate relative loss' and 'severe loss'. According to the user manual the FDT screening C-20-1 and C-20-5 programs employ different baseline normal contrast levels. As a result, they also differ in how they label individual test locations as defective. With the C-20-1 test, points are initially labelled 'mild relative loss' when they reach the $P < 1$ per cent probability significance level (which means that the sensitivity value is found in less than 1 per cent of the normal population). With the C-20-5 test, points are initially labelled when they reach the $P < 5$ per cent probability significance level. Therefore, there is a greater chance that any test location may be deemed as being outside normal limits and, consequently, the C-20-5 test is slightly more sensitive, readily identifying more extensive visual deficits.

Validation of FDT in glaucoma

The majority of research investigations with FDT concentrated on its ability to detect the known visual field loss found using conventional full threshold perimetry. FDT compares favourably in its ability to separate patients with glaucomatous visual field loss, ranging from early to severe found with conventional perimetry, from normal subjects and demonstrates high sensitivity.[22,23] The FDT MD and PSD global indices exhibit a strong correlation with the MD and PSD global indices of the Humphrey field analyser.[24,25] FDT is also reported to exhibit significant correlation with areas of damage on HFA.[24] The FDT visual field instrument used in threshold mode shows a greater ability to detect glaucomatous defects than when used in screening mode.[26] Investigations of test–retest variability in glaucoma have shown that FDT variability does not increase as much with defect severity as it does with conventional perimetry. The

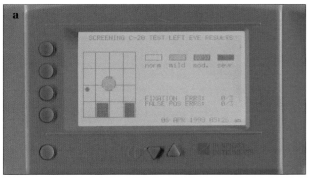

Figure 11.3
The Zeiss Humphrey FDT visual field instrument

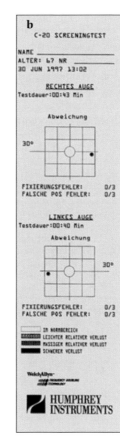

Figure 11.4
(a) The data screen and (b) the printout for the FDT

effects of eccentricity on variability are also less pronounced with FDT than with conventional perimetry. FDT should be able to monitor disease progression effectively.[19]

A number of investigators have developed algorithms for FDT that score the visual loss by location and severity, in an effort to reach a diagnosis on the extent of glaucomatous visual loss.[27,28] One such algorithm[27] weighted FDT deficits according to location and severity of loss on a scale of 0 (no deficit) to 87 (maximum deficit). Results using this algorithm in 137 glaucoma patients indicated that a frequency doubling score of 2 or greater identified more than 80 per cent of individuals with glaucoma, while maintaining specificity greater than 90 per cent. The test was 96 per cent sensitive at identifying patients with moderate or severe visual field loss. This research group concluded that a patient's results may be considered abnormal if he or she possessed deficits in the central five locations. In addition, two or more mild deficits or one moderate or severe deficit in the outer 12 points also qualified as an abnormal test.

A preliminary study reported FDT abnormalities in ocular hypertensive (OHT) patients (46 per cent of 136 patients).[29] SWAP can identify approximately 20 per cent of OHT,[30] so it would appear that FDT may be more effective at detecting glaucomatous damage at an earlier stage than both SWAP and conventional perimetry. To date all of the above studies with FDT have been confined to relatively small sample sizes. The true effectiveness of FDT will only be borne out when large-scale clinical trials are undertaken.

Other clinical applications of FDT

As with perimetry, the use of FDT does not just have to be confined to the investigation of glaucoma. The detection of visual field defects in neuro-ophthalmological conditions is also of importance. In a study of 14 patients with resolved optic neuritis,[31] conventional full threshold perimetry demonstrated visual field depression towards the fovea, whereas FDT demonstrated a general depression and mid-peripheral deficits in function. This suggests that patients with resolved optic neuritis exhibit a loss in M-cell function in the extrafoveal area. A recent report evaluated 103 patients with typical neuro-ophthalmic conditions.[32] These patients had existing visual field defects with conventional perimetry, consistent with these conditions. FDT using the screening program was unable to categorise accurately hemianopic and quadrantanopic defects. However, the study concluded that FDT is a sensitive tool for the rapid detection of neuro-ophthalmic field defects and a useful tool when deciding which patients need further examination using full threshold visual field testing. This suggests that for the investigation of neuro-ophthalmic disorders, FDT is not a substitute for conventional perimetry.

FDT has also been identified as being of potential use for the evaluation of patients with specific reading difficulties (dyslexia). Abnormalities in the magnocellular pathway have been implicated in this condition. Pammer and Wheatley[33] compared the ability to detect the frequency doubling illusion using FDT in a small sample of 21 dyslexic readers with 19 normal controls. The dyslexic group demonstrated a lower sensitivity to the frequency doubling illusion than the normal group. These findings suggest that it may be possible to use FDT to aid in the identification of patients with specific learning difficulties.

Is FDT a replacement for conventional perimetry?

Standard perimetry using a white background and white stimuli is still regarded as the 'gold standard' examination in ophthalmology for the detection and monitoring of chronic primary open-angle glaucoma. The influence of decreased retinal illumination has been shown to reduce significantly the sensitivity to a frequency doubling stimulus.[34] Age-related cataract, however, does not merely reduce retinal illumination, but increases light scatter and impairs contrast sensitivity to low spatial frequencies. As yet there are no published reports of the influence of cataract on FDT. FDT has been validated for the investigation of glaucoma in cases where this is the only underlying condition. The instrument is particularly well suited to non-clinical environments, such as in domiciliary practice, and has an obvious role as a screening tool. However, glaucoma and cataract often coexist and therefore, until the influence of cataract and other variables known to influence the visual field are investigated with FDT, this technique should be regarded as a valuable companion to perimetry, but not as a substitute for it.

References

1 Tielsch JM, Sommer A, Katz J, Royall RM, Quigley HA and Javitt J (1991). Racial variations in the prevalence of primary open-angle glaucoma: the Baltimore Eye Survey. *J Am Med Assoc.* **266**, 369–374.

2 Leibowitz HM, Kruger DE, Mander LR *et al.* (1990). The Framlington eye study monograph: an ophthalmological and epidemiological study of cataract, glaucoma, diabetic retinopathy, macular degeneration, and visual acuity in a general population of 2631 adults, 1973–1975. *Surv Ophthalmol.* **24**(Suppl), 335–810.

3 Sommer A, Katz J, Quigley HA, Miller NR, Robin AL, Richer RC and Witt KA (1991). Clinically detectable nerve fiber atrophy precedes the onset of glaucomatous field loss. *Arch Ophthalmol.* **109**, 77–83.

4 Merigan WH and Maunsell JHR (1990). Macaque vision after magnocellular lateral geniculate lesions. *Vis Neurosci.* **5**, 347–352.

5 Merigan WH, Katz LM and Maunsell JHR (1991). The effects of parvocellular lateral geniculate lesions on the acuity and contrast sensitivity of macaque monkeys. *J Neurosci.* **11**, 994–1001.

6 Quigley HA, Sanchez RM, Dunkelberger GR, L'Hernault NL and Baginski TA (1987). Chronic glaucoma selectively damages large optic nerve fibers. *Invest Ophthalmol Vis Sci.* **28**, 913–920.

7 Quigley HA, Dunkelberger GR and Green WR (1988). Chronic human glaucoma causing selectively greater loss of large optic nerve fibers. *Ophthalmology* **95**, 357–363.

8 de Monasterio FM (1978). Properties of concentrically organised X and Y ganglion cells of the macaque retina. *J Neurophysiol.* **41**, 1394–1417.

9 Dacey DM (1993). Morphology of a small-field bistratified ganglion cell type in macaque and human retina. *Vis Neurosci.* **10**, 1081–1098.

10 Morgan JE (1994). Selective cell death in glaucoma: does it really occur? *Br J Ophthalmol.* **78**, 875–880.

11 Curcio CA, Allen KA, Sloan KR *et al.* (1991). Distribution and morphology of human cone photoreceptors stained with anti-blue opsin. *J Comp Neurol.* **312**, 610–624.

12 Johnson CA, Adams AJ, Casson EJ and Brandt JD (1993). Blue-on-yellow perimetry can predict the development of glaucomatous visual field loss. *Arch Ophthalmol.* **111**, 645–650.

13 Johnson CA, Adams AJ, Casson EJ and Brandt JD (1993). Progression of early glaucomatous visual field loss for blue-on-yellow and standard white-on-white automated perimetry. *Arch Ophthalmol.* **111**, 651–656.

14 Sample PA and Weinreb RN (1992). Progressive color visual field loss in glaucoma. *Invest Ophthalmol Vis Sci.* **33**, 2068–2071.

15 Keltner JL and Johnson CA (1995). Short-wavelength automated perimetry in neuro-ophthalmologic disorders. *Arch Ophthalmol.* **113**, 475–481.

16 Cubbidge RP and Wild JM (2001). The influences of stimulus wavelengths and eccentricity on short-wavelength pathway isolation in automated perimetry. *Ophthalmic Physiol Opt.* **21**, 1–8.

17 Wild JM, Cubbidge RP, Pacey IE and Robinson R (1998). Statistical aspects of the normal visual field derived by short-wavelength automated perimetry. *Invest Ophthalmol Vis Sci.* **39**, 54–63.

18 Johnson CA, Cioffi GA and Van Buskirk EM (1999). Evaluation of two screening tests for frequency doubling technology perimetry. In *Perimetry Update 1998/1999*, p. 103–109, Eds Mills RP and Wall M (Amsterdam: Kugler Publications).

19 Chauhan BC and Johnson CA (1999). Test–retest variability of frequency-doubling perimetry and conventional perimetry in glaucoma patients and normal subjects. *Invest Ophthalmol Vis Sci.* **40**, 648–656.

20 Maddess T, James AC, Goldberg I, Wine S and Dobinson J (2000). A spatial frequency doubling illusion based pattern electroretinogram for glaucoma. *Invest Ophthalmol Vis Sci.* **41**, 3818–3826.

21 Spry PGD, Gibbs ML, Johnson CA and Howard DL (2000). Frequency doubling perimetry using a liquid crystal display. *Am J Ophthalmol.* **131**, 332–338.

22 Johnson CA and Samuels SJ (1997). Screening for glaucomatous visual field loss with frequency-doubling perimetry. *Invest Ophthalmol Vis Sci.* **38**, 413–425.

23 Cello KE, Nelson-Quigg JM and Johnson CA (2000). Frequency doubling technology perimetry for detection of glaucomatous visual field loss. *Am J Ophthalmol.* **129**, 314–322.

24 Serguhn S and Speigel D (2001). Comparison of frequency doubling perimetry and standard achromatic computerized perimetry in patients with glaucoma. *Graefe's Arch Clin Exp Ophthalmol.* **239**, 351–355.

25 Sponsel WE, Arango S, Trigo Y and Mensah J (1998). Clinical classification of glaucomatous visual field loss by frequency doubling perimetry. *Am J Ophthalmol.* **125**, 830–836.

26 Burnstein Y, Ellish NJ, Magbalon M and Higginbotham EJ (2000). Comparison of frequency doubling perimetry with Humphrey visual field analysis in a glaucoma practice. *Am J Ophthalmol.* **129**, 328–333.

27 Patel SC, Friedman DS, Varadkar P and Robin AL (1999). Algorithm for interpreting the results of frequency doubling perimetry. *Am J Ophthalmol.* **129**, 323–327.

28 Trible JR, Schultz RO, Robinson JC and Rothe TL (2000). Accuracy of glaucoma detection with frequency-doubling perimetry. *Am J Ophthalmol.* **129**, 740–745.

29 Sample PA, Bosworth CF, Blumenthal EZ, Girkin C and Weinreb RN (2000). Visual function-specific perimetry for indirect comparison of different ganglion cell populations in glaucoma. *Invest Ophthalmol Vis Sci.* **41**, 1783–1790.

30 Johnson CA, Brandt JD, Khong AM and Adams AJ (1995). Short-wavelength automated perimetry in low-, medium-, and high-risk ocular hypertensive eyes. *Arch Ophthalmol.* **113**, 70–76.

31 Fujimoto N and Adachi-Usami E (2000), Frequency doubling perimetry in resolved optic neuritis. *Invest Ophthalmol Vis Sci.* **41**, 2558–2560.

32 Thomas D, Thomas R, Muliyil JP and George R (2001). Role of frequency doubling perimetry in detecting neuro-ophthalmic visual field defects. *Am J Ophthalmol.* **131**, 734–741.

33 Pammer K and Wheatley C (2001). Isolating the M(y)-cell response in dyslexia using the spatial frequency doubling illusion. *Vision Res.* **41**, 2139–2147.

34 Kogure S, Membrey WL, Fitzke FW and Tsukahara S (2000). Effect of decreased retinal illumination on frequency doubling technology. *Jpn J Ophthalmol.* **44**, 489–493.

12
Visual field defects caused by neurological disease

Geoff Roberson

Neurological lesions that produce visual field defects might be defined as those that affect the intracranial visual pathway (i.e., the pathway from the intracranial part of the optic nerve back to the visual cortex). However, it may be more practical to include the whole of the optic nerve within the definition. Disorders that affect the visual pathway produce characteristic visual loss, which together with the associated neurological deficits, can help identify the location of the problem.

The analysis of visual field defects has an anatomical basis and a topographical classification. A basic working knowledge of the anatomy of the visual pathway is vital to the task of visual field analysis. The major elements that make up the pathway, and particularly the distribution of nerve fibres within them, are the link between the defects you have plotted and your assessment of the position of the lesion producing them.

Anatomy

The visual pathway starts at the receptors in the retina and finishes at the neural cells in the visual cortex. It forms an integral part of the central nervous system (CNS) and, as such, has features that are common to all CNS structures.

The extraocular part of the pathway is made up of a number of distinct and well-recognised anatomical components (*Figure 12.1*). They are the:

*   optic nerve;
*   optic chiasma;
*   optic tract;
*   lateral geniculate nucleus (or body);
*   optic radiations;
*   visual (or striate) cortex;

Optic nerve

The optic nerve is approximately 50mm long and 3mm in diameter. The intraorbital portion is about 30mm long and the intracranial portion of the nerve is about 10mm long. The nerve is made up of about one million fibres, which are divided into approximately 1000 bundles. The intraorbital portion of the nerve is more or less oval in section and, as the distance from the globe to the back of the orbit is only about 18–20mm, it curves in an S shape to pass through the optic canal in the sphenoid bone. The extra length and slight zigzag in the nerve allows for flexing during ocular movements.

In the main the fibres of the optic nerve are afferent visual fibres that comprise the myelinated axons of retinal ganglion cells. There are, however, some afferent pupillary fibres and some efferent fibres, the function of which is not well understood. The organisation of fibres within the optic nerve initially follows the arrangement of nerve fibres at the optic nerve head with the macular fibres from the papillomacular bundle on the lateral or temporal aspect of the nerve (*Figure 12.2*). About one-third of the way along the nerve, at the point where the central retinal artery and vein

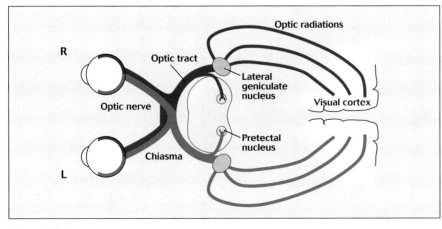

Figure 12.1
Main components of the visual pathway

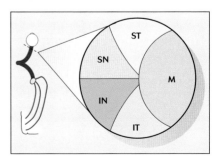

Figure 12.2
Cross-section of the anterior optic nerve showing the distribution of nerve fibres (IN, inferonasal; IT, inferotemporal; M, macular; SN, superonasal; ST, superotemporal)

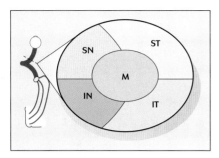

Figure 12.3
Cross-section of the posterior optic nerve showing the distribution of nerve fibres

move into the nerve, the fibres are reorganised so that the macular fibres move into a central position, with the peripheral fibres arranged in the same orientation to the portion of retina where they originated (*Figure 12.3*).

Chiasma
At the chiasma, which is approximately 12mm wide by 8mm deep, the two optic nerves meet and some fibres cross over to the other side of the pathway. The crossing of just over half of the nerve fibres enables the stimulation of corresponding points in the visual field of the two eyes to send signals to the same half of the visual cortex. This arrangement is common in animals with frontward facing eyes, such as cats and primates, and allows binocular vision with the perception of stereopsis. In animals with little overlap of the monocular visual fields, such as rodents, nearly all the fibres (perhaps 90–95 per cent) cross.

At the chiasma, fibres that originate in the temporal retina, relating to the nasal visual field, remain at the outside of the pathway, while those that originate in the nasal retina, relating to the temporal visual field, cross over or decussate. The number of decussating fibres is greater than the number of non-decussating fibres, which reflects the larger peripheral temporal field.

Fibres from the nasal half of the macula also decussate in the same way as the peripheral fibres. The nerve fibres in the chiasma are arranged in a recognisable format and retain groupings based on the area of the retina where they originated (*Figure 12.4*). Fibres that originate from the inferior nasal part of the retina and decussate in the more anterior portion of the chiasma tend to loop slightly forward into the posterior part of the contralateral optic nerve. This forward looping is called the anterior knee or loop of Willebrand. Fibres that pass more posteriorly through the chiasma tend to loop posteriorly into the ipsilateral optic tract.

A number of important structures that do not form part of the visual pathway are situated near to the chiasma. Among these are a number of important blood vessels (see below) and the pituitary gland in its bony fossa. The length of the intracranial optic nerves dictates the position of the optic chiasma in relation to the pituitary fossa. In most case it is underneath and slightly anterior to the chiasma. In about 10 per cent of cases it is further forwards, and in about 10 per cent it is further back.

Optic tract
The optic tract consists of nerve fibres from one-half of the visual field only, but still retain a recognisable organisation, with the macular fibres uppermost, the upper peripheral fibres on the inferior medial aspect and the lower peripheral fibres occupying the inferior lateral aspect (*Figure 12.5*). The optic tract bends the pathway around the brainstem. About 10 per cent of the fibres leave each half of the visual pathway at the posterior end of the optic tract on the medial side (see *Figure 12.1*). These are predominantly fibres that pass to the pretectal nucleus in the brain stem and are associated with the pupillary light reflex. The remainder of the optic tract ends at the lateral geniculate nucleus.

Lateral geniculate nucleus
The lateral geniculate nucleus (LGN), sometimes called the lateral geniculate body, lies on the posterolateral aspect of the brain stem and next to the thalamus. It is generally thought of as a relay station at which nerve fibres that originate from the retinal ganglion cells synapse with fibres that originate from cells in the visual cortex, although there is evidence that some degree of low-level visual processing does go on within it. It has a complex six-layered structure that contains nerve fibres and cell nuclei (*Figure 12.6*).

Fibres from the two eyes are clearly segregated in the LGN. Those that passed through the chiasma uncrossed, that is from the temporal retina on the same side, go to layers 2, 3 and 5, and the fibres from the nasal retina, which have crossed at the chiasma, go to layers 1, 4 and 6.

Each LGN neurone makes contact with a similar number of retinal nerve fibres, always from the same eye, and receives inputs from retinal cells adjacent to each other in a circular pattern. The LGN's prime function is to sort out fibres that have become mixed up in the optic tract so that there is almost perfect 'point-to-point' representation of the retina in the LGN, albeit in adjacent layers.

Optic radiations
The optic radiations continue the visual pathway from the LGN to its end at the neurones of the visual cortex. The fibres leave from the lateral aspect of the LGN and spread out in a fan formation, still retaining a retinotopic projection (*Figure 12.7*). The upper fibres of the optic radiations from the superior peripheral retina move around the lateral ventricle and steadily back to the visual cortex, ending in the area above the calcarine fissure. The fibres from the lower peripheral retina pass underneath and around the bottom of the lateral ventricle, looping backwards and

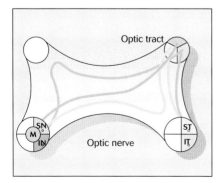

Figure 12.4
General arrangement of fibres at the chiasma. The inferior nasal fibres pass into the contralateral nerve

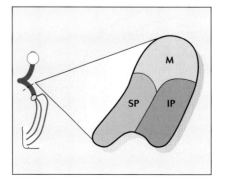

Figure 12.5
Cross-section of the optic tract showing the distribution of nerve fibres. (IP, inferior periphery; SP, superior periphery)

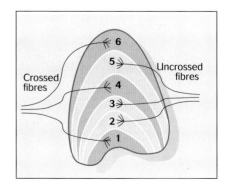

Figure 12.6
Six-layered structure of lateral geniculate nucleus showing the destination of crossed and uncrossed fibres

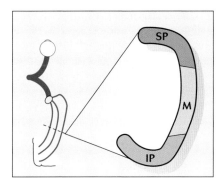

Figure 12.7
Cross-section of the optic radiations showing the distribution of nerve fibres

ending in the area of the visual cortex below the calcarine fissure. The fibres from the macula pass to the cortex in between the upper and lower peripheral fibres.

Visual cortex

Visual information is processed in the cortex in three main areas. The primary visual cortex is Brodmann's area 17 with two secondary areas, Brodmann's areas 18 and 19. The visual cortex, area 17, is situated on the medial aspect of the occipital lobe.

The visual cortex retains the retinotopic organisation seen in the more anterior parts of the pathway. The peripheral parts of the retina are represented in the more anterior parts of area 17, with the upper and lower retina represented either side of the calcarine fissure (*Figure 12.8*). The macular area is represented by a larger portion of the visual cortex occupying the posterior part of area 17 and extending around the posterior pole slightly; again the upper and lower fibres are separated by the calcarine fissure.

In the visual cortex corresponding retinal points finally meet and become perfectly matched by location. The point-to-point relationship between retinal receptors and cortical cells is also maintained. Most corti-

cal cells (about 70 per cent) have directional sensitivity and are also sensitive to a variety of other characteristics, only responding to a particular stimulus (e.g., light or dark edges). Cells in the visual cortex are organised into functional groups, each with a specialised purpose; some only respond to stimuli orientated in one particular direction, others to a specific colour response.

There is some evidence of cross linking of receptive fields in the right and left halves of the visual cortex, either directly or indirectly through the corpus callosum, which might help explain the clinical phenomenon of macular sparing (see below).

Blood supply

An understanding of the blood supply to the visual pathway is important for the clinician. Many of the major blood vessels that supply the visual pathway are physically close to the individual components of the pathway. Thus, not only may clinically significant problems arise if the blood supply is interrupted or disturbed, but a physical abnormality of the blood vessel itself can also cause direct mechanical effects on the pathway.

The blood supply to the visual pathway is derived from three major intracranial vessels, the two internal carotid arteries and the basilar artery, which comes up the front of the brainstem from an anastomosis of the two vertebral arteries. These three vessels are joined by a system of smaller vessels into a complete circuit of interconnecting arteries called the Circle of Willis (*Figure 12.9*). The more anterior parts of the Circle of Willis are very closely situated to the optic chiasma.

The LGN is supplied by branches of the anterior choroidal and posterior cerebral arteries. The anterior parts of the optic radiations are supplied by branches of the anterior choroidal artery and the more posterior parts are supplied by a long branch of the middle cerebral artery, called the deep optic artery.

The visual cortex is supplied mainly by the calcarine artery, which is a branch of the posterior cerebral artery. Some supply is also derived from the middle cerebral artery, which has an anastomosis with the posterior cerebral artery (*Figure 12.10*). This 'dual' blood supply may help to maintain arterial circulation to the visual cortex in the event of a disruption to the supply from one of the vessels, and is also thought to be another possible explanation for macular sparing.

Visual field analysis

Before deciding that a visual field defect results from a neurological lesion, all of the available clinical information must be considered. The importance and relevance of signs, symptoms, history and other findings may be key to the correct interpretation of visual field defects. As in the case of glaucoma, for which the appearance of the optic discs, intraocular pressure and family history are taken into consideration when deciding if field defects are glaucomatous, the presence or absence of other factors may be the key to deciding if a defect is genuinely caused by a neurological abnormality or not. Many non-neurological abnormalities, such as tilted discs, can give rise to 'pseudo' neurological field defects.

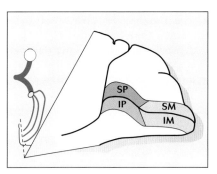

Figure 12.8
Visual cortex showing the general organisation of nerve fibres (IM, inferior macular; SM, superior macular)

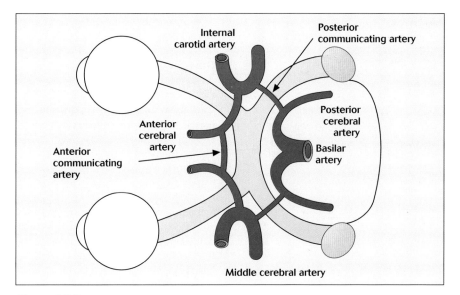

Figure 12.9
Blood vessels of the Circle of Willis seen from underneath

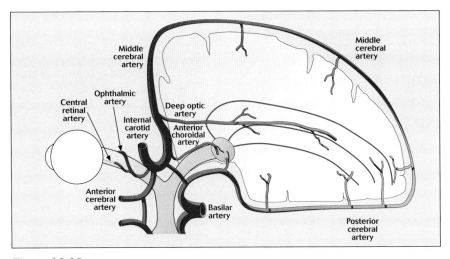

Figure 12.10
Vascular supply to the visual pathway

Ultimately, the diagnosis must be made by a neuro-ophthalmologist or a neurologist with the aid of sophisticated, modern neuro-imaging techniques, but it is important that the correct degree of urgency is attached to the initial referral.

The plots
The results recorded may show genuine abnormalities or artefacts. A stimulus point seen at 1 or 2 decibels below the retinal threshold would not, in normal circumstances, be considered significant. However, a small group of stimuli that are missed close to threshold might, in fact, signify a defect. In comparison, one isolated point seen at a markedly lower setting than all others is probably not a defect despite its low sensitivity, but an anatomical feature such as a blood vessel (an angioscotoma).

Consideration of a specific defect in the field plot should look at four separate components:

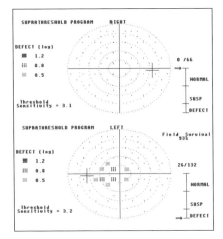

Figure 12.11
Centro-caecal defect caused by an optic nerve lesion

- *Shape*. The shape of the field defect plotted is very important, as it may be directly related to anatomy and physiology. In the case of neurological lesions a comparison of the shape of both defects is an element in judging congruity (see below).
- *Size*. The similarity of size and shape is helpful in neurological defects. Field defects of different size, even if they are the same shape, do not indicate congruity. Size is also important when considering the extent of the lesion and its age.
- *Margins*. The steepness of the margins of a defect gives specific information primarily about the type of causative lesion. Shallow margins suggest a slowly developing lesion, such as a space-occupying lesion, while steep margins are more likely to be found with a vascular accident.
- *Depth*. Deep, almost absolute, scotomata are usually associated with vascular accidents.

Other findings
A number of other clinical findings may need to be taken into account in the analysis of neurological defects, and many of the following are dealt with in detail below:
- symptoms and history;
- visual acuity (VA);
- ophthalmoscopy;
- pupil responses;
- colour vision.
Symptoms of diagnostic value, if present, are either related to the actual field loss, such as mobility problems, clumsiness and positive scotomata, or unrelated, such as headaches. Vascular accidents are of rapid onset and, therefore, the field defects are more likely to be noticeable to the patient, while slowly developing mass lesions are not.

History may indicate the time of onset and duration of a dramatic event like a vascular accident, although history may be so vague as to be of little diagnostic value. Personal history, such as stroke or cranial trauma, may also be directly relevant to findings.

Topographical classification

The topographical classification simply subdivides the extraocular visual pathway into three general sections:
- pre-chiasmal;
- chiasmal;
- post-chiasmal.
The predictable grouping and organisation of the visual pathway nerve fibres, which steadily increases as the pathway moves towards the visual cortex, is helpful for analysis.

Pre-chiasmal
Defects in this category are essentially caused by optic nerve lesions, and are likely to show all or some of the following characteristics:
- *One eye only*. This is true of almost all defects. Classically, a central or centro-caecal defect is found (*Figure 12.11*). A lesion near the posterior end of the optic nerve may produce a defect in both eyes, when anterior looping nasal fibres from the contralateral nerve become affected. In this case a significant defect is present on the affected side, combined with an upper temporal crescent-shaped defect in the periphery on the other side; the so-called 'junction' defect.
- *Reduced VA*. This is likely, as macular fibres are much more susceptible to damage because of their fineness and thinner sheathing.
- *Afferent pupil defect*. A relative afferent pupil defect (RAPD) is highly likely because any lesion serious enough to produce a field defect will affect the pupillary fibres.
- *Colour vision defect*. This is likely to be present if there is reduced VA.
- *Normal ophthalmoscopy*. Retrobulbar optic nerve lesions won't produce any fundus changes. Optic atrophy may give rise to an abnormal disc appearance on ophthalmoscopy. However, the onset of optic atrophy will not occur for many weeks after the initial symptoms.
Defects may be caused by meningiomas (of the optic nerve sheath or the sphenoid bone), arise as a result of previous radiation therapy in the region, or (less commonly) as a result of intrinsic disease such as demyelination.

Chiasmal

The chiasmal part of the pathway is much more likely to be affected by abnormalities than any other pathway, and the vast majority are compressive lesions. Defects caused by lesions that affect the chiasma show the following general characteristics:

- *In both eyes*. As fibres from both eyes are now present in the pathway, there must be a defect of some sort present in both eyes. The 'junction' defect described above is sometimes classified as a chiasmal defect.
- *Heteronymous*. Present in both eyes, but essentially on opposite sides of the field (i.e., both nasal halves, or both temporal halves of the field).
- *Midline not respected*. As a result of the juxtaposition of nasal and temporal fibres, eventually a lesion will have some influence on all the fibres from both of the eyes. Field defects therefore progress from one side to the other across the midline. Chiasmal defects cannot be true hemianopias.

The most common chiasmal lesion is the pituitary tumour. As the chiasma is affected by pressure from underneath, the nasal fibres from each eye are primarily affected and a temporal defect is found in both eyes, the classic bitemporal hemianopia (*Figure 12.12*). The hemianopia is often asymmetrical and may be associated with significant visual loss in one eye from involvement of an optic nerve. In most cases the field defect starts in the upper temporal regions and spreads to the lower temporal quadrants, lower nasal quadrants and eventually the whole field is lost. Patients rarely notice any direct symptoms, but may have general complaints about navigation or problems driving. Pituitary tumours are large by the time they affect

the chiasma, and around two-thirds of them are associated with a variety of hormonal abnormalities including diabetes.

Post-chiasmal

Post-chiasmal neurological lesions affecting the visual pathway may produce defects that are hemianopic, quadrantic, or scotomata. They show the following characteristics:

- *In both eyes*. The defect is present in both eyes.
- *Homonymous*. The defect is always on the same side in both eyes (i.e., the temporal field of the right eye and the nasal field of the left eye).
- *Midline respected*. Defects, if they are big enough, always show perfect demarcation down the vertical midline and not cross over.

Post-chiasmal lesions may produce effects such as reduced VA if macular fibres are affected, and a pupil defect if the lesion is in the optic tract, but not necessarily. It is useful to be able to subdivide post-chiasmal lesions. Although this is more difficult to do, some characteristics of the visual field defect and other clinical findings may help.

Pre lateral geniculate nucleus
- *Incongruous*. The defects are not similar in size and/or shape (*Figure 12.13*).
- *Possible macular splitting*. The VA may be reduced because the macular fibres are affected.
- *Pupil anomalies*. If the lesion is in the tract, then the pupillary fibres may be affected and there will be a RAPD in the contralateral eye because of the greater number of crossed fibres.
- *Possible optic atrophy*. This is likely to take the form of localised rather than general atrophy of the optic disc. Its presence

indicates a slow growing compressive lesion. Isolated optic tract lesions are rare and usually caused by a space-occupying lesion such as a glioma. Occasionally, defects result from demyelination or vascular abnormalities.

Post lateral geniculate nucleus
- *Increasing congruity*.
- *Increasing macula sparing*.
- *Pupil reactions normal*. Even in the presence of cortical blindness.
- *No optic atrophy*.

The optic radiations pass through the parietal and temporal lobes of the cortex, and patients with lesions in these regions tend to present with other neurological deficits that overshadow their visual loss. These include:

- *Parietal lobe*. Agnosia (the loss of the ability to recognise visually), agraphia (the inability to interpret writing), acalculia (the inability to do arithmetic), right and left confusion.
- *Temporal lobe*. Aphasic motor abnormalities (the muscular inability to form words), epilepsy (uncinate seizures characterised by unusual tastes and smells), déjà-vu; hallucinations.

As the superior peripheral fibres are found in the parietal lobe, the visual field defects tend to be found in the lower half, predominantly quadrantic. The inferior peripheral fibres pass through the temporal lobe and the visual field defects are therefore found in the superior half of the field (*Figure 12.14*). This type of defect is described by some authors as a 'pie in the sky' defect.

Parietal lobe lesions may also be characterised by visual neglect, a condition in which if two simultaneous stimuli are presented in the contralateral visual field, only one is seen at a time.

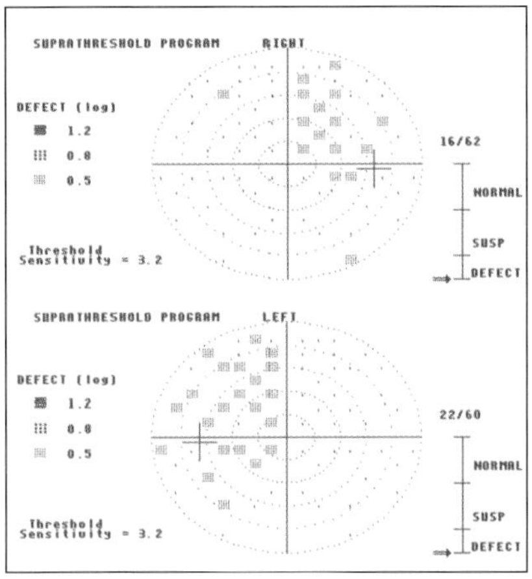

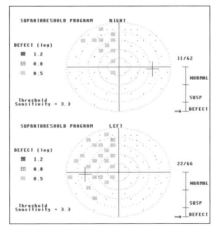

Figure 12.12
Typical bitemporal defect caused by a pituitary tumour at the chiasma

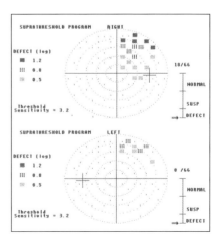

Figure 12.13
Incongruous defect caused by a right optic tract lesion

Figure 12.14
So-called pie in the sky defect caused by a temporal lobe lesion that affects the left optic radiations

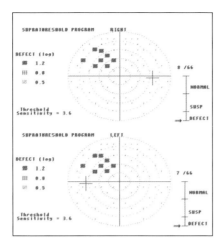

Figure 12.15
Deep congruous homonymous defect caused by a vascular accident in the right occipital cortex

Visual cortex

Lesions in the visual cortex are characterised by:

- *Complete congruity*. Field defects, be they scotomata or hemianopias, show complete congruity because of the exact matching of corresponding retinal points in the visual cortex (*Figure 12.15*).
- *Macular sparing*. The preservation of a small (2–3°) field around the macula. Patients will have normal acuity.

There are a number of possible explanations as to why the clinical phenomenon of macular sparing is found. The dual blood supply to the occipital cortex already mentioned is likely to be a preserving factor. Also, the cross-linking of the right and left halves of the visual cortex and the sheer size of the macular representation in the visual cortex mean that a huge amount of cortex needs to be destroyed before macular function ceases. Some authors have also speculated that psychological factors associated with maintaining fixation are involved.

It is likely that a combination of these mechanisms is responsible for macular sparing found in an individual patient. Most lesions that affect the visual cortex are vascular and present as characteristic visual field loss without other neurological signs.

Conclusion

Neurological visual field defects can be analysed by the application of a simple knowledge of the anatomy of the visual pathway. A range of characteristic visual field defects, together with other clinical findings and specific signs and symptoms, can be used to target the location of the underlying disease process. Although final diagnosis must rest on the use of neuroimaging technology, a confident preliminary identification of neurological lesions that cause visual field defects, leading to an appropriate referral process, can be initiated by optometrists using visual field screeners in their own practice.

13
Visual fields in glaucoma

Chris Steele

Visual field analysis gives essential information about the diagnosis and progress of many diseases that can result in blindness. Fields are a measure of visual function and defects are a measure of functional loss. Of all the conditions that give rise to visual field loss, glaucoma is the most common.

Glaucoma is a group of diseases that share an acquired optic neuropathy, characterised by excavation (cupping) of the optic nerve head and thinning of the neuroretinal rim. When the loss of nerve tissue is significant, patients develop optic nerve-related visual field loss. Glaucoma is often, but not always, associated with a raised intraocular pressure (IOP).[1] It is a leading cause of irreversible blindness, with more than 66.8 million people affected worldwide.[2]

Basic principles of perimetry

The normal visual field extends 100–110° temporally, 60° nasally and superiorly, and approximately 70–75° inferiorly. Most visual field testing concentrates on the central 30°. Visual sensitivity is greatest

Table 13.1 Factors affecting the normal 'hill of vision' resulting in general depression

Ambient light level
Nature of test stimulus, e.g. size
Stimulus duration
Eccentricity
Adaptation level
Age
Media clarity
Pupil size
Refraction

in the centre, the fovea, and decreases towards the periphery. The field of vision is commonly represented as a hill or island of vision. Traquair once described the visual field as 'an island of vision in a sea of darkness'.[3] The height and shape of this normal hill of vision vary among individuals, and many factors affect these parameters (see *Table 13.1*). A field defect can be described simply as any statistically and clinically significant departure from the smooth shape of the normal hill of vision.

Modern perimetry

In recent years there have been significant advances in optic nerve and retinal fibre layer evaluation and studies have addressed these areas with respect to a variety of visual functions in glaucoma.[4]

Perimetry refers to the measurement of the visual field on a curved surface and has all but replaced campimetry (the measurement of visual field on a flat surface, e.g., the Bjerrum screen) in modern clinical practice. Perimetry has progressed from confrontation fields, Bjerrum screens and Goldmann perimetry, all of which use kinetic modes of visual field testing. In kinetic (isopter) perimetry moving targets of different size are presented. As these movements are performed manually they can be open to operator bias.

Static perimetry provides the basis of computerised suprathreshold and threshold perimetry, in which a stationary target is presented and its intensity varied to determine retinal sensitivity. This is now the preferred method of visual field analysis and has been facilitated by the development of automated instruments.

White-light perimetry remains the most reliable and most widely used tool with

which to monitor the functional impairment induced by glaucoma.[5] Perimetry is an invaluable aid to indicating the extent of glaucomatous damage and to determine any deterioration in visual function.[6] It is, however, far from ideal and does have a number of shortcomings.[7]

Modern automated static perimeters

There are several commercially available automated visual field instruments. The Humphrey field analyser has become well established internationally and is the instrument that many clinicians are most familiar with. For this reason much of the discussion in this chapter refers specifically to this instrument.

The Humphrey field analyser has a wide range of both single-stimulus suprathreshold and full threshold programs. The suprathreshold mode is suitable as a screening test and a number of different programs are available. The 120-point and 76-point are perhaps the most popular. However, threshold tests provide much more useful information than suprathreshold tests.

In suprathreshold testing, it is very important to select the appropriate test intensity. If the intensity is set too high then there is a risk that early defects will be missed and there will be too many false-negative responses. Conversely, if the test intensity is set too low, close to the patient's threshold, a large number of patients with normal visual fields will miss stimuli. Therefore, the higher the suprathreshold increment the higher the specificity and lower the sensitivity of the test. The converse applies where the suprathreshold increment is lower.

A full threshold test determines the depth of the scotomata at each point and is more accurate when used to monitor progressive disease over a period of time. This is because thresholds give information regarding the deepening of a field defect as well as the expansion of the defect.

The standard Humphrey test program used for glaucoma patients was the threshold 30-2. The threshold 24-2 program eliminates the most peripheral test locations of the 30-2 program, except for the nasal portion of the field. With Humphrey threshold perimetry a stimulus is presented at a test point and this is increased in intensity in 4dB steps until the threshold is crossed. Once the threshold has been crossed, the stimulus is decreased in intensity in 2dB steps to determine the exact threshold.

Many clinicians now routinely use the 24-2 for glaucoma patients, because it produces as much clinically useful information as the 30-2 program and saves about 2 minutes test time for each eye. The Humphrey 24-2 program tests 54 points and has a 6° spaced grid offset from the vertical and horizontal meridians, unlike the 24-1 strategy, which includes points along the vertical and horizontal meridians. Detection of visual field loss is aided by comparison of the test result to that of a normal standard.

SITA strategies

The SITA (Swedish interactive thresholding algorithm) is one of the most significant developments in modern automated perimetry (also see Chapter 14). There are two SITA strategies available: the standard strategy,[8] which halves the time taken to perform full threshold testing, and the SITA-fast strategy,[9] which halves the time of Fastpac testing. As testing time is significantly reduced, the results are less affected by patient fatigue. SITA is only available on the Humphrey 700 series of instruments and has been demonstrated to be highly accurate and reproducible. This has been achieved by writing a strategy that:

- Takes account of prior knowledge. The starting level is set according to the thresholds of neighbouring locations when these are available. This has made it possible to reduce the number of presentations in certain locations.
- Does away with the need for false-positive catch trials. The SITA algorithm uses the time it takes the patient to press the response button to estimate the false-positive response rate. Usually response times are within a fairly tight time range. However, this range is much broader with false-positive responses, some of which are shorter and others longer. By analysing the number of responses falling outside the patient's normal response range, an estimate is given of the false-positive response rate.
- Speeds up the rate of stimulus presentation in patients who respond quickly. The rate of stimulus presentations is usually constant in full threshold and suprathreshold strategies. Using SITA in this way speeds up stimulus presentation rates, making the complete test time much quicker (up to 50 per cent). The SITA standard test saves approximately 7 minutes per eye in comparison

with the full threshold strategy. Repeatability is as good as, if not better than, the standard full threshold test. SITA-fast is quicker still, as it reduces test time per eye by approximately 10 minutes when compared to standard full threshold testing. SITA-fast does, however, have less repeatability.

If a defect is detected, testing should be repeated to show that the results are reproducible and not artefactual. The Humphrey field analyser also contains powerful software that enables follow-up analysis to confirm any progression in the field loss. The overview facility can present up to 16 fields (four per sheet). The 'Glaucoma Change Probability' option determines change over time by distinguishing random variation from true change.

Glaucoma hemifield test

The glaucoma hemifield test (GHT) is available on the Statpac II software (also see Chapter 14). This innovation is an attempt to provide information about the differences between superior and inferior halves of the visual field by evaluating differences in threshold at mirror-image points on either side of the midline.[10] Often the progression of glaucomatous field defects is asymmetric, with one eye being affected before the fellow eye or advancing faster than the other eye.[11]

Characteristics of glaucomatous field loss

Glaucomatous field defects can occur anywhere, although most do occur in certain regions of the visual field. Most visual field defects seen in glaucoma are the nerve fibre bundle type.[12,13] It has been suggested that the earliest sign of glaucomatous loss is an increased scatter of responses in an area that subsequently develops a defect.[14] Alternatively, there may be a slight asymmetry between the two eyes.

Glaucomatous field defects can be classified as either focal, in which the damage occurs to a specific bundle of fibres, or generalised, in which the entire optic nerve may be involved. These two types have led to different theories being proposed to account for the two apparently separate mechanisms in glaucoma field loss.[15]

Paracentral

The first perimetrically noticeable changes in glaucoma are relatively steep depressions of sensitivity in small, paracentral areas of the visual field (*Figure 13.1*), most

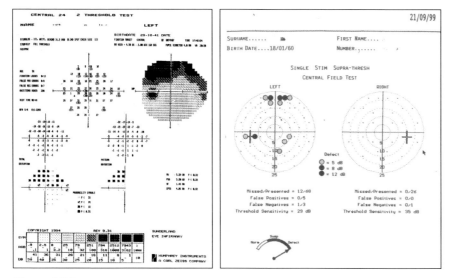

Figure 13.1

(a) A superior paracentral glaucomatous visual field defect – typical in primary open-angle glaucoma (Humphrey). (b) Same eye using a Henson 4000 (note the lower threshold sensitivity in the left compared to the right eye)

commonly superonasally, as opposed to the inferotemporal or macular regions.[16] This type of defect is present in approximately 70 per cent of all early glaucomatous field defects and there may be more than one such defect.[15]

These defects respect the nerve fibre distribution in the retina and often show abrupt changes when they meet the horizontal midline. Nerve fibre bundle defects can be detected by fundoscopy or nerve fibre analysis, and are most easily visualised in younger patients with clear media.

Arcuate

Paracentral scotomata may increase progressively in density, elongating along the course of the damaged retinal nerve fibres. This represents a more advanced stage of glaucomatous visual field loss (*Figure 13.2*). Most glaucoma field defects progress quite slowly and may take years to become repeatable on perimetric investigation. These can then coalesce to produce arcuate scotomata that are more common in the superior hemifield compared to the inferior field, as with paracentral defects. These defects respect the horizontal midline because the retinal nerve fibres terminate at the horizontal raphe.[17] They are depicted by a more irregular pattern on static perimetry, which may also exhibit significant variation from one session to another. For example, in threshold perimetry there may be large differences in thresholds between examinations, whereas in suprathreshold perimetry a particular location might seem defective at one visit, but quite normal during the next.

Nasal step

Nasal step is a characteristic defect associated with a difference in the sensitivity above and below the horizontal midline in the nasal field (*Figure 13.3*). The sensitivity loss associated with this type of field is more frequent in the superior field.[18] A nasal step can be seen in a normal field. However, if greater than 5–10°, this would be considered to be significant and not just a variation of a normal field. Although a nasal step may occur in a number of other conditions that affect the optic nerve head, up to 40 per cent of patients with glaucomatous field loss have a demonstrable nasal step.[19] A nasal step is rarely seen in isolation.

Overall depression

Overall depression represents a gradual sinking of the island of vision resulting in reduced sensitivity measures (*Figure 13.2*). Early glaucomatous visual field loss frequently involves a diffuse component[20] and is thought to be caused by diffuse loss of retinal nerve fibres throughout the optic nerve.

Other causes, such as media opacities (cataracts) or miosed pupils, can also give rise to an overall depression of the visual field.[15]

Baring of the blind spot

If retinal sensitivity below the optic disc is slightly lower than the corresponding area above, it is possible to demonstrate baring of the blind spot with kinetic perimetry. Its significance in glaucoma diagnosis nowadays is much less important, mainly because it can be demonstrated in many normal patients.

Enlargement of the blind spot

Enlargement of the blind spot is found in isolation only rarely and is very difficult to differentiate from the normal disc, which may vary significantly in its parameters. It is no longer considered to be an important factor in the early diagnosis of glaucomatous field loss.

Development of glaucomatous fields

As the glaucomatous visual field progresses, defects become more extensive, both in size and depth, until the whole hemifield is involved (*Figure 13.3*). It is not until the final stages of glaucomatous field loss that both hemifields become affected. The asymmetry between inferior and superior hemifields can be a very specific sign of glaucomatous field loss. Indeed, this type of asymmetry is, for example, what the Humphrey field analyser glaucoma hemifield test is based on.[10]

Field differences in normal tension and high-tension glaucoma

Both high-tension glaucoma (HTG) and normal-tension glaucoma (NTG) produce characteristic field defects. NTG patients often have paracentral defects that are a significant risk to central fixation. Nasal steps and arcuate loss are common patterns of early glaucomatous loss. The superior visual field is affected preferentially in NTG, with depressions in sensitivity that are more localised, closer to fixation and with steeper gradients compared with HTG eyes[21] (*Figure 13.4*).

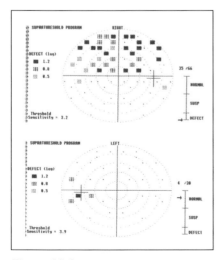

Figure 13.2
Henson 3000 fields: right superior arcuate defect with overall depression in sensitivity. Note the threshold sensitivity is 3.2dB and 3.9dB, right and left, respectively

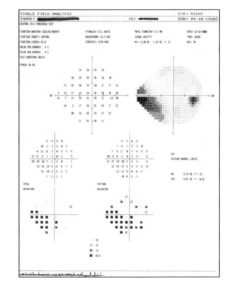

Figure 13.3
Localised glaucomatous nasal step. Note the GHT is outside normal limits

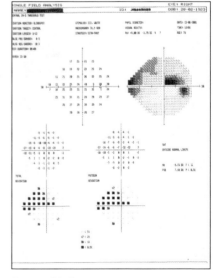

Figure 13.4
Deep superior paracentral scotoma, close to fixation. A typical visual field defect in NTG

Reliability indices

Interpretation of the visual field results can be difficult because of the amount of information these instruments provide and its significance can be easily missed unless a systematic approach is applied to their interpretation (also see Chapter 14).

In threshold and single-stimulus suprathreshold perimetry, patient test reliability is monitored by the determination of fixation losses; false-positive and false-negative responses. The reliability indices are an indicator of the extent to which a

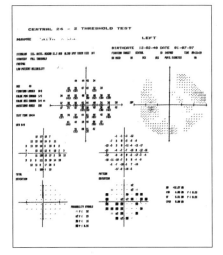

Figure 13.5
Areas of 'white out' on the Humphrey grey scale. This is caused by a typical 'button presser' with significant false positives and false negatives. The positive mean deviation is very high (note the black pattern-deviation plot)

particular patient's results may be compared reliably with the normal range of values stored in the computer memory. Reliability indices are often misinterpreted as an indicator of how accurate and believable a patient's test results are. Often, many patients who are flagged by the perimeter as having low reliability appear to have very accurate and reproducible field results. Conversely, some patients who appear to be very reliable have highly variable results. The measurement of reliability indices takes up a significant proportion of total test time and is based on small catch of samples of the total points tested.

Fixation losses

The instrument determines the location of the blind spot and periodically rechecks its location. The quality of fixation is often estimated by the Heijl–Krakau technique (also see Chapters 14 and 16), in which a bright stimulus is presented in the blind spot. If points in the blind spot are seen at subsequent representations, a false-positive response is recorded. If the fixation loss rate exceeds 33 per cent the Humphrey indicates this. This criterion is really quite arbitrary as it depends on how well the blind spot has been located in the first place. Simply checking how well the blind spot shows up on the printout is also useful.

False-positive errors

The machine makes a noise as if a stimulus has been presented, but no stimulus is projected on to the screen. If the button is pressed, this counts as a false positive

(also see Chapter 14). This detects 'button-pressers' or 'trigger-happy' patients who occasionally confuse the background noise of the visual system with stimulus presentations. A high false-positive rate gives rise to increased sensitivity estimates in threshold estimates and to misleadingly normal results on suprathreshold field tests. In such a 'button-presser', 'white out' on the grey scale can often be seen because of abnormally high decibel thresholds, with a positive mean deviation and a black printout on the pattern deviation (*Figure 13.5*).

False-negative errors

Once the threshold for a given locus has been determined, the machine increases the stimulus intensity by 9db. If this presentation is missed, a false-negative response is recorded (also see Chapter 14). False-negative responses may indicate an unreliable observer or an observer who is fatiguing, but they may also reflect the short-term fluctuation associated with scotomata (*Figure 13.6*). Other indications of a fatiguing observer are 'clover-leaf' or 'Mickey-Mouse' fields (*Figure 13.7*).

Some types of visual field defects are themselves associated with changes in reliability indices. For example, glaucoma causes an increase in the false-negative response rate[22,23] (*Figure 13.8*), while very large defects may be associated with low rates of fixation loss. Much useful information may still be obtained from many patients, even though they give high fixation loss and high false-negative rates.

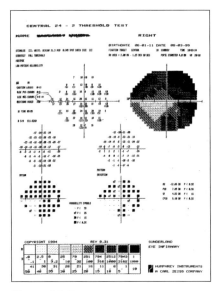

Figure 13.6
Humphrey field plot with a high degree of false-negative responses. These are from a fatiguing patient and the resultant lack of attentiveness

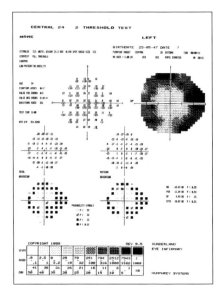

Figure 13.7
Humphrey field of fatiguing patient. The resultant field is often referred to as a 'clover leaf'

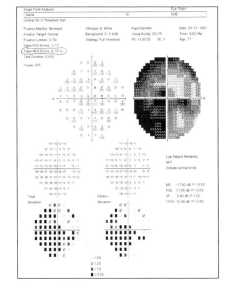

Figure 13.8
Advanced glaucomatous visual field loss. Note the high false-negative rate.

Raw data and grey scales

The simplest way to examine visual field results from a threshold examination is to look at the grey scale, in which varying sensitivity is linked to the grey-scale tones (also see Chapter 14). Grey-scale maps should not be used to monitor change with time alone, as they can overemphasise reduced sensitivity in the periphery of the visual field and miss small, but nevertheless significant, changes in areas close to the fixation.

The numerical printout on the top left of the Humphrey printout gives the actual threshold values and the right side gives the grey-scale map. Thus, the top-left part of the Humphrey printout provides the unprocessed threshold data that have not been compared to norms for age (total deviation plot) or processed to allow for overall changes in the hill of vision (pattern deviation).

Analysis of threshold values

Statpac II is a popular statistical package incorporated into the software of the Humphrey field analyser, and in this section the significance and interpretation of the data provided is discussed.

Total deviation

The Humphrey field analyser contains normal thresholds for age, together with their standard deviations. The data about the 'normal' population were gathered from subjects with no history of eye disease, a normal eye examination and a refractive error in the range ±5.00DS spherical equivalent.[24] This allows comparison of the raw data with age matched norms. Situated in the lower left of the printout are the numerical values and probability (P) symbols. The probability symbols take into account the greater variance in the periphery of the visual field and the values represent the likelihood of a defect occurring by chance, and as a result indicate the significance of a defect (also see Chapter 14). A probability symbol of <0.5 per cent, however, does not necessarily mean the threshold value is clinically significant, even though it shows statistical significance.

Pattern deviation

Glaucoma, unless very advanced and extensive, mainly causes localised loss. The pattern deviation aims to separate out the localised field defects that may be hidden by a generalised depression that affects the whole hill of vision, such as that caused by

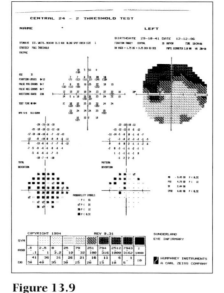

Figure 13.9
Lens opacity causing a general reduction of sensitivity in the total deviation plot. A superior arcuate visual field defect is revealed in the pattern deviation plot

cataracts and other media opacities (*Figure 13.9*). This is achieved by ranking the thresholds in order. The threshold of the seventh-highest threshold location is adjusted to zero and the same correction factor is applied to all points. The threshold of this seventh-highest value is termed the 'general height value'. A probability plot again provides the associated values for each point and their variation from the norm. Visual defects of varying conditions are thus identified from a single analysis.

Global indices

Global indices aim to give a set of simple numbers that can be used to compare fields plotted on different occasions (also see Chapter 14).[25,26] Calculation of the global indices is weighted to give greater importance to the test locations near fixation and less importance to more peripheral locations.[27]

The mean deviation (MD) is the overall departure of the average deviation of the visual field result from that expected of a normal field of the same age group. It therefore measures the average height of the hill of vision. In normal fields this value is low and in abnormal fields the value is high. Positive values suggest a 'button-presser', whereas negative values represent a depression. This value is insensitive to small localised depressions of the sort seen in glaucoma, but is strongly affected by general trends.

Pattern standard deviation (PSD) represents the unevenness of the hill of vision or how much spread there is between sensitivity values. A normal hill of vision, with a 'regular' surface, will give a low PSD value. Where there is a localised loss of vision, such as with paracentral scotomata or glaucomatous arcuate defects, the hill of vision will be deviated from the norm and a high PSD value will be obtained. It is not so affected by generalised depressions.

Short-term fluctuation (SF) is monitored throughout the test and 10 preselected points are checked twice to determine the reliability of response. This gives an estimate of the repeatability of the measured thresholds. When both values at one point are within 4db of each other, the response is taken as reliable. However, when values are greater than 5db in difference, the reliability at this point is questionable. The reason may be poor fixation or lack of concentration, but occasionally it may be early or progressive visual field loss that also results in false-negative responses. SF values are usually between 1db and 2.5db in a normal field result.

Variability of the threshold estimates is mainly dependent on the sensitivity. In the centre of the visual field, where sensitivity is highest, variability is low and threshold estimates are relatively repeatable. In areas of visual loss, or even in the normal periphery of the field, where sensitivity is lower, variability is increased. Arguably the usefulness of summarising this variability is limited.

Corrected PSD (CPSD) takes into consideration any intra-test variability as noted by the SF. It is probably the best measure of variation across the field. This will highlight any suspicious points that, although they may be within the normal decibel values for that point, may indicate the early onset of visual deficit and therefore should be observed for possible progression. Both PSD and CPSD return to lower values as visual field loss increases in severity. When the entire field becomes involved, the hill of vision is then depressed as a whole. Change analysis gives a statistical evaluation of the change in visual field with time.[28]

Visual field tests can provide a great deal of information about the state of a patient's visual function. The challenge for the practitioner is to enable the patient to do as well as possible, to guard against artefacts and to examine all of the information obtained (*Figures 13.10* and *13.11*). Certainly, the perimetrist's instructions can significantly affect the results obtained with automated perimetry.[29]

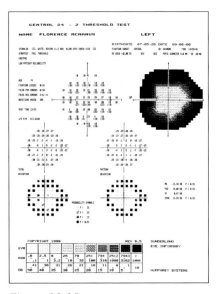

Figure 13.10
High plus lens artefact demonstrating concentric contraction of the visual field

Newer psychological techniques

Despite the developments in perimetry in recent years, there was still a real need for a quick and simple screening and/or early detection test that combined ease of use with high sensitivity and specificity. There were also potential benefits if the instru-

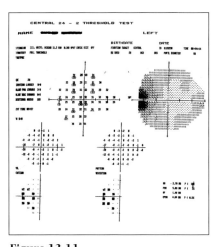

Figure 13.11
High minus lens artefact where the blind spot is shifted temporally. Courtesy of K Gales, RVI, Newcastle

mentation was portable, with results independent of refractive error and room illumination. The relatively recently introduced visual field screener/analyser, called the Frequency Doubling Perimeter (FDP), which is produced by Welch Allen and distributed by Zeiss, achieves these goals (also refer to Chapter 11).[30] The FDP uses the illusion that when a low spatial frequency sinusoidal grating flickers at a high temporal frequency, the grating

appears to be twice its actual spatial frequency.[31] This is thought to originate from the magnocellular (M) cells. M-cells may be involved in the detection of low-contrast, achromatic stimuli and may be specialised for temporal resolution. M-cells have a relatively large diameter. It is thought that these cells are selectively damaged first in the early stages of glaucoma.[32] Motion-detection perimetry has also been advocated as a useful glaucoma screening technique.

Another subset of retinal ganglion cells, the parvocellular (P) pathway, is responsible for the transmission of colour-specific neural impulses and spatial acuity at high contrasts. The P-cell function is targeted in short-wavelength automated perimetry (SWAP). This form of perimetry displays a blue stimulus on a yellow background and is claimed to detect visual field defects earlier than conventional white-on-white perimetry. This technique produces high inter-subject variability and is affected adversely by media opacities, thus making it practically useless in older patients with cataract. These limitations mean that this technique remains very much a research tool.

Acknowledgement
Figure 13.8 with permission from AB Litwak, *Glaucoma Handbook*, Butterworth–Heinemann (2001).

References

1 American Academy of Ophthalmology (1996). *Preferred Practice Pattern: Primary Open Angle Glaucoma* (San Francisco: American Academy of Ophthalmology).
2 Tielsch JM, Sommer A, Katz J, *et al.* (1991). Racial variations in the prevalence of primary open angle glaucoma. *JAMA* **266**, 369–374.
3 Henson DB (2000). *Visual Fields*, Second edition, Chapter 1 (Oxford: Butterworth–Heinemann).
4 Logan JFL and Rankin SJA (2000). Glaucoma: moving with the times? *Optom Practice* **1**, 5–16.
5 American Academy of Ophthalmology (1996). Ophthalmic procedures assessment: automated perimetry. *Ophthalmology* **103**, 1144–1151.
6 Quigley HA, Tielsch JM, Katz J, *et al.* (1996). Rate of progression in open angle glaucoma estimated from cross-sectional prevalence of visual field damage. *Am J Ophthalmol.* **122**, 355–363.
7 O'Brien C and Wild JM (1995). Automated perimetry in glaucoma – room for improvement? *Br J Ophthalmol.* **79**, 200–201.
8 Bengtsson B, Olsson J, Heijl A, *et al.* (1997). A new generation of algorithms for computerised threshold perimetry, SITA. *Acta Ophthalmol.* **75**, 368–375.

9 Bengtsson B and Heijl A. SITA fast, a new rapid perimetric threshold test. Description of methods and evaluation in patients with manifest and suspect glaucoma. *Acta Ophthalmol Scand.* **76** (4), 431–437.
10 Asman P and Heijl A (1992). Glaucoma hemifield test. Automated visual field evaluation. *Arch Ophthalmol*, **110**, 812–819.
11 Chen PP and Park RJ (2000). Visual field progression in patients with initially unilateral visual loss from chronic open angle glaucoma. *Ophthalmology* **107**(9), 1688–1692.
12 Caprioli J (1990). Automated perimetry in glaucoma. In *Visual Fields Examination and Interpretation*, p. 71–90. Ed. Walsh TJ (San Francisco: American Academy of Ophthalmology).
13 Anderson DR (1992). *Automated Static Perimetry*, p. 40–68 (St Louis: Mosby–Year Book).
14 Armaly MF (1971). Visual field defects in early open angle glaucoma. *Trans Am Ophthalmol Soc.* **69**, 147–162
15 Henson DB (2000). *Visual Fields*, Second edition, Chapter 7 (Oxford: Butterworth–Heinemann).
16 Heijl A and Lundvist L (1984). The frequency distribution of earliest glaucomatous visual field defects documented by automated perimetry. *Acta Ophthalmol.* **62**, 658–664.

17 McNaughton J. Visual field defects in glaucoma. In *Glaucoma Module Parts 1–12*; p. 38–42. Continuing Professional Development Series (London: AOP and City University).
18 Hart WM and Becker B (1982). The onset and evaluation of glaucomatous visual field defects. *Ophthalmology* **89**, 268–279.
19 Caprioli J and Spaeth GL (1985). Static threshold estimation of the peripheral nasal field in glaucoma. *Arch Ophthalmol.* **103**, 1150–1154.
20 Henson DB, Artes PH and Chauhan BC (1999). Diffuse loss of sensitivity in early glaucoma. *Invest Ophthalmol Vis Sci.* **40**(13), 3147–3151.
21 Samuelson TW and Spaeth GL (1993). Focal and diffuse visual field defects: their relationship to intra-ocular pressure. *Ophthalmic Surg.* **24**(8), 519–525.
22 Katz J, Sommer A and Witt K (1991). Reliability of visual field results over repeated testing. *Ophthalmology* **98**(1), 70–75.
23 Bengtsson B and Heijl A (2000). False-negative responses in glaucoma perimetry: indicators of patient performance or test reliability? *Invest Ophthalmol Vis Sci.* **41**(8), 2210–2214.
24 Heijl A, Lindgren G and Olsson J (1989). Visual field interpretation with empiric probability maps. *Arch Ophthalmol.* **107**, 204–208.

25 Heijl A, Lindgren G, Olsson J, *et al.* (1992). On weighted visual field indexes. *Graefe's Arch Clin Exp Ophthalmol.* **230**, 397–398.

26 Rowe FJ (1998). Visual fields in glaucoma. *Eye News* **5**(1, Jun/Jul), 13–20.

27 Flanagan JG, Wild JM and Trope GE (1993). The visual field indices in primary open angle glaucoma. *Invest Ophthalmol Vis Sci.* **34**, 2266–2274.

28 Griffiths P and Gales K (2000). *Visual Fields Refresher Course Notes Handbook.* Form meeting held at The Royal Victory Infirmary, Newcastle, March 2000.

29 Kutzko KE, Brito CFC and Wall M (2000). Effect of instructions on conventional automated perimetry. *Invest Ophthalmol Vis Sci.* **41**(1), 2006–2013.

30 Johnson and Samuels SJ (1997). Screening for glaucomatous visual field loss with frequency doubling perimetry. *Invest Ophthalmol Vis Sci.* **38**, 413–425.

31 Kelly DH (1966). Frequency doubling in visual responses. *J Opt Soc Am Acad.* **56**, 1628–1633.

32 Quigley HA, Addicks EM, Green WR, *et al.* (1981). Optic nerve damage in human glaucoma, II: the site of injury and susceptibility to damage. *Arch Ophthalmol.* **99**, 635–641.

14
Analysis of visual field data

Robert Cubbidge

In perimetry, sensitivity (the reciprocal of threshold) is defined as $L/\Delta L$, where L is the background luminance, and ΔL is the minimum light energy necessary to evoke a visual response. The background luminance determines the state of retinal adaptation and therefore influences ΔL. The dynamic range corresponds to the range of the maximum stimulus luminance of the perimeter, and to the threshold stimulus luminance of an eye with normal sensitivity.[1] The measurement unit used for sensitivity in perimetry is the decibel (dB). A value of 0dB corresponds to the maximum stimulus luminance of the perimeter. Increasing sensitivity to light is denoted by an increasing value in decibels. One decibel is equal to 0.1 log unit; accordingly, 10dB is equal to a 1 log unit and 20dB is equal to a 2 log units attenuation of the maximum possible stimulus luminance (e.g., a 10-fold and a 100-fold reduction). The variations in the background and the maximum stimulus luminance between perimeters mean that decibels are relative units and cannot be compared easily between instruments.

The threshold is defined in terms of a psychometric function, the frequency-of-seeing curve (*Figure 14.1*), which describes the probability of seeing a stimulus. The stimulus luminance at which the probability of perception is 50 per cent is defined as the threshold. Visual field testing necessitates determining the threshold at a large number of locations in the visual field. In full threshold examination, threshold algorithms employ staircase procedures to estimate the threshold at a given location in the visual field. In psychophysical experimentation, a large number of crossings of the threshold are made so that the threshold is precisely estimated. However, in perimetry, a trade-off must occur between the number of crossings of the threshold and the accuracy of the estimate, as the number of stimulus presentations is directly proportional to the examination time. The staircase is therefore truncated, and only crosses the threshold once or twice. A number of algorithms have been developed to estimate the threshold in perimetry.

Threshold determination

The full threshold (4-2dB) algorithm initially estimates the threshold at four 'seed' points (*Figures 14.2* and *14.3*). The initial stimulus presentation is above threshold, based on the expected threshold for the patient's age. If the patient sees

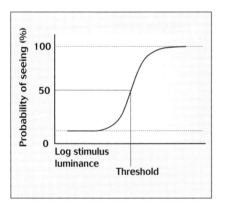

Figure 14.1
The threshold is defined as 50 per cent probability of seeing on the frequency-of-seeing psychometric function

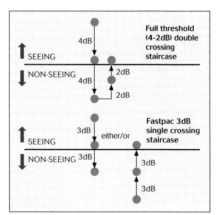

Figure 14.2
Full threshold (4-2dB) double crossing staircase

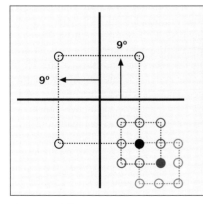

Thresholds are initially determined at four 'seed' points, one in each quadrant of the visual field (open black circles ○).
Once the threshold is determined (closed black circle), thresholding begins at adjacent locations (red open circles ○).
Similarly, as thresholds are competed at these locations (red closed circles ●), more locations are 'opened' for thresholding (blue open circles ○). At all open locations, the stimulus presentations occur randomly, but as a whole thresholds at more peripheral stimulus locations are estimated later in the test.

Figure 14.3
Pattern of thresholding on the HFA 4-2dB and Fastpac algorithms

this stimulus, the next stimulus presentation is 4dB dimmer. Each subsequent presentation is decreased in 4dB steps until the threshold is passed and the patient no longer sees the stimulus. Further stimulus presentations are made at 2dB brighter than previously and continue to brighten in 2dB steps until the patient responds to the stimulus. The threshold is recorded as the last seen stimulus. Threshold determination then begins at adjacent locations and each estimated threshold opens up adjacent stimulus locations, such that the order of threshold determination gradually spirals out towards the edge of the visual field. It can be seen that, because the smallest staircase step is 2dB, if the true threshold lies between the step there will be an error in the estimated threshold of 1dB. The 4-2dB algorithm is recognised as the clinical 'gold standard' for perimetry, but a typical examination takes approximately 12–15 minutes per eye.

The Fastpac algorithm (*Figures 14.2 and 14.3*) was developed to reduce the testing time with respect to the 4-2dB algorithm (also refer to Chapter 13). Staircase steps are 3dB and initially presented above threshold at 50 per cent of locations and below threshold at the remainder. The staircase only crosses the threshold once and the threshold is recorded as the last-seen stimulus. Fastpac offers a saving in time of approximately one-third over the 4-2dB algorithm,[2] but since the staircase step sizes are greater and the threshold is only crossed once, the number of threshold errors is higher.[3] Consequently, Fastpac yields greater variability in measurement and the algorithm should not be used in cases where a critical diagnosis is required.[4]

In the mid-1990s, Swedish interactive threshold algorithms (SITA) was developed to reduce the testing time without altering the accuracy of the threshold estimate. Models of normal and glaucomatous visual field behaviour are constantly updated during the test. Bayesian probability is used to calculate the maximum probability (MAP) estimate, which is a threshold distribution, the peak of which indicates the threshold and the width the accuracy. Accuracy is determined by the size of the measurement error selected: low for SITA-standard and greater for SITA-fast. Once a predefined level of accuracy is reached, testing is terminated. SITA-standard has a greater accuracy than SITA-fast and, therefore, takes longer to complete. The speed of the examination is dictated by the patients, based on their response times to the presentation of the stimuli.

After the examination is complete, post-processing occurs; the frequencies of false-positive and false-negative responses are

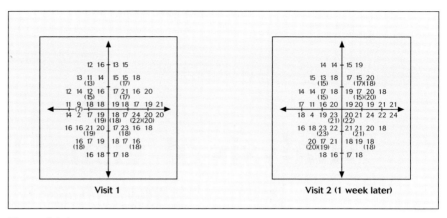

Figure 14.4
The learning effect whereby an improvement in visual field sensitivity occurs over successive examinations

incorporated into the model and thresholds altered where necessary. SITA-standard is approximately 50 per cent faster than the 4-2dB full threshold algorithm, while SITA-fast is approximately 50 per cent faster than the Fastpac algorithm. The accuracy of SITA-standard is slightly greater than that of the 4-2dB algorithm, and it is likely that it will become the 'gold standard' algorithm for the detection of glaucoma.

Another approach to reducing testing time without affecting accuracy has been developed by Interzeag (Haag–Streit Group) for use in the Octopus perimeters in a threshold algorithm named tendency oriented perimetry (TOP). As visual field defects occur in patterns, there is a relationship or 'tendency' between thresholds in neighbouring regions. Unlike conventional algorithms in which each staircase procedure at a given stimulus location occurs in isolation of adjacent locations, in TOP each stimulus location is adjusted five times, once by a direct stimulus presentation and four times from the patient responses at presentations in neighbouring locations. The visual field grid is divided into four evenly interspaced grids that are examined in succession. The thresholds at locations in adjacent matrices are adjusted by interpolation and staircase steps varied according to a series of mathematical rules. Using this approach, the G1 program can be completed in approximately 3 minutes, compared to a typical 12–15 minutes using the 4-2dB strategy.

Regardless of the method by which thresholds are estimated, as the number of stimulus locations increases, so does the examination time, since more stimulus presentations are required. Therefore, the spatial grid needs to be optimised so that the minimum number of stimulus locations yields the greatest chance of detecting a visual field defect.

Visual field loss in glaucoma primarily occurs in the central field.[5,6] In the Humphrey field analyser, the default stimulus separation in full threshold examination is 6°, and is based upon the findings of Fankhauser and Bebié,[7] who reported that the probability of detecting an 8.4° diameter scotoma with a square grid of 6° separation was 100 per cent. The 6° stimulus separation employed in the Humphrey field analyser and Octopus perimeters is entirely sufficient to detect early glaucomatous visual field loss.[8]

In macular conditions, a higher density sampling of the visual field is desirable and the 10-2 program of the Humphrey field analyser is 2°. The default program G1 of the Octopus perimeter differs from the 30-2 and 24-2 programs of the Humphrey field analyser in that the stimulus separation is not constant throughout the visual field. Stimulus separation is 2° centrally, increasing to 8° in the periphery. The grid is denser around fixation to detect paracentral scotomas.[9]

Data analysis

The imprecision in the staircase and the large number of locations for which thresholds need to be found create a degree of noise in the data gathering process that must be filtered out as much as possible to enable statistical interpretation. Factors such as the learning effect (*Figure 14.4*), whereby a patient's visual field sensitivity improves over successive examinations, and the fatigue effect (which reduces sensitivity during the course of an examination) also need to be considered when evaluating a visual field. A number of approaches are used in a typical visual field printout to aid the practitioner in interpretation. Two visual fields are provided here

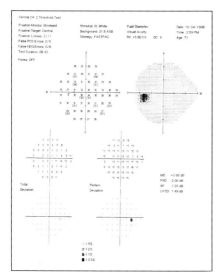

Figure 14.5
Patient A

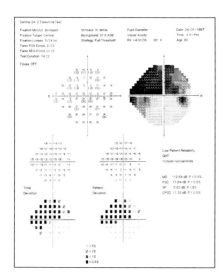

Figure 14.6
Patient B

to assist in understanding the interpretation of these methods (patients A and B in *Figures 14.5* and *14.6*, respectively).

Numeric data

The simplest form of data presentation is to represent the threshold values in decibels arranged in the spatial locations of the test grid. Double determinations of threshold at any given stimulus location are illustrated by the two values of sensitivity (the latter in brackets). Presentation in this form permits the display of the raw data prior to statistical manipulation. However, the disadvantage is that the large amounts of such data hinder interpretation of the visual field.

Greyscale

The greyscale aims to display perimetric data in a map so that it can be interpreted more readily than by viewing the numeric data. Sensitivity values are represented by shades of grey, ranging from black to white. Sensitivity values are generally banded into 5dB groupings, with increasing greyness denoting decreasing sensitivity. Regions between the locations tested in the visual field are illustrated by interpolation. The disadvantage of the greyscale is that a location may have high sensitivity but may still be abnormal, and thus will not readily appear as a defect. Patient A shows a greyscale of normal appearance, but has two defective locations in the inferior nasal visual field.

Probability plots

To understand probability plots (also see Chapter 13), it is necessary to understand the normal age-related decline in sensitivity that occurs across the visual field.

Figure 14.7 illustrates the decline in sensitivity with age for a central and a peripheral stimulus location. The normal sensitivity of the peripheral visual field declines at a faster rate than centrally (i.e., the hill of vision changes shape with advancing age, becoming steeper in profile). It can be seen that there is a range in sensitivity, which is wider at the more peripheral locations. The red lines indicate the 95 per cent confidence interval (i.e., 95 per cent of normal values fall within this region). Therefore, if a sensitivity value falls outside this range, it will gain a $P<5$ per cent probability level (i.e., the sensitivity is normal in less than 5 per cent of the normal population). Thus, probability plots graphically illustrate the level of statistical significance associated with a given visual field abnormality compared with the normal reference field.

There are two types of probability plots, total deviation and pattern deviation (*Figure 14.8*). In the total deviation plot, the differences between the measured visual field sensitivity and the expected normal visual field sensitivity are plotted as a numeric map. A second plot illustrates those locations at which the deviation is significantly different from the normal population, at the $P<0.5$ per cent, $P<1$ per cent, $P<2$ per cent, or $P<5$ per cent levels. The pattern deviation probability map separates the general reduction in sensitivity that may arise through media opacities, optical defocus, or pupillary miosis (i.e., the total deviation) from the localised reduction in sensitivity. To calculate the pattern deviation probability map, all locations within 24° of fixation are ranked according to the deviation in sensitivity

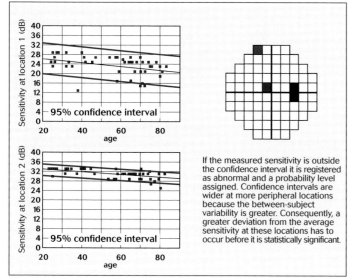

Figure 14.7
Confidence intervals

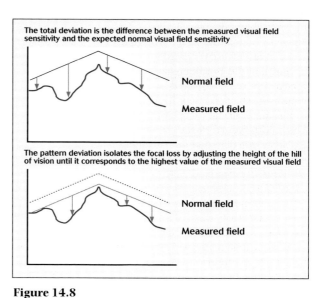

Figure 14.8
Representation of the distinction between pattern and total deviation

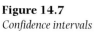

compared to the age-matched normal population. The general height of the hill of vision is calculated from the measured value of the seventh-highest deviation (85th percentile) in sensitivity.[10]

Patient B (see *Figure 14.6*) clearly shows large areas of focal loss on the pattern deviation consistent with a superior arcuate scotoma cause by glaucoma. Over time, these locations are likely to worsen with both the level of significance and the number of locations increasing. The probability map is therefore of use when monitoring a patient over time. Caution with these plots should be applied, however, when small isolated areas of loss are found, such as in patient A (see *Figure 14.*5). These locations may be of significance merely because of noise generated in the data. The patient's fundus should be examined to see whether there is a pathological cause for the visual field loss. If none can be found, then the patient's visual field should be repeated at a later date. Only if the visual field defect is repeatable should the patient be considered for referral to a specialist.

The glaucoma hemifield test

The glaucoma hemifield test (GHT) was introduced in the Humphrey field analyser to decide whether visual field loss was compatible with a diagnosis of glaucoma.[11] Ten anatomical sectors in the visual field are superimposed on the program 30-2 test grid, selected according to the normal arrangement of retinal nerve fibres. Five sectors in the upper hemifield mirror five sectors in the inferior field (also refer to Chapter 13).

Probability scores are calculated for each location within the ten sectors according to the pattern deviation probability map. Within each sector, the sum of the probability scores is calculated and the difference compared to the mirror-image sector. A visual field is classed as 'outside normal limits' if the difference in any of the five corresponding pairs of sectors falls outside the 0.5 per cent or 99.5 per cent confidence limits for that pair of sectors. Visual fields are classified as 'borderline' if any sector-pair difference exceeds the 3 per cent confidence limit. If the general height of the field is below the 0.5 per cent limit, the GHT evaluates the field as a 'general reduction in sensitivity'.

A classification of 'abnormally high sensitivity' is associated with a high level of false-positive responses. The general height test is not performed if the visual field has already been classified as 'outside normal limits'. Sensitivity and specificity of 80.8 per cent and 81.4 per cent, respectively, have been reported for the GHT.

Bebié curve

The Bebié curve is a cumulative distribution of the defect depth at each location and is designed to separate normal visual fields from those with early diffuse loss.[12] The defect depth is sorted into ascending order of severity and plotted as a function of rank. A shaded zone is employed to aid interpretation of the resultant curve. The enclosed region corresponds to the 5th and 95th percentiles. A normal visual field yields a curve above or closely following the 95th percentile line. A curve falling below (i.e., outside) the 95th percentile line indicates visual field loss. A visual field with purely diffuse loss mimics the shape of the curve associated with normality, but at a greater overall defect depth. Focal loss is indicated by a steepening of the curve. A clear boundary does not separate diffuse from focal loss on the curve.[13]

Furthermore, the Bebié curve does not yield information about the spatial characteristics of the visual field loss[14] and may not detect central visual field depressions in early glaucoma.[15]

Global visual field indices

Graphic displays such as greyscales suffer from a number of disadvantages, namely that they inadequately define diffuse visual field loss and changes between a series of visual fields.[16] Statistical interpretation of perimetric data does not suffer from these disadvantages. Global visual field indices are a useful method of data reduction, since they yield a single number that is an indication of the degree of diffuse or focal loss in the visual field. They are also of use when evaluating visual field change over time. A wide variety of visual field indices have been developed for the Octopus and Humphrey field analyser perimeters to summarise the visual field data.

Mean sensitivity

Mean sensitivity (MS) represents the arithmetic mean of the sensitivity of all stimulus locations tested in the visual field. Since there is no reference to the patient's age, this index is of little use clinically (also see Chapter 13).

Mean defect and mean deviation

The mean defect (MD) is the arithmetic mean of the difference between the measured values and the normal values at the different test locations. This statistic is employed in the Octopus and Henson perimeters. A positive MD represents a loss of sensitivity. The index is sensitive to diffuse visual field loss, but is relatively unaffected by focal loss. Thus, in the presence of cataract, the MD is increased. The equivalent index used in the Humphrey

field analyser is mean deviation, which is also abbreviated to MD. Mean deviation is a weighted average deviation from the normal reference visual field. A negative mean deviation represents a loss in sensitivity. Thus, care should be taken to check whether the MD index represents mean defect or mean deviation. In the presence of large areas of focal loss, the MD is also increased (Patient B, see *Figure 14.6*).

Loss variance and pattern standard deviation

The loss variance (LV) statistic of the Octopus perimeter describes non-uniformity in the height of the visual field. It is small if visual field damage is diffuse (e.g., in cataract) and high in the presence of focal loss [e.g., in glaucoma (see Chapter 13) or hemianopia]. The pattern standard deviation (PSD) statistic of the Humphrey field analyser is a weighted standard deviation of the differences between the measured and normal reference visual field at each stimulus location. It is analogous to LV on the Octopus perimeters. Patient A (see *Figure 14.*5) has a very small isolated area of focal loss and the PSD is unaffected. However, Patient B (see *Figure 14.6*) has a large area of focal loss reflected by the magnitude of the PSD.

Short-term fluctuation

The variability in the sensitivity that occurs when a threshold is estimated repeatedly during a single visual field examination is termed the short-term fluctuation (SF). In the Octopus perimeter, this is the average of the local scatter over the entire visual field, determined from the square root of the sum of the local standard deviations averaged over the visual field[16] (*Figure 14.9*). Calculation of SF in this way assumes that the variance is constant at all locations in the visual field. However, the variance is known to increase with eccentricity.[17] In the Humphrey field analyser, double determinations of threshold obtained at ten locations in the visual field are used to calculate a weighted mean of the standard deviations. The G1 program of the Octopus perimeter estimates the SF from double determinations of threshold at each location in the visual field, obtained over two phases. The 30-2 and 24-2 programs of the Humphrey field analyser estimate SF from double determinations of threshold obtained from ten locations within 21° eccentricity. The SF is greater around the borders of a scotoma,[18] since small movements in fixation may result in the first and second threshold determination falling within and outside a scotoma, respectively.[19] Therefore, a high SF may indicate a pathological visual field.

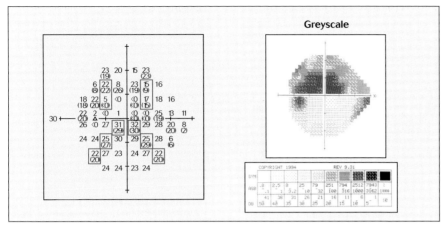

Figure 14.9
Numeric printout showing the locations used in the determination of short-term fluctuation

Corrected loss variance and corrected pattern standard deviation

Corrected loss variance (CLV) and corrected pattern standard deviation (CPSD) represent the LV and PSD corrected for the SF. They are, therefore, indices sensitive to focal loss that separate real deviations from those deviations due to variability. Since SITA adjusts thresholds for variability, the SF and CPSD indices are not calculated.

Reliability parameters

Automated static perimetry is time-consuming and demanding of the patient. Patient inattention during the examination may produce unreliable results. A number of criteria are useful in assessing patient reliability and are adopted easily into the threshold programs of automated static perimeters.

Fixation losses

Fixation can be monitored during the course of a perimetric examination by a variety of means. The crudest method is to observe the fixating eye through a telescope or on a television monitor. In the Heijl–Krakau method[20] of fixation monitoring, a stimulus of maximum luminance is periodically positioned in the blind spot (also refer to Chapter 16). If the patient sees this stimulus then a fixation loss is recorded. For the 30-2 program of the Humphrey field analyser, the number of blind spot stimulus presentations may be as many as 10 per cent of the total number of stimulus presentations in a perimetric examination.[21]

The visual field is usually classed as unreliable if the number of fixation losses exceeds 20 per cent. This value was derived during development of strategy software for the Humphrey field analyser threshold, because at higher rates of fixation losses, the sensitivity and specificity of the test began to deteriorate.[22] Fixation losses greater than 20 per cent have been shown to account for the largest number of unreliable tests in normal subjects, and those with ocular hypertension and glaucoma.[23] Consequently, it has been suggested that the percentage of fixation losses permitted before a visual field examination is classed as unreliable be increased from 20 per cent to 33 per cent.[24]

Methods that constantly measure fixation during the perimetric examination have been devised for the Octopus 1-2-3 and the Humphrey field analyser II perimeters. The Octopus 300 employs infrared ocular illumination to produce four corneal reflexes, two on each side of the pupil. Deviations of gaze and blinking are immediately registered by the perimeter during the course of the examination. If any deviation or prolonged closure of the lids occurs, the examination is temporarily interrupted automatically until the problem is rectified.

The Humphrey field analyser 'gaze tracking' system employs real-time image analysis to measure the distance between the centre of the pupil and the first corneal reflex (Purkinje I), produced by infrared lights in the perimeter bowl. Head movement does not affect this distance. A gaze graph is generated for the complete examination and shows upward and downward spikes deviating from a base line. Upward deviations indicate the eye deviated from the fixation target at the time of stimulus presentation, with the magnitude of the spike indicating the degree of deviation, up to an angle of 10°. Small downward deviations indicate that the gaze tracking system was unable to detect the patient's gaze, whereas large downward deviations illustrate patient blinking. To date, the clinical utility of the gaze-tracking system has not been determined.

False-positive and false-negative errors

To monitor the patient's responses, a number of catch trials are carried out by the perimeter during the course of an examination (also see Chapter 16). The perimeter regularly presents stimuli. In a false-positive catch trial the perimeter does not present a stimulus, as expected, and the patient pressing the response button indicates patient inattention and a false-positive error is recorded. In a false-negative catch trial, a stimulus is presented at a suprathreshold (brighter) level at a location in the visual field at which the threshold has already been established. If the patient fails to respond to this stimulus a false-negative error is recorded. A false negative may also be registered when the catch trial occurs within the physiological blind spot, since the patient would be unable to detect any stimulus.[25]

A visual field is usually classed as unreliable if the number of false-positive or false-negative answers exceeds 33 per cent, as it has been found that above this rate the sensitivity and specificity of the test begin to worsen.[22] High false-positive rates may give rise to higher MS and therefore reduce the magnitude of any focal loss. It has been demonstrated that high false-positive rates occur in inexperienced perimetric observers.[26] A positive correlation between false-positive rates and fixation losses has been demonstrated.[27] A high false-negative rate may result in reduced MS and, therefore, in an overestimation of focal loss. Katz and Sommer[28] found that in glaucoma patients who exhibited high false-negative rates, the number of false negatives is higher in glaucomatous eyes.[21]

The SITA algorithm assesses false-positive responses from knowledge of the reaction time of the patient. False-positive and -negative answers are incorporated into the final estimations of threshold given after the test has completed.

Statistical interpretation of the visual field aids the practitioner when deciding whether or not visual field loss is present and, in the case of serial examination, when determining whether or not visual field progression has occurred. However, a degree of clinical judgement is also required when evaluating visual fields and the results must be used in conjunction with other clinical data when making decisions regarding patient management.

References

1 Fankhauser F (1979). Problems related to the design of automatic perimeters. *Doc Ophthalmol.* **47**, 89–138.

2 Flanagan JG, Moss ID, Wild JM, Hudson C, Prokopich L, Whitaker D and O'Neill EC (1993). Evaluation of FASTPAC: a new strategy for estimation with the Humphrey Field Analyser. *Graefe's Arch Clin Exp Ophthalmol.* **231**, 465–469.

3 Glass E, Schaumberger M and Lachenmayr BJ (1995). Simulations for FASTPAC and the standard 4-2 dB full-threshold strategy of the Humphrey Field Analyzer. *Invest Ophthalmol Vis Sci.* **36**, 1847–1854.

4 O'Brien C, Poinoosawmy D, Wu J and Hitchings R (1994). Evaluation of the Humphrey FASTPAC threshold program in glaucoma. *Br J Ophthalmol.* **78**, 516–519.

5 Werner EB and Drance SM (1977). Early visual field disturbances in glaucoma. *Arch Ophthalmol.* **95**, 1173–1175.

6 Caprioli J and Spaeth GL (1985). Static threshold examination of the peripheral nasal visual field in glaucoma. *Arch Ophthalmol.* **103**, 1150–1154.

7 Fankhauser F and Bebié H (1979). Threshold fluctuations, interpolations and spatial resolution in perimetry. In *Proceedings of the Third International Visual Field Symposium*, p. 295–309, Ed. Greve EL. Documenta Ophthalmologica Proceedings Series 19 (The Hague: Dr W Junk Publishers).

8 Heijl A and Drance SM (1983). Changes in differential threshold in patients with glaucoma during prolonged perimetry. *Br J Ophthalmol.* **67**, 512–516.

9 Flammer J, Bebié JH and Keller B (1987). The Octopus glaucoma G1 program. *Glaucoma* **9**, 67–72.

10 Heijl A, Lindgren G, Lindgren A, Olsson J, Asman P, Myers S and Patella M (1991).

Extended empirical statistical package for evaluation of single and multiple fields in glaucoma: Statpac 2. In: *Perimetry Update 1990/91. Proceedings of the IXth International Perimetric Society Meeting*, p. 303–315, Eds: Mills RP and Heijl A (Amsterdam and Milan: Kugler & Ghedini).

11 Asman P and Heijl A (1992). Glaucoma hemifield test. Automated visual field evaluation. *Arch Ophthalmol.* **110**, 812–819.

12 Bebié H, Flammer J and Bebié T (1989). The cumulative defect curve: separation of local and diffuse components of visual field damage. *Graefe's Arch Clin Exp Ophthalmol.* **227**, 9–12.

13 Funkhouser AT, Fankhauser F and Weale RA (1992). Problems related to diffuse versus localized loss in the perimetry of glaucomatous visual fields. *Graefe's Arch Clin Exp Ophthalmol.* **230**, 243–247.

14 Asman P and Heijl A (1992). Weighting according to location in computer-assisted glaucoma visual field analysis. *Acta Ophthalmol (Scand)* **70**, 671–678.

15 Asman P and Olsson J (1995). Physiology of cumulative defect curves; consequences in glaucoma perimetry. *Acta Ophthalmol (Scand)* **73**, 197–201.

16 Flammer J (1986). The concept of visual field indices. *Graefe's Arch Clin Exp Ophthalmol.* **224**, 389–392.

17 Heijl A, Lindgren G and Olsson J (1987). Normal variability of static perimetric threshold values across the central visual field. *Arch Ophthalmol.* **105**, 1544–1549.

18 Flammer J, Drance SM and Zulauf M (1984). Differential light threshold. Short- and long-term fluctuation in patients with glaucoma, normal controls, and patients with suspected glaucoma. *Arch Ophthalmol.* **102**, 704–706.

19 Henson DB and Bryson H (1991). Is the variability in glaucomatous field loss due to poor fixation control? In: *Perimetry Update 1990/91. Proceedings of the IXth International Perimetric Society Meeting*, p. 217–220, Eds: Mills RP and Heijl A (Amsterdam and Milan: Kugler & Ghedini).

20 Heijl A and Krakau CET (1975). An automatic static perimeter, design and pilot study. *Acta Ophthalmol (Scand)* **53**, 293–310.

21 Katz J and Sommer A (1988). Reliability indexes of automated perimetric tests. *Arch Ophthalmol.* **106**, 1252–1254.

22 Sanabria O, Feuer WJ and Anderson DR (1990). Pseudo-loss of fixation in automated perimetry. *Ophthalmology* **98**, 76–78.

23 Katz J, Sommer A and Witt K (1991). Reliability of visual field results over repeated testing. *Ophthalmology* **98**, 70–75.

24 Johnson CA and Nelson-Quigg JM (1993). A prospective three-year study of response properties of normal subjects and patients during automated perimetry. *Ophthalmology* **100**, 269–274.

25 Fankhauser F (1993). Influence of missed catch-trials on the visual field in normal subjects. *Graefe's Arch Clin Exp Ophthalmol.* **231**, 58–59.

26 Bickler-Bluth M, Trick GL, Kolker AE and Cooper DG (1989). Assessing the utility of reliability indices for automated visual fields. *Ophthalmology* **96**, 616–619.

27 Reynolds M, Stewart WC and Sutherland S (1990). Factors that influence the prevalence of positive catch-trials in glaucoma patients. *Graefe's Arch Clin Exp Ophthalmol.* **228**, 338–341.

28 Katz J and Sommer A (1990). Reliability of automated perimetric tests. *Arch Ophthalmol.* **108**, 777–778.

15

Common errors in visual field analysis

Andrew Franklin

Perimetry is not an entirely straightforward process. In addition to the genuine detection of anomalies, a proportion of all field plots show significant errors. Points that in reality have reduced sensitivity may be found to be normal. In this case, the diagnosis of significant pathology may be delayed, with potentially unpleasant consequences to the vision or general health of the patient. Spurious field anomalies found for normal patients may simply waste time and money as tests are repeated, but they can also cause avoidable distress to the patient through continued investigation or referral. The precise way in which errors appear depends on the method used to assess the field of vision.

The Humphrey perimeter is a sophisticated automatic instrument, where the patient responds by pushing a button when a stimulus is seen. The Henson instrument is a semi-automated field screener that, in general, is used with multiple suprathreshold strategies, the patient reporting how many stimuli were seen. The Bjerrum or Tangent screen is an example of kinetic perimetry, in which a target of known size is moved until it is reported by the patient. Where a high degree of participation on the part of the perimetrist is called for (e.g., Bjerrum screen), an experienced practitioner may spot potential errors as they occur and modify the test to eliminate them. In automated strategies (e.g., Humphrey, Octopus) where the patient's are left largely to their own devices, certain types of error are more likely to occur, but strategies are incorporated to assist in their detection.

Operating errors

Operating errors arise as a result of incorrect testing methods and are largely avoidable.

Defocus spreads the image of the target over a wider area, changing the luminance gradient at the edge of the image and in smaller targets depressing the luminance at the centre. The effects appear to be more marked for smaller targets[1] and less marked with increasing eccentricity.[2] Fortunately, for small errors in focus the effect is fairly constant over the central 30° commonly screened. Henson[3] recommends that all errors over 1.00D should be corrected, and this correction should be that employed when reading. Where bifocal or varifocal corrections are worn, some practitioners prefer to check fields without correction, though this is a dubious strategy when subtle relative anomalies are sought. Ready-glazed reading spectacles of similar power, or clip-in lenses such as those described by Henson and Earlam,[4] may be employed, though neither bifocals nor varifocals usually cause problems with screening tests.

It is important that the patient understands the task and that the perimetrist listens carefully to the answers. Poor communication may result in the threshold being set too high or too low, or individual points being assessed incorrectly. When dealing with elderly patients, allowance must be made for reduced hearing and longer reaction times. Lapses of attention may also reduce the apparent sensitivity, as may illness, fatigue or anxiety.

In some older instruments (e.g., Friedmann mark 1), threshold setting may be set according to the age of the patient. While it is known that there is a relationship between age and declining sensitivity, it has also been shown that the variability increases as well, possibly through variations in media transmission. Setting threshold by age is therefore not reliable where subtle anomalies (e.g., as in glaucoma) are being sought. In automatic perimetry, the

age of the patient is used to decide whether the response of the patient is within normal limits. If the age is entered wrongly, this calculation is inappropriate and false positives or negatives may occur.

It is possible to manually override the normal semi-automatic strategies on some instruments (e.g., Henson). While this is a useful feature in experienced hands, it could be abused either inadvertently, through ignorance, or even deliberately to avoid work. The author has heard of an optical assistant who routinely changed the threshold setting if any points were missed, though this was apparently done in the belief that this was helping the patient! When techniques are passed on between members of staff a form of 'Chinese whispers' can result and remarkably whimsical strategies can evolve with the best of intentions. Any practitioner who is liable for the consequences of delegated perimetry should periodically ensure that the work of all members of staff stays within acceptable guidelines, to avoid unpleasant surprises. After all, if you remembered everything you were told about fields, why would you be reading this article?

Physical artefacts

Physical artefacts are genuine scotomata or limitations of the visual field caused by physical features integral to the patient or to the instrument. Examples are the limitation caused by lid ptosis, or the scotoma associated with a retinal blood vessel, but we can also include rim defects caused by refractive corrections and temporary field anomalies associated with ophthalmoscopic after-images and migraine.

Angioscotomata are caused by the veins and arteries of the retina. As they branch out from their central vessels on the optic disc, they overlie receptor cells and can reduce or eliminate their response to a stimulus. Using dynamic perimetry, it is possible to plot these scotomata if a suitably small target is used, provided that the subject has very stable fixation and the perimetrist a very high boredom threshold. It has been claimed by Evans[5] that these represent more than the shadows cast by the blood vessels and that they may widen as a result of digital pressure on the eyes, fright, suspension of expiration, jugular vein compression, cervical sympathetic stimulation and menstruation. It has been suggested that the technique is valuable in the detection of early glaucoma, but it is little used, probably because it is so time-consuming.

With static perimetry, angioscotomata appear as missed points, either singly or, more rarely, as more than one point along a line that corresponds to the path of the vessel on the retina (*Figure 15.1*). These are most likely to be near the blind spot, as the vessels are thicker and more frequent there. Angioscotomata are more likely to occur with small stimuli, and is a common finding with screening instruments such as the Friedmann or Henson.

Rim defects are produced by spectacle frames, or by trial lenses in the lens holders provided on some instruments. In the latter case the defect is concentric, in the former it varies according to the shape of the frame; when smaller frames are fashionable, these artefacts become more common. In general, the defects are dense with sharp edges, though variations in head position and fixation may modify this. They can be reduced by the use of purpose-designed frames with clip-in lenses, such as those described by Henson and Earlam, or more simply in practice by the use of large ready-readers of suitable prescription. If the use of spectacles is unavoidable, the field can be repeated without them to confirm that there is a rim defect.

The eyelids and lashes produce characteristic upper field defects (*Figure 15.2*), usually dense, but often with a gradual edge because of the lashes.

Bushy eyebrows may produce similar anomalies. The defect tends to have a straight or down-curved lower edge, but not invariably. Marked ptosis may produce an alarming field defect, which may mimic either retinal detachment or glaucoma, especially as non-contact tonometers also often read high on such patients. It may be necessary to repeat the field with the lid raised, surgical tape being a useful adjunct in such cases. It is also worth remembering that real life imitates artefact sometimes. Retinal detachments may appear similar to lid defects on occasion (*Figure 15.3*).

When plotting fields wider than the 30° usually screened, the facial features of the patient limit the field. If this is forgotten the results may look ominous, and occasionally patients are referred because they have a large nose and the apparent binasal defect produced causes alarm (*Figure 15.4*).

The nose, cheekbones and brow are all capable of misinterpretation, particularly in elderly patients with deep-set eyes. If in doubt, the head may be re-positioned so that the absolute, rather than the relative, field can be plotted. Even the 30° field may be affected in this way, and many practitioners prefer to screen smaller (24°) areas routinely.

Inappropriate head positions or fixation may exaggerate the effects of both facial features and spectacle rims. If the head is turned temporally, the nose may present a considerable obstacle, even to a central 30° plot. If the head is tilted, the blind spot may be elevated. If the patient does not fixate at the correct point, the blind spot may relocate in any direction (*Figure 15.5*). In automated perimeters, this also tends to elevate both fixation errors and false-positive rates.

Aphakia is of little consequence if the patient has either intraocular lens implant or contact lenses. However, a spectacle correction can magnify the image size by approximately 30 per cent. The field contracts, the blind spot is smaller and nearer to fixation and the

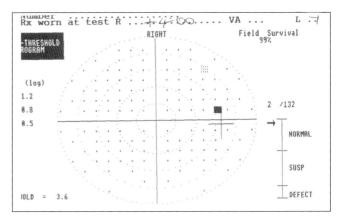

Figure 15.1
Angioscotoma

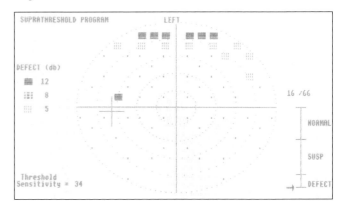

Figure 15.2
Lid defect

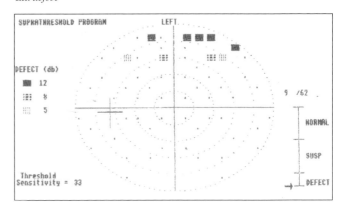

Figure 15.3
Retinal detachment

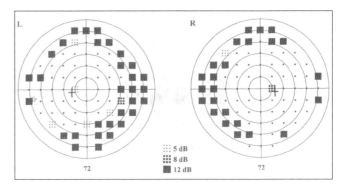

Figure 15.4
Plot of nose, brow and spectacle rim

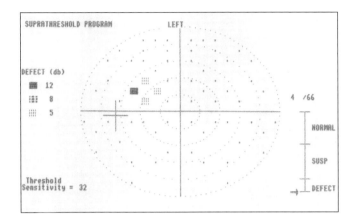

Figure 15.5
*Inappropriate
fixation displaces
the blind spot*

peripheral sensitivity is reduced. The smaller the back vertex distance of the correction the smaller the effect.

Miosis occasioned by the use of pilocarpine reduces the total amount of light that reaches the retina. However, the luminance of both the stimulus and its background are reduced and it is the contrast between them that largely determines whether the target will be seen. Weber's law states that $\Delta I / I$ = constant, where I is the intensity of the background and ΔI is the difference between the stimulus and the background. Unfortunately, this only applies at photopic levels. At lower photopic to mesopic levels the relationship breaks down. Instruments such as the Goldmann, which employ relatively high background luminances, are affected less by pupil size than those instruments, such as the Friedmann and Henson, that employ lower background luminances. It has been reported that the effect of pupil size is greater in the periphery than the centre of the visual field, and that miosis increases the variability of threshold measurement.[6] When tracking the progress of glaucoma, it is important to minimise the effects of variation in pupil size, as they may mimic real progression.

Media opacities act as a filter, and so reduce the level of light that reaches the retina, and scatter the light, which reduces contrast. The latter has the greater effect. Media opacities may produce a generalised depression of sensitivity or more localised effects, depending on their nature and position. When present with glaucoma this can cause considerable difficulties when attempting to plot the progression of visual loss. Large vitreous floaters may also cause localised scotomata. These tend to migrate when fields are repeated, though the rate of change depends upon the mobility of the floater and tends to be higher in the elderly. Automatic perimeters employ programs to filter out generalised depression of sensitivity (e.g., the pattern deviation plot on the Humphrey).

Ophthalmoscopy produces an afterimage that could appear as a localised central scotoma if the fields are plotted too soon afterwards. Suppression fields may also produce central scotomata. While these are normally a feature of binocular vision, they may persist (e.g., in microtropia) in monocular viewing.

Migraine produces a range of visual field disturbances. Many patients find having their eyes examined a stressful process, and migraines are relatively common in optometric practice. A scintillating scotoma may start near fixation and be perceived initially as whirls of light or jagged streaks, or a ripple effect or heat haze. This may develop into a homonymous hemianopia. Micropsia, macropsia, metamorphopsia diplopia, and polyopia are all possible and may all affect the visual field plotted. The usual effect on the visual field, however, seems to be a generalised random loss of sensitivity. In general, the best policy is to plot the field on another day, when it will be found to have normalised, unless there is serious underlying pathology.

Functional artefacts

Patients sometimes fail to respond to stimuli that they can see, or respond to ones that they cannot see, for a variety of reasons. Modern automated perimeters monitor patient reliability in a number of ways. The Humphrey perimeter is used as an example here.

Fixation errors are monitored by projecting approximately 5 per cent of the stimuli within the blind spot, which is located at the beginning of the test (also refer to Chapters 14 and 16). A high rate of fixation losses (over 20 per cent) results in a 'low patient reliability' message on the printout, and may result in underestimation of the field loss in glaucoma patients.[7] However, poor fixation itself is probably not the most common reason for a high fixa-

tion-loss score.[8] The same result may occur if the blind spot is incorrectly located, or if the patient has a high false-positive rate, as in either case responses to targets presumed to be invisible will occur. For this reason, fixation error rates up to 33 per cent are often accepted.[9] When the fixation alarm sounds, yet the patient appears to be fixating correctly to the perimetrist via the telescope or video monitor, the blind spot can be replotted, or the blind-spot check-size reduced or turned off altogether, and fixation monitored by direct observation. Newer Humphrey perimeters have a continuous infrared tracking system, though this may be disrupted by eyelid ptosis or drooping lashes.

Genuine difficulty with fixation may occur with a central scotoma, in which case the central target may be replaced by a diamond of lights, or by a white cross, as in the Henson instrument. Fixation is difficult to monitor in this type of perimeter, and should be encouraged by periodically reminding the patient to 'look at the white spot'. Unreliable fixation tends to make the number of stimuli seen variable. If fixation is consistently off-target (i.e., the patient fixates the wrong point), the blind spot may be plotted out of position.

False-positive errors are detected on the Humphrey by setting it up to project a stimulus, with all the appropriate mechanical noises, but not actually projecting one. If the rate of false-positive responses exceeds 33 per cent a 'low patient reliability' message appears on the printout, though scores below this should also create doubts. 'Trigger-happy' patients may respond to the time delay or to sounds produced by the instrument rather than the stimulus itself, or may respond to the stimulus before it goes off (i.e., within 0.2 seconds), producing two responses to a single stimulus (*Figure* 15.6). They usually produce both a high false-positive rate and a high fixation-error rate, since they respond to targets they cannot see (also see Chapter 14).

The equivalent situation on the Henson is when patients report more stimuli than they can see. This can have a variable effect on the final field plot. The threshold may be set abnormally high, in which case false scotomata may be plotted. Alternatively, genuine field losses may be missed. The only clue the perimetrist is likely to find is that the patient either sets an unfeasibly high threshold (e.g., over 3.8 on the Henson), or counts more targets than are actually presented. In such cases, it may be helpful to ask the patient where the stimuli are seen.

False negatives are found when the perimeter presents suprathreshold stimuli in locations that have already been found to be of a greater sensitivity. High scores may be produced by inattentiveness, fatigue (especially in fields with large relative scotomata), poor fixation or malingering. False negatives produce fields that appear artificially abnormal. False negatives manifest as inconsistent responses in semi-automated multiple-stimulus instruments. For this reason, if a point is missed the first time it is presented this is rarely noted unless the response is repeatable.

Learning and fatigue may affect the outcome of perimetry. It is known that sensitivity tends to increase with experience of the test. In normals, the effect is variable, and often greater in the periphery and in the superior parts of the field. The latter effect may result from the patient learning to keep the upper lid raised.[6] The effects are similar in glaucoma sufferers,[10] but in both cases are largely confined to the first eye examined. As the test proceeds, loss of attention becomes an increasing factor, with similar effects to those of defocus. The effect may be greater when patients exert an excessive accommodative effort. In glaucoma patients, the effects are greatest in areas of abnormality, which makes the plot more variable. Semi-automated strategies may have an advantage here, as the verbal feedback given may help to maintain attention.[11] The Humphrey instrument, because of the order in which it presents its targets, produces characteristic patterns for both (*Figure 15.7*).

With kinetic perimetry, learning produces a progressive widening of the isopter and fatigue gives a narrowing, which can produce spiral fields if adjacent meridians are tested successively.

Hysteria and malingering are examples of 'functional loss' when the visual pathway appears to be structurally normal. The distinction between malingering, in which visual loss is deliberately feigned, and hysteria, in which the effect is involuntary, may be difficult in practice, and is often best left to those with appropriate training in psychology. Using static methods, the results are unpredictable, and may mimic genuine field defects (*Figure 15.8*).[12]

Methods that have no regular sequence of presentations tend to scramble those characteristics that suggest functional loss, and the reliability indices built into these instruments are rarely helpful. False positives are uncommon (malingerers are unlikely to admit to seeing extra stimuli), false negatives are increased, but no more than they would be in severe organic loss, and fixation losses are within normal lim-

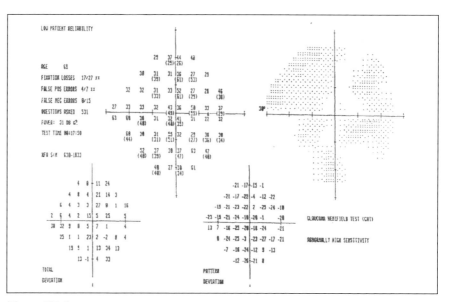

Figure 15.6
Trigger-happy patient. Note the characteristic white scotomata on the greyscale plot. High false-positive and fixation-loss scores and an abnormally high sensitivity message are also typical

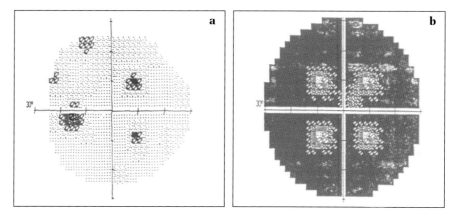

Figure 15.7
(a) Learning and (b) fatigue fields obtained with the Humphrey instrument, showing characteristic 'maple leaf' or 'four leaf clover' patterns in the greyscale plot. Courtesy of A Diddams

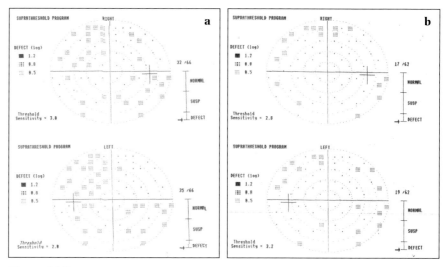

Figure 15.8
Field obtained with a Henson CFA 3000 on a malingering child. The plots were taken two days apart. (a) There is at first sight a possible homonymous quadrantopia. (b) On the later plot, there is a reduction in the more peripheral points, which suggests a rim defect or a tubular field

its. Provided that urgent referral is not indicated by the findings, repetition of the field after a few days may be useful, as functional defects tend to be highly variable. In general, functional losses do not mimic well those produced by organic disease. True hemianopias and nerve fibre bundle defects are rarely functional in origin.

The most typical finding is a 'tubular field', a concentrically reduced field, usually with sharp edges.[13] If the testing distance is changed, but the stimulus is unchanged, then the diameter of the field in millimetres does not change, whereas normally it is the angular subtense that remains the same and the diameter of the field varies with the testing distance for a given target. This is an important characteristic of functional loss.

With the Bjerrum screen, a common finding is the 'fatigue' or spiral field. If the test object is move slowly inwards along successive meridians, initially the target is seen in the normal position, or nearly so. However, as each meridian is examined the target is seen later and later, so the field seems to spiral in, eventually becoming a small tubular field. The second eye typically shows a tubular field (*Figure 15.9*).

If the target is presented centrifugally (i.e., from the centre outwards), the field may spiral outwards. In normal subjects, if the target is presented centrifugally, the isopter plotted is usually larger than that plotted centripetally. In functional loss this may be reversed. One variation of the functional field loss is the 'missing half' loss reported by Keane,[14] which is best seen with confrontation testing. The patient complains of poor vision in one eye. There is a temporal hemianopia in the 'affected' eye, and a full field in the other. Binocularly, the hemianopia reappears.

Kinetic testing is the preferred strategy when functional defects are suspected, and the tangent screen is probably the instrument of choice, as the testing distance may be varied easily. It also lends itself to subterfuge. Hysterics are highly suggestible, and bizarre field plots may be produced as a result of remarks by the perimetrist. If the field is marked by pins or chalk that are in the view of the patient, and the patient is taken to another room for another test, the markings can be moved. A frequent finding is that when the field is retested, the new field plotted will conform to the changed markings. The fixation point may be moved, which sometimes fools the malingerer into an eccentric field.

Hysterics believe in their condition, so tend to co-operate, sometimes ad nauseam. Malingerers often co-operate poorly with any clinical test, and tend to be surly and defensive, and look for excuses to avoid discovery. They may complain that the ophthalmoscope light produces photophobia, refraction gives them a headache, etc.

Harrington and Drake[13] suggest placing a wastepaper basket between the examining room door and the chair (having first ensured that third party cover was up to date). Organically blind patients usually move carefully. If they brush against the obstacle they will move round it slowly or ask for help. Hysterics will often walk around the basket. Malingerers will often walk straight up to the basket and kick it. So the moral to the story is: if the patient kicks the bucket, they were probably malingering.

Finally, a useful way to detect hysterical blindness, in the rare case of a patient reporting total loss of vision, is to look for an oculokinetic nystagmus movement by presenting a moving linear target, such as that created by a Catford drum.

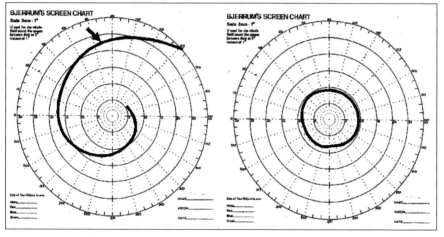

Figure 15.9
Bjerrum plot showing a spiral in one eye and a tubular field in the other

References

1 Sloan LL (1960). Area and luminance of test object as variables in examination of visual field by projection perimetry. *Vis Res.* **1**, 121–138.
2 Atchison DA (1987). Effect of defocus on visual field measurement. *Ophthalmol Physiol Opt.* **7**, 259–265.
3 Henson DB (1993). *Visual Fields*, p. 47 (Oxford: Oxford University Press).
4 Henson DB and Earlam RA (1995). Correcting lens system for perimetry. *Ophthalmol Physiol Opt.* **15**, 387–390.
5 Evans JN (1948). Angioscotometry. In *Modern Trends in Ophthalmology* Ed. Sorsby A (London; Butterworths).

6 Wood JM, Wild JM, Smerdon DL and Cres SJ (1987). The role of intraocular light scatter in the attenuation of perimetric response. *Doc Ophthalmol Proc Ser.* **49**, 51–59.
7 Katz J and Sommer A (1990). Screening for glaucomatous visual field loss. *Ophthalmology* **97**, 1032–1037.
8 Sanabria O, Feuer WJ and Anderson DR (1991). Pseudo-loss of fixation in automated perimetry. *Ophthalmology* **98**, 76–78.
9 Budenz DL (1997). *Atlas of Visual Fields* (Philadelphia: Lippincott–Raven).
10 Wild JM, Dengler-Harles M, Searle AE, O'Neill EC and Crews SJ (1989). The influence of the learning effect on automated perimetry in patients with suspected glaucoma. *Acta Ophthalmol.* **67**, 537–545.
11 Henson DB and Anderson R (1988/89). Thresholds using single and multiple stimulus presentations. In *Perimetry Update, 1988/89* Ed. Heijl A. (Amsterdam: Kugler & Ghedini).
12 Smith TJ and Baker RS (1987). Perimetric findings in functional disorders using automated techniques. *Ophthalmology* **94**, 1562–1566.
13 Harrington DO and Drake MV (1990). *The Visual Fields*, 6th edn (St. Louis: Mosby).
14 Keane JR (1977). Hysterical hemianopia: the 'missing half' field defect. *Arch Ophthalmol.* **97**, 865.

16
Catch trial responses, fixation errors and test intensities

David Henson

Introduction

Catch trial responses, fixation errors and test intensities have each recently been the subject of one or more research papers, the findings of which have important clinical implications for the practitioner. The first two areas are measures of patient reliability. They help the clinician decide whether any changes in the visual field are significant. The sceptics among us may say that they do not need a computer to tell how reliable the patient is, as it is frequently obvious from the moment their chin is placed on the chin rest. However, the trouble with these subjective assessments is that they are rarely documented and when they are it is done in a qualitative way that may not be understood by others. Of course, there is the reverse problem, namely those that believe the computer's estimate of reliability is error free. The final topic deals with establishing the suprathreshold test intensity. This is a continuing problem that, if not carefully done, can easily lead to false-positive referrals.

Catch trials

Most automated perimetric programs include a number of catch trials that are used to estimate the false-positive and false-negative response rates (see *Table 16.1*). Catch trials are intended to give the perimetrist an estimate of patient reliability. Clearly, if the patient makes a high proportion of errors then the results must be viewed with a certain amount of suspicion.

The number of catch trials and catch trial errors are normally included on the printout in the form of a fraction in which the numerator represents the number of errors and the denominator represents the number of trials (*Figure 16.1*).

One of the encouraging findings of modern perimetry is that most patients give very few false-positive or false-negative responses. Katz and Sommer[1] reported that 72 per cent of patients gave no false-positive response errors and 54 per cent no false-negative response errors. An unexpected finding of this study was that the number of false-negative responses increased with the extent of glaucomatous field loss. This is likely to be an artefact produced by the algorithm used to test for false negatives and the increased variability of responses seen in locations with reduced sensitivity.

Table 16.1 False-positive and false-negative catch trials
False-positives catch trials
On occasions the program goes through the motions of presenting a stimulus, but does not actually present one. If the patient presses the button, indicating the non-existent stimulus as seen, this is classified as a false positive.
False-negatives catch trials
After the program has established the threshold at a number of locations, it occasionally goes back and re-presents a stimulus at an intensity that is above the already established threshold. If the patient fails to respond positively to this presentation, this is classified as a false negative.

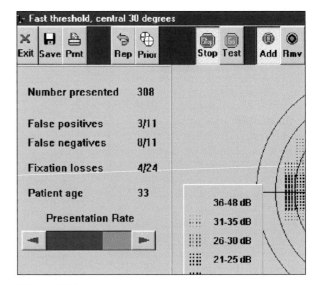

Figure 16.1

Part of the display from a Henson Pro perimeter showing the number of catch trials and number of catch trail errors

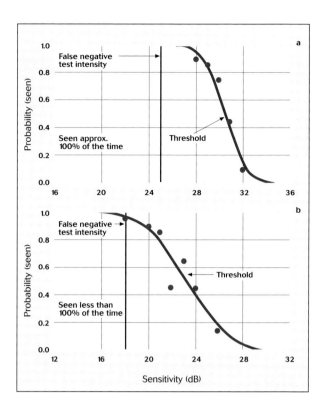

Figure 16.2
Frequency-of-seeing curves from (a) a test location with normal sensitivity and (b) a test location with reduced sensitivity. The vertical line represents the intensity of a false-negative catch trial (5dB above the threshold). Note that in (b) the chance that the patient will miss the catch trial is increased because the frequency-of-seeing curve has a shallow slope

Figure 16.2 illustrates this in more detail. It shows two frequency-of-seeing curves (*Table 16.2*) from a patient with glaucoma. Curve (a) refers to a test location at which there was no glaucomatous damage (the sensitivity being within the normal range), while curve (b) refers to a test location with reduced sensitivity. In the location where the sensitivity is lowered the curve is shallower. This means that the patient's responses are more variable at this test location, a finding noted by several research groups.[2–5]

Importantly, the increased variability only occurs at the damaged location; the patient's responses have not become more variable across the whole visual field, but only at the damaged locations. Most perimeters test for false negatives by presenting stimuli at a fixed intensity above the threshold estimate. Assume that the false-negative test increment is 5dB, represented by the bold vertical line drawn on the two frequency-of-seeing curves. *Figure 16.2* shows that, while the increment for the normal location is well into the approximately 100 per cent seeing level, it is a little short of this at the damaged location, that is there is a greater chance of the patient not seeing the stimulus at the damaged location.

As a visual field defect becomes larger, there are more and more damaged locations with shallow frequency-of-seeing curves and hence an increasing chance of one of these being used for a false-negative trial. We should, therefore, expect the number of false negatives to go up with the extent of loss. It is not the patient who has changed. The patient's responses are always more variable at test locations with a reduced sensitivity (e.g., in the peripheral field). It is simply a matter of there being more locations with a reduced sensitivity. One way forward would be for perimetric routines to test only for false-negative responses at locations where the sensitivity is close to normal.

Surprisingly, no published results give the relationship between the number of errors and reliability. In fact, given that the cut-off for excluding data, through unreliability, is normally set at 20 per cent of

catch trial presentations, the value of these catch trials has been questioned.[1,6]

The situation is further complicated by the recent work of Vingrys and Demirel,[7] who pointed out that the precision of catch trial estimates is very low, especially when the number of errors is relatively high. For a true false-positive rate of 33 per cent (33 per cent chance that the patient will press the button when no stimulus is presented) estimates derived from catch trials could lie anywhere between 7 and 57 per cent. This wide range of values arises simply because of the low number of catch trials conducted within a perimetric examination. While increasing the number of catch trials within the perimetric examination would increase the reliability of the estimate, the number needed for a precise estimate is very high and beyond the practical limit for routine perimetry.

What is the clinical implication of this finding? Well, it rather makes a mockery of the current policy of using a single cut-off value for accepting the visual field test as being 'reliable'. Clinicians need to interpret these findings with some caution and not simply throw out results if they happen to exceed some threshold value. However, they should not automatically assume that when the response error rates are low, the patient is a perfect observer.

In suprathreshold perimetry, including drivers' tests, false-positive trials have an additional function. They help to stop the patient slipping into the habit of automatically responding even when they do not see anything. Patients need to be made aware that some of the trials are blank and that they should wait until they see the stimulus before pressing the button. While there has not been any published research on this topic, it is generally accepted that in suprathreshold perimetry the false-positive response trial rate should be fairly high (approximately 25 per cent). The high rate has the additional advantage of giving a more precise estimate of reliability.

The poor precision of catch trial estimates in threshold perimetry has been the subject of some research by Olsson *et al.*[8] They devised a technique based upon the patient's response times to perimetric stimuli. Unbeknown to the patient, they logged the time it takes for the patient to press the button after every 'seen' stimulus. They established that patients normally respond to a stimulus within a particular response-time window.

This research was extended[9] and showed that false-positive response times follow a very different distribution (*Figure 16.3*). Rather than occur within a relatively narrow response window, false-pos-

---

Table 16.2 Frequency-of-seeing curves

Frequency-of-seeing curves represent how patients respond at given locations in the their visual fields. They are obtained by making a large number of presentations at a series of intensity levels that straddle the threshold. The large numbers of presentations at the test location are often mixed with presentations at other test locations, so that the patients cannot predict where the next presentation will be made. From the fitted curve you can establish, for any particular test intensity, the likelihood that the patient will see the stimulus (probability of being seen).

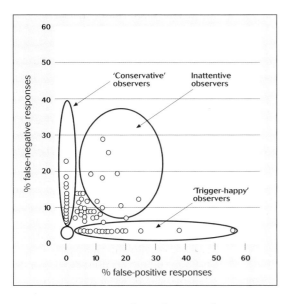

Figure 16.3
Distribution of transformed latencies from responses to false-positive catch trials and suprathreshold stimuli. Courtesy of Paul Artes

itive responses occur with a wide range of response times – some shorter than the normal response window and some longer. The upshot of this is that responses with very short or long latencies are much more likely to be errors than true responses.

Looking at the number of responses that fall outside the normal response window might be a better way to estimate patient reliability than using catch trial responses. There are several reasons for this:

- This method gives a more precise estimate, as it uses all the patient responses rather than just those from catch trials.
- It does not require any false-positive trials (i.e., it shortens the examination time).
- It could lead to strategies that exclude data with abnormal response times, and thereby increase the quality of the visual field data.

This technique of estimating false-positive responses on the basis of response times has been incorporated into the SITA program.[10,11]

Response-time analysis is also incorporated in the multisampling suprathreshold program of the Henson perimeters. In this program the computer stores all the response times and, at the end of the test, calculates which ones fall outside the normal range for that patient. It then deletes any suspect responses and retests them. The power of modern computers means that it can do all this within a single interstimulus interval (i.e., there is no break in the timing between collecting the initial set of data and any retesting).

The way in which a patient responds to perimetric stimuli is dependent upon the instructions given at the onset of the test. If the perimetrist emphasises that patients should not press the button until they are absolutely sure they have seen the stimulus, then the patients will be more 'con-

servative' responders. This highlights an important and little discussed point about automated perimetry – the value of the instructions given to the patient.

A colleague who is involved in the collection of a large amount of visual field data from elderly patients tells the patients not to worry if they occasionally press the button in error, because the machine will come back and check any funny findings. This comment really helps the patients. Elderly patients can become worried and confused after they have made a mistake, so this little extra comment at the onset of the examination can make a vital difference. Interestingly, however, there is no relationship between the variability of responses and the age of the patient. Maybe now is the time to check on how your patients are being instructed.

Accuracy of fixation

Fixation errors are another means by which automated perimetric test strategies derive an estimate of the patients' reliability. During an examination of the visual field, it is important that patients keep looking at the fixation target. If they do not, the results are likely to be more variable.

While at the beginning of the examination the importance of accurate fixation can be emphasised to the patient, it is also important to be able to monitor fixation throughout the examination. If the patient starts to make lots of eye movements (*Figure 16.4*), then appropriate action can be taken (e.g., telling the patient to keep the eye still). The current generation of perimeters incorporates a variety of fixation-monitoring devices.

Fixation monitoring by observation
The simplest technique for monitoring fixation is observation by the perimetrist. This can be direct, as is the case in most tangent-screen instruments, or with the aid of a telescope or camera, as is the case in most bowl perimeters. Such techniques are totally dependent upon the perimetrists judgement and continued vigilance. The fact that the perimetrist needs to be present to make this judgement is an obvious disadvantage, as is the lack of any formal way for the perimetrist to comment on the accuracy of fixation.

The technique is, however, much better than some of the more sophisticated techniques, and has been shown to correlate better with precise measures of fixation than some of the techniques described below.[12]

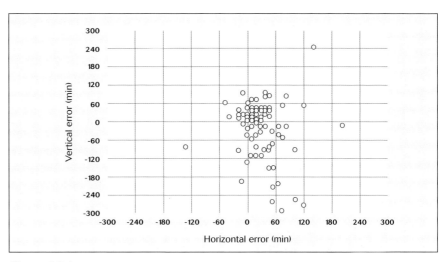

Figure 16.4
Example of the fixation errors made by a patient who, despite being told to keep the eye still, produced a large number of errors. Note how the patient is often several degrees away from the fixation point at the time the stimuli are presented

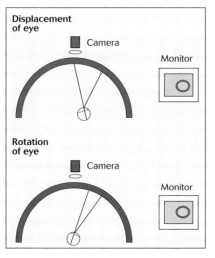

Figure 16.5
The difference between a displacement of the eye (top) with continued fixation and rotation of the eye (bottom) with loss of fixation

Automatic monitoring of fixation

The perimeter itself can incorporate a fixation monitor that either indicates to the perimetrist when fixation is inaccurate or, in the more sophisticated instruments, automatically repeats any measurements made while fixation was inaccurate. This is a very attractive option, as it is both totally objective and does not require the perimetrist to be continually vigilant. However, most fixation monitors cannot differentiate between rotations of the eye, which occur when the patient looks away from the fixation target, and translations of the eye, which occur when the patient fidgets (*Figure 16.5*). A translation of the eye, such as a slight sideways movement of the head, does not necessarily mean that fixation has been lost or that the angular subtense of the perimetric stimuli has been changed by a large amount. A 10mm lateral displacement of the eye only changes the angular subtense of a stimulus at 30° by 1.7%.[13]

In addition to the problems associated with differentiating between rotation and translation, automatic fixation monitors are generally insensitive to small, but significant, fixation errors (1%). Some of the early computerised perimeters had automatic fixation monitors with sensitivity that could be varied. It was soon evident, to anybody who used these instruments, that if the fixation monitor was set to be sensitive to small fixation inaccuracies (≤3%), then the incidence of fixation errors became so great that it was almost impossible to record any data. The solution was to either turn the fixation monitor off or to lower its sensitivity. While the latter approach may have given the perimetrist a sense of well being, in the belief that fix-

ation was being monitored, in reality it was so crude as to be practically worthless.

In the research laboratory we can differentiate between rotations and translations by looking at the relative positions of the first and fourth Purkinje images. However, the problem is that a clear lens, a large pupil and a stack of computer hardware are needed. The first two requirements are rare in the typical population of patients scheduled for perimetry.

Heijl–Krakau technique for sampling fixation.

With this technique stimuli are occasionally presented in the region of the patient's blind spot (also see Chapters 13, 14 and 15). If fixation is accurate during these presentations the stimulus will not be seen. If, on the other hand, fixation is inaccurate then the stimulus is likely to fall outside the blind spot and elicit a response. The results of this technique are usually presented in the form of a fraction in which the numerator represents the number of times the patient reported seeing the blind spot stimulus and the denominator gives the number of times it was presented (*see Figure 16.1*).

As the position of the blind spot varies from one individual to another it is necessary, at the onset of the examination, to have a little routine that establishes the blind spot's location. The accuracy of this routine is important, as errors may later manifest themselves as numerous fixation errors in a patient who has maintained good fixation.

In a study that utilised an accurate eye-position monitor during perimetric testing,[12] a poor correlation was found between the reported accuracy of fixation using the Heijl–Krakau technique and true error. The perimetrist's opinion, derived from watching the patient's eye on a fixation monitor, was found to be a better estimate of fixation accuracy.

Figure 16.6 shows an optic nerve head upon which has been superimposed the standard Goldmann size III target (angle of subtense ≈ 0.5%). As can be seen from *Figure 16.6*, the target is quite small in comparison to the optic disc. The patient's fixation must be quite a long way out for the stimulus to fall outside the blind spot. In other words, this technique is not going to be very sensitive to small fixation errors.

The major advantage of the Heijl–Krakau technique is its simplicity. Its disadvantages are:
- It only samples fixation. Ideally, fixation should be monitored every time a stimulus is presented.
- It increases the examination time.
- It is unlikely to detect small fixation errors.

It appears that, at present, the best fixation monitor is the perimetrist looking at an image of the eye displayed on a monitor. This technique is not only sensitive, but also, via verbal feedback, can result in an improvement in the fixation accuracy for subsequent presentations. There is nothing worse than reaching the end of a long visual field examination and then finding that the patient's eye has been moving about so much that the results cannot be relied upon. It is helpful if the perimetrist's judgement is backed up by an objective measurement, such as the Heijl–Krakau technique. Perimetrists should be encouraged to write on the record chart when they believe that the 'automatic' system has given an erroneous impression of the patient's fixation accuracy.

Selection of the test intensity at the onset of suprathreshold perimetry

Selecting a suitable test intensity is an important part of a suprathreshold test. If the intensity is set too high, there is a danger that early defects will be missed. The test is insensitive to early loss, and produces too many false negatives. On the other hand, if the test intensity is set too low, close to the threshold of the patient, a large number of patients with normal visual fields miss the stimuli. In this case, the test has a low specificity and produces too many false positives. *Figure 16.7* gives the results from two tests carried out on the same patient. In one the test intensity was correctly set, while in the other it was set too close to the threshold, with the result that many missed stimuli were scattered across the visual field:

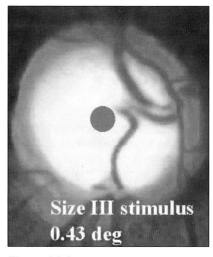

Figure 16.6
Relationship of standard perimetric stimulus to optic disc

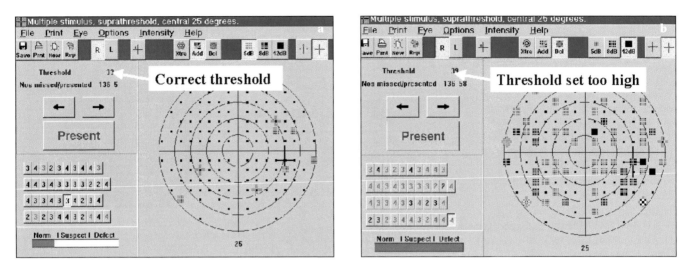

Figure 16.7

Two visual field results from the same eye of the same patient. (a) The first is with the threshold correctly set at 33dB, while (b) the second is with the threshold incorrectly set at 39dB. Setting the threshold too high results in many scattered misses that do not follow any recognisable pattern

- The higher the suprathreshold increment, the higher the specificity and the lower the sensitivity.
- The lower the suprathreshold increment, the lower the specificity and the higher the sensitivity.

Chauhan[14] used a mathematical technique called information theory to look at the effects of varying the test intensity with respect to the patient's threshold. He found that information peaked when the test intensity was 6dB above the patient's threshold and concluded that the ideal suprathreshold increment was 6dB. The majority of instruments currently being used recommend tests at intensities calculated to be between 4 and 6dB above the patient's threshold. At these levels, the number of false positives does not appear to be a great problem.

Currently, two techniques are widely used to set the suprathreshold test intensity, the age-related technique and the threshold-related technique.

Age-related technique

It is well known that the sensitivity of the eye decreases with age, declining at a rate of approximately 0.6dB/decade (*Figure 16.8*). It is, therefore, fairly simple to attach or incorporate a set of tables into the instrument that can be used to calculate the test intensity on the basis of the patient's age. The advantages of this technique are its simplicity and speed. A disadvantage is that within any particular age group not all have the same sensitivity (*Figure 16.8*). This is particularly so in the older age groups, in which factors such as cataracts can affect the threshold. It is the older age groups that most frequently

develop visual field loss and are, therefore, most frequently subjected to visual field examination.

Threshold-related technique

The threshold-related technique, which is currently the most popular, compensates for any variations in sensitivity within a particular age group by deriving an estimate of the patient's sensitivity at the onset of the test. Clearly, there are many ways to derive this estimate.

Three studies have looked at the accuracy of deriving the sensitivity estimate. In the first study, Henson and Anderson[15] looked at the accuracy of an age-related technique and a simple multiple-stimulus staircase technique (stepping the intensity down in 1dB steps until the patient cannot see any of the stimuli). They compared

the estimate of the patient's sensitivity with a 'gold standard' measure and calculated the errors. They found the standard deviation of the errors to be 1.7dB for the age-related technique and 0.8dB for the staircase technique (i.e., the simple staircase technique was found to give much more accurate estimates).

The second study[16] looked at the technique that is currently incorporated in the Humphrey range of perimeters. This uses a full-threshold algorithm at four locations in the visual field and takes the second most sensitive as a basis for calculating the suprathreshold test intensity. The researchers found that the SD of the errors was anywhere between 1.4 and 1.9dB (depending upon whether or not there was a visual field defect). This result is only marginally better than the age-related

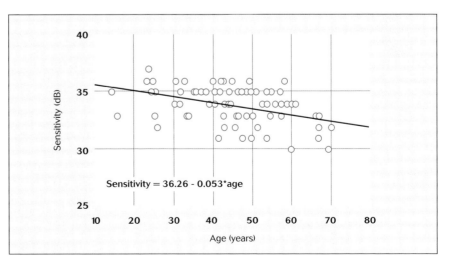

Figure 16.8

Relationship between sensitivity and age. Results collected with the Henson Pro perimeter

technique, and is actually worse in eyes with some pre-existing damage.

The third study attempted to find an alternative and more precise technique for single-stimulus perimetry. The final result, which is known as the HEART algorithm and is incorporated in the Henson range of perimeters, again uses four test locations. It differs from previous techniques by combining the data from all four locations and by using 1dB steps and a fixed number of presentations. The standard deviation of the errors is about 0.7dB. *Figure 16.8* gives threshold-versus-age data collected with the Humphrey and the HEART techniques. It can be seen that there is much less variability with the HEART algorithm. The correlation between the two eyes is also much higher with the HEART algorithm, which indicates it is a more precise technique.

Results from age-related and threshold-related techniques

The age-related approach gives a result that shows how the patient responds in comparison to an age-matched normal. In cases that have an overall loss in the visual field, a large number of stimuli are likely to be missed.

Threshold-related techniques adopt one of two strategies. The first is to allow unlimited adjustment of the sensitivity, so if the threshold estimate is 20dB below the expected value then the stimulus intensity is incremented by 20dB. The second limits the adjustment to some predetermined value (e.g., 4dB). In the above example the stimuli would have been presented at the maximum increment allowed, 4dB above the age-matched normal value.

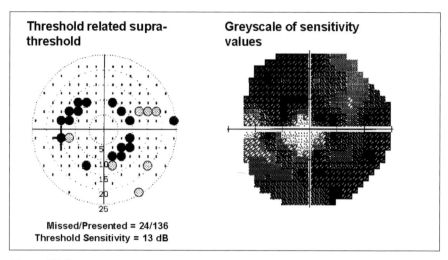

Figure 16.9
Two results from the same eye. The one on the left is from a threshold-related suprathreshold test with unlimited adjustment of the test intensity, while the one on the right is a greyscale result from a full threshold test in which the greyscale represents sensitivity values. Note that the threshold sensitivity of the suprathreshold result was only 13dB. This compared to 31dB in the other eye

With the first technique the visual field chart shows areas of localised loss, while the 'threshold sensitivity' value indicates the overall extent of (diffuse) loss. The importance of this is highlighted in *Figure 16.9*, which shows two results from the same eye.

The field result on the left of *Figure 16.9* is from a threshold-related suprathreshold test, with unlimited adjustment, while the one on the right is the greyscale result from a full-threshold test. The greyscale represents threshold values. The threshold-related result looks far less alarming than the greyscale one because the test intensity was set very high. The patient has advanced glaucomatous loss that affected the test locations used to set the suprathreshold test intensity. Note the threshold setting for this eye was 13dB, 18dB below that for the other eye. The threshold-related result presents localised defects and minimises the effects of diffuse or widespread loss.

The results from a threshold-related suprathreshold test, with limited adjustment (such as the HEART algorithm), would present findings similar to that of the threshold test. While a case can be made for both approaches it is important, especially when using strategies with unlimited adjustment, that clinicians take account of the threshold sensitivity value, otherwise the danger is that they might underestimate the extent of damage.

References

1 Katz J and Sommer A (1988). Reliability indexes of automated perimetric tests. *Arch Ophthalmol.* **106**, 1252–1254.
2 Weber J and Rau S (1992). The properties of perimetric thresholds in normal and glaucomatous eyes. *German J Ophthalmol.* **1**, 79–85.
3 Chauhan B, Tompkins J, LeBlanc R and McCormick T (1993). Characteristics of frequency-of-seeing curves in glaucoma in normal subjects, patients with suspected glaucoma, and patients with glaucoma. *Invest Ophthalmol Vis Sci.* **34**, 3534–3541.
4 Henson DB, Chaudry S, Artes PH, Faragher EB and Ansons A (2000). Response variability in the visual field: comparison of optic neuritis, glaucoma, ocular hypertension and normal eyes. *Invest Ophthalmol Vis Sci.* **41**, 417–421.
5 Henson DB (1998). Variability in the visual field responses of patients with glaucoma. *Optom Today* **July 31**, 40–42.
6 Bickler-Bluth M, Trick GL, Kolker AE and Cooper DG (1989). Assessing the utility of reliability indices for automated visual fields. *Ophthalmology* **96**, 616–619.
7 Vingrys AJ and Demirel S (1998). False-response monitoring during automated perimetry. *Optom Vis Sci.* **75**, 513–517.
8 Olsson J, Bengtsson B, Heijl A and Rootzen H (1997). An improved method to estimate frequency of false positive answers in computerized perimetry. *Acta Ophthalmol.* **75**, 181–183.
9 Artes PH, McLeod D and Henson DB (2002). Response time as a discriminator between true- and false-positive responses in suprathreshold perimetry. *Invest Ophthalmol Vis Sci.* **43**, 129–132.
10 Bengtsson B, Olsson J, Heijl A and Rootzen H (1997). A new generation of algorithms for computerised threshold perimetry, SITA. *Acta Ophthalmol.* **75**, 368–375.
11 Bengtsson B and Heijl A (1998). SITA fast, a new rapid perimetric threshold test. Description of methods and evaluation in patients with manifest and suspect glaucoma. *Acta Ophthalmol.* **76**, 431–437.
12 Henson DB, Evans J, Chauhan BC and Lane C (1996). Influence of fixation accuracy on threshold variability in patients with open angle glaucoma. *Invest Ophthalmol Vis Sci.* **37**, 444–450.
13 Henson DB and Earlam RA (1995). Correcting lens system for perimetry. *Ophthalmic Physiol Opt.* **15**, 59–62.
14 Chauhan B (1987). PhD Thesis, University of Wales.
15 Henson DB and Anderson R (1991). Threshold related suprathreshold field testing: which is the best technique of establishing the threshold? In *Perimetry Update 1990/91*, p. 367–372. Eds Mills RP and Heijl A (Amsterdam: Kugler Publications).
16 Henson DB, Artes PH, Chaudry SJ and Chauhan BC (1999). Suprathreshold perimetry: establishing the test level. In *Perimetry Update 1998/1999*, p. 243–255. Eds Wall M and Wild J (Amsterdam: Kugler Publications).

17
Amsler assessment of visual fields

Andrew Franklin

Disturbance to the central area of the retina can cause both localised loss of vision (scotoma) and distortion of vision (metamorphopsia). After staring at the sun, Thomas Reid, the philosopher, experienced and wrote of the latter in 1764. The painter Edvard Munch made drawings of the effects of his intraocular haemorrhage and used a grid of lines to document them. Lines or grids have appeared in textbooks of ophthalmology for over a century, but the routine use of them to check for maculopathy only occurred after Marc Amsler's charts became widely available in the middle of the 20th century.[1]

The *Amsler Charts Manual*[2] contains a number of charts designed to detect changes in the central visual field (*Figures 17.1* and *17.3*). For the most part, these charts are based on a grid pattern that allows both scotomata (detected by missing or blurred lines) and metamorphopsia (bowed or distorted lines) to be detected,

and the likely position on the retina of the associated pathology to be determined readily. By the strictest definition of the word, metamorphopsia refers to a changing or shimmering distortion. The nature of the distortion can be useful in predicting whether the underlying cause is an active disease process as opposed to a longstanding static lesion. The basic grid is printed in white on a dull black background. It is intended for use at 28–30cm, at which distance each square subtends an angle of 1°, and the whole chart 20°. According to its author, a larger chart would be of no benefit as beyond this central area the detection of anomalies of the grid would be poor.

How the grid relates to the retina

It is worth considering the area covered by the grid in relation to the retina (*Figure 17.2*).

The optic disc is centred fractionally higher than the midpoint, about five squares outside the temporal side of the square, and about 6° (corresponding to 1.5mm) in diameter. The terminology applied to the posterior pole of the eye is somewhat variable in the literature, so the terminology adopted here is that used in Kanski's *Clinical Ophthalmology*, as it is likely to be familiar to most readers. On that basis, the macula refers to an oval area at the posterior pole that contains xanthophil pigment and has more than one layer of ganglion cells.[3] It is about 5mm in diameter, so it subtends an area that corresponds roughly to the area of the grid. The fovea

is a depression of the inner surface of the retina in the centre of the macula. It has a similar size to the optic disc. An avascular zone of variable diameter surrounds the foveola, which is the thinnest part of the retina as it is devoid of ganglion cells. The diameter of the foveola is 0.35mm (i.e., about a square on the Amsler grid). At the centre of the foveola is the umbo, a tiny depression that forms the bright reflex seen through the ophthalmoscope.

Conditions

Originally, it was intended that the chart should be used with the same lighting as for a reading test, but more recently the development of the 'threshold Amsler' test makes some means of reducing illumination desirable. Cataract patients may not be able to see the standard grid and a modified, transilluminated grid has been used to increase contrast. The test should be car-

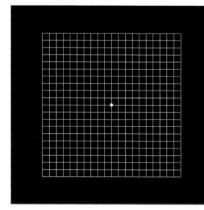

Figure 17.1
Amsler chart 1 is used first

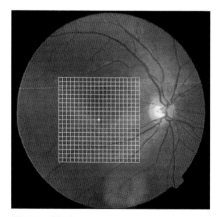

Figure 17.2
Grid superimposed on the retina

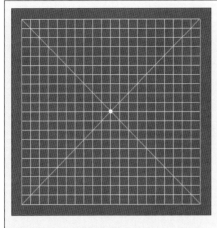

Chart 2 has a diagonal cross incorporated to assist correct fixation in cases with a central scotoma

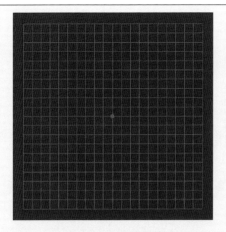

Chart 3 is identical to chart 1, but red on black. It was designed to detect colour scotoma, particularly in optic nerve disease. While it may in some cases assist in the detection of relative scotoma, sensitivity to metamorphopsia is curtailed by the use of a red grid[4]

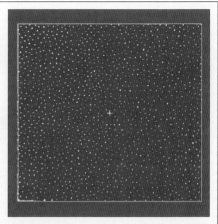

Chart 4 has no lines, only a random pattern of dots. It was intended to differentiate areas of scotoma and metamorphopsia. Since it has no regular forms, this chart does not detect metamorphopsia. However, it is no more sensitive than the standard chart for relative scotoma and defects are more difficult to locate precisely

Charts 5 and 6 allow investigation of metamorphopsia along specific meridians, especially horizontal, to examine difficulties with reading. A version of these charts has been described that is designed to make the self-monitoring of the progression of disease more reliable. It is wider than the Amsler version and has a red diamond positioned so that when the patient is holding the chart at the right distance, it disappears into a blind spot[5]

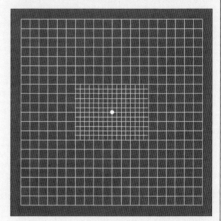

Chart 7 has a more central area with a 0.5° grid for a more precise location within the central area. It can also be used at the far point of high myopes, where the standard grid would subtend too great an angle

Figure 17.3
Amsler charts

ried out with the refractive error of the eye corrected accurately for the testing distance. For a fully presbyopic patient this would, strictly speaking, require a reading addition of +3.25 if used at 30cm, although in optometric practice it is usual to employ the patient's own reading spectacles and trust to depth of focus to do the rest. Mydriasis and ophthalmoscopy should be avoided immediately prior to examination, especially with suspected maculopathy, as persistent after-images may give rise to spurious scotomata. This is more likely in general practice, where Amsler charts are usually employed after ophthalmoscopy has revealed cause for concern.

Method

In all cases Chart 1 is used first (see *Figure 17.1*), and is usually employed alone in general optometric practice.

The test is almost invariably used monocularly, but occasionally binocular tests are performed when investigating suppression scotomata or reading difficulties in maculopathy patients. The series of six questions suggested in the accompanying manual allows a systematic analysis of the results, though slavish adherence to the precise wording is discouraged in the interests of better communication with a variety of patients.

Question 1 establishes that the central fixation spot is visible clearly. A central scotoma is indicated by either the absence of the spot or, in the case of a relative scotoma, blurring of the spot. However, patients with central scotomata may fixate eccentrically, which creates the impression of a paracentral defect.

Question 2 determines whether the outer limits of the square are visible. Chronic glaucoma may cause arcuate defects, which can affect the temporal angles of the grid, or nasal defects that may extend into the grid field. Late-stage glaucoma or retinitis pigmentosa may result in an annular field in which all of the corners may be missing. Toxic amblyopia may cause a scotoma that extends from the optic disc to the fovea. Defects that continue outside the area covered by the grid are referred to as 'exterior' defects.

Question 3 looks for holes or areas of blur within the network, which correspond to absolute or relative scotomata. Either may be caused by organic lesions, such as haemorrhages, exudates or areas of oedema. In addition, they may be functional anomalies. Suppression scotomata generally show up better if both eyes are open, but in microtropia there may be a persistent central defect (Lang's one-sided scotoma) under monocular conditions.[6]

Question 4 investigates the phenomenon of metamorphopsia, which shows up as bowing or distortion of the lines of the grid. Metamorphopsia is associated with changes in macular topography, generally caused by oedema, but not with either ischaemia or haemorrhages alone.[7] It is therefore particularly important as an indicator of macular oedema in both 'wet' age-related macular degeneration (ARMD) and diabetic maculopathy (DM). Where the lines are seen to bow, micropsia (lines converge) or macropsia is often reported. The lines frequently appear to have been crudely penned in and the term 'handdrawn' is descriptive. Foveolar oedema often presents as a distorted central 5° or so in diameter, with micropsia.

Question 5 invites the patient to describe entoptic phenomena, such as movement of lines, vibration, shining, or colours. To quote the manual: 'If this question is systematically asked one is astonished by the frequency of affirmative replies' ... or perhaps not. While such phenomena may be the precursors to more definite defects, the potential for artefacts seems almost limitless, given a sufficiently imaginative patient. Without corroborative evidence from the ophthalmoscope, colour vision test or contrast sensitivity, referral on the basis of such findings is rare, though a note for future reference is in order.

Question 6 seeks to use the grid to measure the angular subtense and position of any anomalies found. In many cases this is done by encouraging the patient to draw the anomalies on a recording chart, which is a reversed (i.e., printed black on white) replica of chart 1 (*Figure 17.4*).

Threshold Amsler grid

The standard (number 1) chart is high contrast (see *Figure 17.1*), and so is chart 4 (see *Figure 17.3*). Even the red chart 3 is the equivalent of a 2/1000 white target. Consequently, relative scotomata are rarely found when the charts are used in normal light conditions. Wall and colleagues suggested reducing the luminance of the target by using cross-polarising filters,[8,9] although similar results should be possible by using a dimmer switch to control the illumination. The increasing use of computers within the consulting room should enable a whole range of grids of different contrasts, colours and line widths to be generated. The luminance is reduced progressively and, just before the target disappears altogether, relative scotomata become readily apparent, usually with a coincident resolution of metamorphopsia (i.e., the lines straighten, but some disappear). Large haemorrhages, dense hard exudates and areas of leakage and any cotton-wool spots that may be present can be monitored in this way. In addition, areas of non-perfusion invisible to ophthalmoscopic examination may be revealed. However, neither the standard nor threshold versions appear to be particularly good at detecting scotomata under 6° in diameter, compared to conventional perimetry.[10] The 'completion phenomenon', by which we perceptually fill small gaps in line stimuli, appears to have some bearing on this.[11]

Indications for use

Any patient with unexplained visual loss should be tested with the Amsler grid, even if no anomalies are detected ophthalmoscopically. Patients who are at risk from choroidal neovascularisation (including ARMD, myopic degeneration) or macular oedema (diabetes, retinal vascular disease) should be tested, as should patients at risk from disruption of the Bruch's membrane photoreceptor or retinal pigment epithelium (RPE) complex.[12]

A number of common systemic and topical drugs have been reported to cause macular anomalies detectable with the Amsler charts (*Table 17.1*).

Any patient with macular disease in one eye should monitor the other eye regularly.

Self-diagnosis by patients

It has become common practice to issue patients who have maculopathy with Amsler grids, usually in the form of the recording sheets, so that they can monitor their own eyes regularly at home. As an alternative, the patient can use a version the size of a credit card,[13] with detailed instructions on the back, which the patient can carry in a wallet.

There are now several websites that offer Amsler-type grids for self-examination.

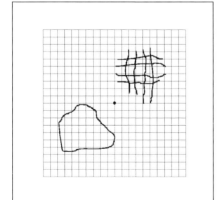

Figure 17.4
Amsler recording chart on which a patient has drawn to indicate metamorphopsia and a relative scotoma

Table 17.1 Drugs that may cause anomalies detectable with the Amsler charts

Medication	*Uses*
Allopurinol	Gout
Beta-blockers (topical)	Glaucoma
Carbonic anhydrase inhibitors	Used as diuretic and in glaucoma
Chloroquine/hydroxychloroquine	Anti-malarials, also used in arthritis
Epinephrine and derivatives (e.g., dopamine)	Parkinson's disease
Hexamethonium	Hypertension
Iodine and iodide compounds	Thyroid dysfunction
Nonsteroidal anti-inflammatory drugs (e.g., naproxen, ibuprofen)	Rheumatoid arthritis
Niacin, niacinamide	Lipid disorders
Quinine	Anti-malarial, anti-spasmodic
Tamoxifen	Breast cancer, infertility

Unfortunately, compliance is an issue[14] and the most common presenting symptom with early maculopathy is blurred vision and distortion with reading, rather than changes on the Amsler chart, even in patients who are supposed to be self-monitoring.

Conclusion

The Amsler grids provide a convenient way to detect and monitor macular and some optic nerve diseases in optometric practice. The system is particularly useful when applied to those patients with diabetic or age-related maculopathies, and those who take certain commonly prescribed systemic drugs.

It is not entirely reliable, and should be regarded as a screening device rather than one that will give definitive answers. Several useful modifications have been made to the original designs, and with the widespread use of computers within the consulting room it is likely that a whole range of grids of various contrasts, colours and designs will become available to the practitioner.

References

1 Marmor MF (2000). A brief history of macular grids: From Thomas Reid to Edvard Munch and Marc Amsler. *Surv Ophthalmol.* **44**(4), 343–353.
2 Amsler M. *The Amsler Charts Manual* (London: Hamblin Instruments Ltd).
3 Kanski JJ (1994). *Clinical Ophthalmology*, p. 382, Third edn (London: Butterworth–Heinmann).
4 Wall M and Sadun AA (1989). *New Methods of Sensory Testing*. (Berlin: Springer).
5 Potter JW and Wild BW (1986). A new self assessment test for age-related macular degeneration patients. *South J Optom.* **4**, 482–486.

6 Eperjesi F and Evans B (1999). Binocular vision, Part II – microtropia. *Optician* **218**(5724), 23.
7 Arrifin A, Hill RD and Leigh O (1992). *Diabetes and Primary Eye Care*, p. 147–151 (Oxford: Blackwell Scientific Publications).
8 Wall M and Sadun AA (1986). Threshold Amsler grid testing. Cross-polarising lenses enhance yield. *Arch Ophthalmol.* **104**(4), 520–523.
9 Wall M and May DR (1987). Threshold Amsler grid testing in maculopathies. *Ophthalmology* **94**(9), 1126–1133.
10 Scuchard RA (1993). Validity and interpretation of Amsler grid reports. *Arch Ophthalmol.* **111**(6), 76–80.
11 Archard OA, Safran AB, Duret FC and Ragama E (1995). Role of the completion

phenomenon in the evaluation of Amsler grid results. *Am J Ophthalmol.* **120**(3), 322–329.
12 Cavallerano AA and Oshinskie LJ (1997). Additional tests of macular function. In *Macular Disorder: An illustrated diagnosis guide*, p. 29–36, Eds Cavallerano AA, Gutner RK and Oshinskie LJ. (Boston: Butterworth–Heinmann).
13 Yannuzzi LA (1982). A modified Amsler grid. A self-assessment test for patients with macular disease. *Ophthalmology* **89**(2), 157–159.
14 Fine AM, Elman MJ, Ebert JE, Prestia PA, Starr JS and Fine SL (1986). Earliest symptoms caused by neovascular membranes in the macular. *Arch Ophthalmol.* **104**(4), 513–514.

Multiple-choice questions, Section 3

There is one correct answer per question. The answers are given at the end of the book.

1 **Fibres from the superior peripheral nasal retina pass through the chiasma:**
   A   Decussating anteriorly.
   B   Decussating posteriorly.
   C   Laterally and inferiorly.
   D   Laterally and superiorly.
   E   Decussating centrally.

2 **In the lateral geniculate nucleus (LGN) corresponding retinal points are arranged:**
   A   In the same layers.
   B   In adjacent layers.
   C   Always in even layers.
   D   Always in odd layers.
   E   Randomly.

3 **What proportion of cells in the visual cortex have directional sensitivity?**
   A   About 30 per cent.
   B   About 50 per cent.
   C   About 70 per cent.
   D   About 80 per cent.
   E   About 95 per cent.

4 **Which of the following are not components of the Circle of Willis?**
   A   The internal carotid arteries.
   B   The anterior communicating arteries.
   C   The anterior cerebral arteries.
   D   The middle cerebral arteries.
   E   The ophthalmic arteries.

5 **If a lesion is affecting one optic tract, which of the following will not be an associated finding?**
   A   A field defect in one eye only.
   B   An ipsilateral relative afferent pupil defect (RAPD).
   C   Congruous homonymous defects.
   D   An acquired colour-vision defect.
   E   A contralateral RAPD.

6 **Which of the following statements is false?**
   A   Homonymous defects are found in visual cortex abnormalities.
   B   Homonymous defects may be found with pupil abnormalities.
   C   Homonymous defects will not be found with optic atrophy.
   D   Homonymous defects are on the opposite side to the lesion.
   E   Homonymous defects can be scotomata.

7 **Incongruous, heteronymous field defects and optic atrophy describe a lesion:**
   A   Near the optic tract.
   B   Near the visual cortex.
   C   Near the chiasma.
   D   Near the optic radiations.
   E   Near one optic nerve.

8 **A centrocaecal field defect is found in one eye. Which of the following is unlikely to be an associated finding?**
   A   RAPD.
   B   Optic atrophy.
   C   Colour-vision defect.
   D   Observable fundus lesion.
   E   Reduced visual acuity.

9 **Incongruous, homonymous field defects and a RAPD describe a lesion:**
   A   Near the optic tract.
   B   Near the visual cortex.
   C   Near the chiasma.
   D   Near the optic radiations.
   E   Near one optic nerve.

10 **Which of the following statements is false?**
   A   Optic nerve defects may arise as a result of radiation therapy in the region.
   B   The majority of optic nerve defects result from demyelinating disease.
   C   The chiasma is more likely to be affected by abnormalities than any other part of the visual pathway.
   D   The vast majority of chiasmal lesions are compressive.
   E   Isolated optic tract lesions are rare.

11 **Which of the following is a characteristic associated with temporal lobe abnormalities?**
   A   Agnosia.
   B   R and L confusion.
   C   Defects in the lower half of the field.
   D   Visual neglect.
   E   Déjà-vu.

12 **Which of the following statements is true?**
   A   Many visual cortex lesions are associated with hormonal abnormalities.
   B   Many visual cortex lesions cause observable optic atrophy.
   C   Most visual cortex lesions are vascular in origin.
   D   Most visual cortex lesions result from space-occupying lesions.
   E   Many visual cortex lesions give rise to colour-vision abnormalities.

13 **The earliest perimetrically detectable sign of glaucomatous visual-field loss is relatively steep depressions of sensitivity in small, paracentral areas of the visual field, most commonly:**
   A   Inferotemporally.
   B   Superonasally.
   C   Inferonasally.
   D   Superotemporally.
   E   Close to the blind spot.

14 Causes of overall depression of the visual field in glaucoma include all of the following except:
- A Media changes.
- B Beta-blocker therapy.
- C Pilocarpine therapy.
- D Incorrect spectacle prescription.
- E Age.

15 Compared to high-tension glaucoma (HTG), visual-field defects in normal-tension glaucoma (NTG) tend to be:
- A Localised, paracentral, inferior depressions that are closer to fixation with steeper gradients.
- B Localised, paracentral superior depressions that are closer to fixation with steeper gradients.
- C Localised, paracentral superior depressions that are closer to fixation with shallower gradients.
- D Localised, paracentral inferior depressions that are closer to fixation with shallower gradients.
- E Localised, paracentral inferior depressions that are away from fixation with shallower gradients.

16 In suprathreshold testing, if the intensity of the stimulus is set too high this results in:
- A Low test-specificity and high sensitivity.
- B Low false-negative response rate and detection of early defects.
- C High false-negative response rate and early defects missed.
- D High test-specificity and low test-sensitivity.
- E High false-positive response rate and early defects missed.

17 The SITA (Swedish interactive thresholding algorithm) strategy has been developed and achieved by including all the following except:
- A Taking more account of prior knowledge of neighbouring test locations.
- B Speeding up the rate of stimulus presentation in patients who respond quickly.
- C Doing away with the need for false-negative catch trials.
- D Analysing the number of responses that fall outside the patient's normal response range.
- E Employing frequency-of-seeing curves to shorten the time required to threshold each point.

18 The Heijl–Krakau technique is:
- A A technique to establish the threshold increment.
- B A new laser-tracking system to monitor fixation.
- C A means of estimating the accuracy of fixation using response times.
- D A means of estimating the accuracy of fixation by presenting stimuli towards the blind spot.
- E A new way to combine false-negative and false-positive responses to monitor fixation losses.

19 High false-positive errors:
- A May indicate an observer who is fatiguing.
- B Give rise to decreased sensitivity estimates in threshold tests.
- C Produce 'white out' on the grey scale in 'trigger-happy' patients.
- D Give rise to a high negative mean deviation.
- E Are produced when the patient fails to respond to a previously seen stimulus.

20 The threshold of the seventh-highest threshold location or 'general height value' is used to calculate:
- A Total deviation.
- B Short-term fluctuation.
- C All global indices.
- D Glaucoma hemifield test estimates.
- E Pattern deviation.

21 'Clover leaf' and 'Mickey mouse' fields are associated with a:
- A 'Button presser'.
- B Fatiguing patient.
- C Low false-negative rate.
- D Low false-positive rate.
- E High false-positive rate.

22 As field loss increases in severity:
- A Both pattern standard deviation (PSD) and corrected PSD (CPSD) return to lower values.
- B Both PSD and CPSD return to higher values.
- C Both PSD and CPSD remain approximately the same.
- D PSD reduces as CPSD increases.
- E PSD increases as CPSD reduces.

23 Corrected PSD:
- A Takes into consideration any intra-test variability, as noted by the short-term frequency fluctuation (SF), and is probably the best measure of variation across the field.
- B Will separate out any localised field defects that may be hidden by generalised depression.
- C Is the overall departure of the average deviation of the visual field result from that expected of a normal field of the same age group.
- D Determines change over time by distinguishing random variation from true change.
- E Detects asymmetry between inferior and superior hemifields.

24 Frequency-doubling perimetry:
- A Is thought to involve the parvocellular (P) pathway.
- B Involves detection of short wavelengths.
- C Involves detection of high-contrast, chromatic stimuli.
- D Is thought to involve the magnocellular (M) pathway.
- E Is dependent on the patient wearing an appropriate refractive correction.

25 The threshold is defined as:
- A $\Delta L/L$.
- B L.
- C $L/\Delta L$.
- D ΔL.
- E $L\Delta L$.

26 Which of the following is false?

A   30dB is a 10,000 times reduction in stimulus luminance relative to the maximum stimulus luminance.

B   0dB represents the maximum stimulus luminance of the perimeter.

C   The decibel scale is a linear scale.

D   A threshold of 36dB on the Henson perimeter is equivalent to a 36dB threshold on the Humphrey field analyser.

E   30dB is equal to 3 log units.

27 Which of the following is true?

A   50 per cent of the stimuli presented with the Fastpac threshold algorithm are presented from below threshold.

B   The 4-2dB threshold algorithm is 50 per cent faster than the SITA standard.

C   The Fastpac threshold algorithm yields lower variability than the 4-2 dB algorithm.

D   The 4-2dB threshold algorithm crosses the threshold once.

E   The 4-2dB threshold algorithm initially monitors two 'seed' points.

28 Using a stimulus separation of 6°, an 8.4° diameter scotoma has a probability of detection of:

A   0 per cent.

B   50 per cent.

C   75 per cent.

D   100 per cent.

E   150 per cent.

29 The 10-2 program of the Humphrey field analyser has a stimulus separation of:

A   2°.

B   4°.

C   6°.

D   8°.

E   10°.

30 The pattern deviation plot is calculated from which percentile of the total deviations?

A   95th.

B   85th.

C   75th.

D   50th.

E   5th.

31 Which of the following is a false statement?

A   A false-positive rate of 25 per cent classes the visual field as unreliable.

B   A high number of false positives decreases the mean defect.

C   In SITA, false negatives are calculated using the patient's reaction time.

D   False positives and negatives can be used to grade the reliability of the visual-field data.

E   Patient reliability is a significant variable in field assessment.

32 Which of the following statements is true of the mean deviation index:

A   It is sensitive to focal loss in the visual field.

B   It is increased in the presence of a cataract.

C   A high positive value indicates diffuse loss in the visual field.

D   A high positive value indicates widespread focal loss in the visual field.

E   It is of little consequence, so not employed in modern screeners.

33 Which of the following statements about the normal visual field is false?

A   The sensitivity of the visual field decreases with age.

B   The hill of vision becomes steeper with increasing age.

C   Peripheral stimulus locations exhibit lower variability than central locations.

D   If a sensitivity value falls within a given confidence interval, it is deemed to be normal.

E   Visual fields are useful indicators of ocular health.

34 In the Glaucoma Hemifield Test, how many sectors is the inferior visual field split into?

A   3

B   5

C   7

D   10

E   18

35 Which of the following statements is false for the Bebié curve analysis?

A   A normal visual field would yield a curve that closely follows the 95th percentile line.

B   The curve gives information regarding the location of any visual-field loss.

C   The curve gives information about focal and diffuse loss in the visual field.

D   Focal loss is indicated by a steepening of the curve.

E   The curve represents a cumulative distribution of a defect.

36 Which of the following is not likely to be the case in a patient who has a hemianopia?

A   The PSD will be high.

B   The mean defect (MD) will be high.

C   The pattern deviation probability plot will show significant probability symbols in either the temporal or nasal visual field respecting the vertical midline.

D   The MD will be low.

E   Fixation may be a problem.

37 Which of the following statements about angioscotomata is true?

A   They are caused by peripapillary nerve fibres.

B   They are only detectable by static perimetry.

C   They are more likely near to the blind spot.

D   They represent evidence of poor fixation by the patient.

E   There are never more than one in any single eye.

38 Which of the following statements concerning head position of the patient during field analysis is true?

A It is of no significance.

B A head tilted nasally exaggerates loss because of the nose.

C Head position is a considerable cause of artefactual field loss within the central 24°.

D A head tilt may result in an apparent relocation of the blind spot.

E Facial features cause absolute as opposed to relative scotomata.

39 Which one of the following field disturbances is unlikely to result from migraine?

A Heteronymous hemianopia.

B Macropsia.

C Metamorphopsia.

D Polyopia.

E Scintillating scotoma.

40 Which one of the following statements concerning the relationship between the stimulus and the background within a field screener is incorrect?

A Weber's law is only applicable at photopic levels.

B Weber's law represents the relationship between the background intensity and the difference between background intensity and stimulus .

C Miosis will affect the results achieved by instruments that employ lower background luminances.

D Weber's law will not be followed in mesopic conditions.

E Miosis will primarily affect the results from the central field.

41 Which of the following is least likely to cause an upper field defect?

A Ptosis.

B Superior retinal detachment.

C Coloboma.

D Eyebrows.

E Glaucoma.

42 High scores of false negatives are not associated with which of the following?

A Glaucoma.

B Malingering.

C Poor fixation.

D Fatigue.

E Inattentiveness.

43 'Trigger-happy' patients on the Humphrey perimeter:

A Have a high false-negative rate.

B Have a high false-positive rate and high fixation-error rate.

C Produce a maple-leaf field.

D Have a high false-negative rate and a high fixation-error rate.

E Have a low fixation-error rate and a high false-negative rate.

44 Which characteristic pattern in the greyscale plot of the Humphrey perimeter is produced by fatigue?

A Tubular field.

B Maple-leaf field;

C Spiral field.

D Altitudinal defect.

E Paracentral scotoma.

45 Ophthalmoscopy may produce after-images that:

A Can be detected with both Amsler and static perimetry.

B Can only be detected with the Amsler grid.

C Can only be detected with static perimetry.

D Affect neither Amsler nor static perimetry.

E Only affect coloured targets.

46 Which one of these statements is false? A tubular field:

A Has the same angular subtense regardless of testing distance.

B Has the same diameter regardless of testing distance.

C Is a characteristic of functional field loss.

D Is a concentrically reduced field.

E May be found in the second eye tested with a spiral field in the first eye tested.

47 Which of the following statements is true? In aphakic patients:

A An intraocular lens (IOL) contracts the visual field.

B A contact lens gives a smaller field than a spectacle lens.

C A spectacle correction magnifies the image size by approximately 30 per cent.

D The blind spot is enlarged with a spectacle correction.

E Peripheral sensitivity increases with a spectacle correction.

48 Which of the following statements is true?

A Defocus has no effect on visual fields.

B Refractive errors over 1.00D should be corrected.

C Defocus results in an artificially high threshold setting.

D Defocus causes increased false positives.

E Defocus has less effect with smaller targets used.

49 What is the approximate percentage of patients who have no false-positive responses to catch trial presentations?

A 30 per cent.

B 40 per cent.

C 50 per cent.

D 60 per cent.

E 70 per cent.

50 The variability in a visual-field test is not dependent on:

A The test location's threshold.

B The test strategy.

C Fixation errors.

D The age of the patient.

E The size of the test stimulus.

51 Which of the following is not a measure of patient reliability?

A   False-positive response errors.

B   False-negative response errors.

C   Fixation losses.

D   The global index mean deviation or mean defect.

E   Patient responses that fall outside the normal response window.

52 Which is the best technique for monitoring fixation?

A   Direct observation by the perimetrist.

B   A built-in eye movement recorder.

C   A built-in eye movement recorder with feedback that excludes results collected while fixation was inaccurate.

D   Blind spot sampling, the Heijl–Krakau technique.

E   Direct observation backed up by objective measurement.

53 A false-positive catch trial response is:

A   When the patient presses the response key to a non-existent stimulus.

B   When the patient fails to respond to a previously seen stimulus.

C   When the patient presses the response key too late.

D   When the patient presses the response key too early.

E   When the patient presses the response key twice.

54 The Heijl–Krakau technique:

A   Uses response times to estimate patient reliability.

B   Is a new technique for establishing the suprathreshold increment for suprathreshold perimetry.

C   Is a means of estimating the accuracy of fixation that involves presentations directed towards the blind spot.

D   Is a new way of integrating false-positive and false-negative responses to catch trials.

E   Is an automatic fixation monitor that uses an eye-movement recorder.

Multiple-choice answers, Section 1

1 **A patient reads all the letters on a logMAR chart down to the 0.1 line and two letters on the line below. Their logMAR score would be:**
   A   0.3
   B   0.12
   C   0.06
   D   0.14
   E   −0.2

The correct answer is C. The letter size on a logMAR chart changes in steps of 0.1 logMAR units per row. As there are five letters on each row, each can be assigned a score of 0.02. If a patient reads all the letters on the 0.1 line and two letters on the line below, the score would be $0.1 − (2 \times 0.02) = 0.06$.

2 **The logMAR equivalent of 6/9 is:**
   A   0.176
   B   0.214
   C   0.182
   D   0.122
   E   0.163

The correct answer is A. A letter on the 6/9 line subtends 7.5 minutes of arc. The minimum angle of resolution (MAR) for such a letter is therefore 1.5 minutes of arc and the logMAR is 0.176.

3 **Visual acuity obtained using a letter chart (90 per cent contrast) can be estimated from the contrast sensitivity function (CSF; see *Figure 1.4*) by examining:**
   A   The intersection of the CSF with the *x*-axis.
   B   The peak of the CSF.
   C   The intersection of the CSF with the *y*-axis.
   D   The intersection between the CSF and a horizontal line passing through 1.11 on the contrast sensitivity scale.
   E   The intersection between the CSF and a horizontal line passing through 0.90 on the contrast sensitivity scale.

The correct answer is D. Visual acuity obtained using a letter chart (90 per cent) can be estimated from the CSF by examining the intersection between the CSF and a horizontal line passing through 1.11 on the contrast sensitivity scale, 1.11 being the contrast sensitivity that corresponds to a contrast of 0.9 (1/0.9). Letters, in fact, contain a range of other spatial frequencies and so the correlation between grating and letter acuity is less than perfect.

4 **The contrast of a sine wave grating (as defined by the Michelson equation) ranges from:**
   A   0 to 10
   B   0 to 1
   C   1 to 100
   D   0 to 100
   E   0 to 1000

The correct answer is B. Michelson contrast is defined as $(L_{max} − L_{min})/(L_{max} + L_{min})$, where L_{max} and L_{min} are the maximum and minimum luminances, respectively. For a uniform field $L_{max} = L_{min}$ and therefore the contrast is 0. The maximum contrast (1) occurs when $L_{min} = 0$.

5 **The Pelli–Robson chart measures:**
   A   Visual acuity at low contrasts.
   B   Contrast sensitivity for one spatial frequency.
   C   A contrast sensitivity function.
   D   Contrast sensitivity for one contrast.
   E   Two points on the contrast sensitivity function.

The correct answer is B. The letters on a Pelli–Robson chart are all the same size, but have decreasing contrast. The chart therefore measures contrast sensitivity for one spatial frequency. In fact, letters contain a range of spatial frequencies and some caution is required when directly equating letters and gratings.

6 **A contrast sensitivity function shows a loss of sensitivity at low spatial frequencies and normal sensitivity at high spatial frequencies. State which of the following is true:**
   A   High-contrast visual activity (VA) and Pelli–Robson contrast sensitivity (CS) will be reduced.
   B   High- and low-contrast VA will be reduced.
   C   High-contrast VA will be reduced, but low-contrast VA will be normal.
   D   High-contrast VA will be reduced, but Pelli–Robson CS will be normal.
   E   High-contrast VA will be normal, but Pelli–Robson CS will be reduced.

The correct answer is E. If a patient has normal contrast sensitivity at high spatial frequencies, high-contrast VA will usually be normal, but Pelli–Robson contrast sensitivity will be reduced. For such a patient, high-contrast VA would overestimate their visual capability.

7 **State which of the following statements is true:**
   A   Cathode ray tube (CRT) monitors are capable of producing 100 per cent contrast.
   B   Eye movements cause raster-scanned screens to appear to flicker.
   C   The luminance of CRT monitors is not high enough to present test-chart stimuli.
   D   CRT monitors do not have adequate resolution to present test-chart stimuli.
   E   CRT monitors cannot display coloured images.

The correct answer is B. Raster-scanned displays can be thought of as a series of horizontal lines that move very rapidly from the top to the bottom of the screen. If the eyes are moved downwards across the screen, the velocity of these lines on the retina is reduced momentarily and a burst of flicker may be perceived. This is particularly apparent when viewing a display from several metres away. For this reason, raster-scanned displays are not ideal for displaying optometric test stimuli.

8 State which of the following is true:
   A Thin-film transistor (TFT) flat panel liquid-crystal displays (LCDs) are raster scanned.
   B TFT flat panel LCDs can only produce low contrast images.
   C TFT flat panel LCDs do not flicker.
   D TFT flat panel LCDs cannot display coloured images.
   E Eye movements cause TFT flat panel LCDs to appear to flicker.

The correct answer is C. Each pixel on a TFT flat panel LCD has its own transistor which holds it at a particular luminance value until the image is changed. Therefore, TFT displays do not need to be refreshed in the same way as raster-scanned displays and so do not flicker.

9 The logMAR equivalent of 6/6 is:
   A 0
   B 1
   C 0.1
   D −1
   E 0.6

The correct answer is A. A 6/6 letter subtends five minutes of arc. To read such a letter the subject must resolve the gaps between the 'limbs' of the letter that subtend one minute of arc. The minimum angle of resolution (or MAR) for such a letter is therefore one minute of arc and the logMAR = 0 ($\log_{10}1$).

10 A patient reads all of the letters on the 0 logMAR row and three letters on the line below. Their logMAR score would be:
   A 3
   B 0.6
   C −0.03
   D 0.06
   E −0.06

The correct answer is E. The letters on a logMAR chart increase in steps of 0.1 logMAR from the bottom to the top of the chart. As there are five letters on each row, each letter can be assigned a value of 0.02. The row below the logMAR 0 row is logMAR −0.1. Therefore, if a patient reads three letters on this row, their logMAR score will be −0.06.

11 A patient has reduced contrast sensitivity (CS) for high spatial frequencies, but normal CS for low spatial frequencies. State which of the following statements is true:
   A High-contrast visual acuity (VA) will be normal and Pelli–Robson CS will be reduced.
   B High-contrast VA will be normal and Pelli–Robson CS will be normal.
   C High-contrast VA will be reduced and Pelli–Robson CS will be reduced.
   D High-contrast VA will be reduced and Pelli–Robson CS will be normal.
   E High-contrast VA will be normal, but the patient will report poor vision.

The correct answer is D. High-contrast VA can be estimated from the high spatial frequency cut-off of the contrast sensitivity function. The Pelli–Robson chart gives a measure of contrast sensitivity at lower spatial frequencies. A patient who has reduced CS for high spatial frequencies, but normal CS for low spatial frequencies will therefore tend to have reduced high-contrast VA and normal Pelli–Robson CS. In these cases, high-contrast VA gives an adequate indication of visual function.

12 Patients with various neurological conditions, such as glaucoma, optic neuritis and multiple sclerosis, sometimes show a reduction in contrast sensitivity to low and intermediate spatial frequencies while maintaining good sensitivity to high spatial frequencies. In these cases, state which of the following statements is false?
   A High-contrast visual acuity (VA) will be normal.
   B Low-contrast VA will be normal.
   C Pelli–Robson contrast sensitivity will be reduced.
   D Low-contrast VA will be reduced.
   E High-contrast VA will be normal, but the patient will report poor vision.

The correct answer is B. Patients who have reduced contrast sensitivity at low and intermediate spatial frequencies, but good sensitivity to high spatial frequencies, will tend to have good high-contrast VA, but reduced low-contrast VA and Pelli–Robson CS. The false statement is therefore 'low-contrast visual acuity will be normal'. High-contrast VA on its own will not give a good indication of visual function for these patients.

13 What is the prevalence of protan colour deficiency in females?
   A 0.01 per cent.
   B 0.03 per cent.
   C 0.04 per cent.
   D 0.10 per cent.
   E 0.30 per cent.

The correct answer is C.

14 Which combination of colour vision tests are recommended to implement CIE colour vision Standard 3?
   A The Ishihara plates and the Farnsworth D15 test.
   B The Ishihara plates and the Holmes–Wright Lantern Type A.
   C The Farnsworth D15 test and the Holmes–Wright Lantern Type A.
   D The Ishihara plates and the Holmes–Wright Lantern Type B.
   E The Farnsworth Munsell 100-hue test and the Holmes–Wright Lantern Type.

The correct answer is A. The draft CIE Standard 3 applies to personnel in low-risk activities in transport services who need to identify pigment colour codes correctly. The required standard is the same as that approved by the UK Home Office for firefighters and also applies to some workers in the electrical and electronics industries. Applicants who fail the Ishihara plates, and who are identified as colour deficient, must be able to pass the Farnsworth D15 test without error. The Ishihara plates is a screening test that is not designed to grade the severity of colour deficiency. The D15 is a well-documented grading test. People with slight colour deficiency pass and people with moderate or severe colour deficiency fail.

15 Which of the following colour combinations are not confused by protanopes?
- A Yellow and red.
- B Purple and grey.
- C Brown and green.
- D Orange and yellow.
- E Green and violet.

The correct answer is C.

16 Which of the following statements is false?
- A Women who are mixed-compound heterozygotes have normal colour vision.
- B Specificity is the percentage of normals correctly identified as normal.
- C Typical monochromats rarely have nystagmus.
- D John Dalton was a deuteranope.
- E Neutral colours are used to classify types of colour deficiency.

The correct answer is C.

17 Which of the following statements is true?
- A The Farnsworth Lantern shows pairs of signal colours.
- B Congenital tritan defects are inherited as an autosomal recessive trait.
- C The majority of fovea cones contain middle wavelength sensitive (green) photopigment.
- D Colours specified within a specific isochromatic zone are confused.

- E Fifty percent of the daughters of females who are heterozygous for X-linked traits are also heterozygous.

The correct answer is E.

18 Which of the following statements concerning the Nagel anomaloscope is untrue?
- A The Nagel anomaloscope is used to grade the severity of colour deficiency.
- B The Nagel anomaloscope is the reference test for diagnosing all different types of colour deficiency.
- C The Nagel anomaloscope is used in clinical trials to ensure that colour-deficient people taking part are representative of the colour-deficient population as a whole.
- D The Nagel anomaloscope is sometimes used as part of a battery of colour vision tests used to select recruits to the UK fireservice.
- E The Nagel anomaloscope presents a Rayleigh match (red + green = yellow).

The correct answer is E. The Nagel anomaloscope is the standard reference test for red–green colour deficiency. Normal and abnormal red–green colour vision can be identified. Protans and deutans are distinguished, and dichromats and anomalous trichromats are distinguished. The Nagel anomaloscope has no facility to identify or categorise tritan (blue) colour deficiency.

Multiple-choice answers, Section 2

1 Which of the following factors does not govern the resolution of the microscope on a slit lamp?
A   Its numerical aperture.
B   The diameter of the objective lens.
C   The diameter of the eyepiece lenses.
D   The working distance.
E   The wavelength of light.

The correct answer is C. The resolution of the microscope on a slit lamp is governed by its numerical aperture, which in turn depends on the:
• diameter of the objective lens (the larger the better);
• working distance (the shorter the better);
• refractive index between the objective lenses and the eye under examination (the greater the better);
• wavelength of light (the shorter the better).
The diameter of the eyepiece lenses has no effect.

2 Which statement on focusing and setting up a slit lamp is false?
A   Both the illumination system and the microscope have a variable focus.
B   The illumination system has a fixed focus while the microscope has adjustable eyepieces.
C   Ideally, the slit lamp should be focused with a focusing rod.
D   When setting the focus of the instruments the magnification of the microscope should be high.
E   Focusing the microscope on the patients' eyelids is inaccurate.

The correct answer is A. The slit lamp consists of two systems that should have a common focal plane that lies in the same plane as the mechanical pivot of the two systems. In most slit lamps this is the centre of the hole of the pivot.

3 Which one of these statements about sclerotic scatter is true?
A   A wide beam should be used.
B   The technique relies on total internal reflection.
C   The slit height should be 8mm.
D   The illumination and observation systems should be set at 90°.
E   Scarred corneal areas do not scatter light and so are difficult to detect.

The correct answer is B. The principle of this technique is total internal reflection. A narrow focused slit of about 1–2mm is directed temporal to the limbal area at an angle of 40–60° to the normal to the patient's corneal apex. The height of the beam should be 4 or 5mm. Scarred or oedematous areas of the cornea scatter light and facilitate their detection.

4 Which of the following statements about specular reflection is true?
A   The corneal endothelium cannot be visualised using this technique.
B   This technique is completely independent of Purkinje images.
C   The corneal endothelium can be viewed by utilising the second Purkinje image.

D   It is essential that the illuminating system and microscope are placed either side of the centre of the eye.
E   It is not possible to view the anterior surface of the lens (orange peel effect) using the technique.

The correct answer is C. The basis of specular reflection is to form an image utilising Purkinje images. With this technique the corneal epithelium (see *Figure 4.4*), anterior and posterior crystalline lens surface can be viewed.

5 Which statement on assessment of the anterior chamber depth is false?
A   Van Herick's method is the technique most commonly used to assess the anterior chamber depth.
B   Van Herick's method is based on forming a section at the limbal/corneal boundary.
C   The ratio between corneal thickness and aqueous space is assessed in van Herick's technique.
D   The ratio between the aqueous space and the corneal thickness is assessed in van Herick's technique.
E   An alternative to the van Herick technique was described by Smith in 1979.

The correct answer is D. The van Herick technique is the method most commonly used to assess the anterior chamber angle. It essentially uses the thickness of the cornea as a ruler to measure the depth of the anterior chamber angle. It is done by forming a section of the cornea just at the limbal/corneal boundary and deciding the ratio of the thickness of the cornea and the optical space between the section and the reflection off the iris.

6 Which of these statements about conic sections is true?
A   This technique is useful for assessing the presence of inflammatory material in the anterior chamber.
B   The technique should be performed in a brightly illuminated room.
C   The area between the reflex of the cornea and the lens should always appear bright.
D   The slit height should be no less than 8mm for this technique.
E   The microscope should always be decoupled when performing this technique.

The correct answer is A. This technique directs a conical beam of light into the eye and is most frequently used by practitioners to assess inflammatory activity in the anterior chamber. A small slit of 3–4mm in height is directed into the eye and should be focused in the anterior chamber. In a coupled instrument the microscope should also focus in this plane.

7 The anterior chamber can only be viewed with a goniolens because:
A   Other instruments cannot focus enough light in this part of the eye.
B   The iris prevents a clear view with any other procedure.
C   The cornea is milky white with other techniques.
D   Scleral limbal overhang and total internal reflection by the cornea prevent a clear view with any other procedure.

E   The critical angle of the cornea is too high.

The correct answer is D. The anatomy of the anterior chamber angle is obscured by opaque scleral tissue, which is often found to occur at the corneal limbus. In the eye, the light rays from the anterior chamber strike the anterior corneal surface at an angle greater than the critical angle, estimated at 46° to 49°, and as such are totally internally reflected.

8   In gonioscopy the critical angle of the cornea is eliminated by:
A   The anaesthetic.
B   Slit-lamp magnification.
C   Light refracted by the steep curved outer surface of the contact lens.
D   The small thumbnail mirror.
E   The tear film.

The correct answer is C. When a goniolens is placed on the eye, the air interface with the anterior cornea is replaced by the lens surface with an index of refraction similar to the index of refraction of the corneal tissue. The critical angle is eliminated because the light is refracted by the steep curved outer surface of the contact lens. Light from the anterior chamber can then be reflected by a mirror into the examiner's eyes (see *Figure 6.2*). This is the basic concept by which indirect goniolenses, used in conjunction with a slit lamp, allow visualisation of the anterior chamber angle.

9   The most important part of the anterior chamber angle is the posterior portion of the trabecular meshwork because:
A   Behind it lies the canal of Schlemm.
B   It can easily be occluded by the iris.
C   It can often fill with blood.
D   It is involved in uveoscleral outflow.
E   It is a site often involved in neoplastic activity.

The correct answer is A. The trabecular meshwork can be arbitrarily divided into anterior and posterior portions. The former runs from Descemet's membrane to the area anterior to Schlemm's canal. This is considered to be the non-filtering portion of the meshwork because it has no contact with Schlemm's canal. The other portion is the filtering portion and overlies the canal. The filtering portion has a grey, translucent appearance. In older or in heavily pigmented eyes, the filtering portion of the trabecular meshwork is often pigmented and darker than the remainder of the meshwork. This helps to identify the portion of the meshwork involved in filtration and in localisation of the canal of Schlemm, which lies internal to the meshwork at this point. In eyes without pigmentation, the filtering portion can be identified by its known location from the scleral spur and Schwalbe's line, as well as by its grey, granular appearance in comparison to the white scleral spur.

10   The Thorpe four-mirror lens has:
A   One mirror angled for the anterior chamber and three for the retina.
B   Does not need any viscous coupling gel.
C   Has four mirrors angled for the anterior chamber.
D   Is useful in children and those with small palpebral apertures.
E   Has to be rotated through 270° for the optimum viewing angle.

The correct answer is C. The Thorpe four-mirror goniolens is designed to provide a view of the angle in each mirror. The mirrors are angled at 62° and show the anterior chamber angle in normal size. This is useful in that the lens has to be rotated only slightly for the complete angle to be observed. This lens is the preferred choice of many practitioners for assessing the integrity of the angle. The mirrors are housed in a large cone, which is easier to manipulate by those practitioners with large fingers and hands who might find the smaller lens types difficult to control once on the eye. It does, however, require an optical coupling gel.

11   Optimum initial magnification and slit beam dimensions are:
A   ×15, 2mm width and 5mm height.
B   ×6, 1mm width and 4mm height.
C   ×10, 3mm width and 5mm height.
D   ×10 to ×15, 3mm width and 5mm height.
E   ×10 to ×15, 2mm width and 2–4mm height.

The correct answer is E. Slit-lamp magnification should be set at approximately ×10 to ×15 and the illuminating slit beam to 2mm width and 2–4mm in height, with the rheostat at a medium setting. If light enters the pupil, pupillary constriction may make the angle appear more open than it is under general lighting conditions. The microscope is positioned straight ahead and the light source is directly in front of the microscope so that neither eye is occluded.

12   Prior to dilation, for what van Herick's grade is gonioscopy recommended:
A   1
B   2
C   3
D   4
E   0

The correct answer is B. If the angle appears narrow with the van Herick procedure (typically grade 2) gonioscopy is recommended. Van Herick grade 2 corresponds to an anterior chamber to corneal thickness ratio of 1 to 4, respectively. This type of angle could result in a closed angle, especially following dilation.

13   Aqueous is secreted at which of the following rates?
A   2ml per minute.
B   2ml per hour.
C   2µl per minute.
D   2µl per hour.
E   20ml per hour.

The correct answer is C. Aqueous is secreted at 2µl per minute. This rate is variable, as should be clear from the very many variables that influence aqueous production listed in Chapter 7 (see *Figure 7.1*).

14   Which of the following is not associated with a rise in intraocular pressure (IOP)?
A   Age.
B   Systemic beta-blockers.
C   Cardiac systole.
D   Blinking.
E   Winter time.

The correct answer is B. There is a link between several groups of systemic drugs and the IOP. A topically introduced beta-blocker is one of the methods employed to manage IOP in glaucoma patients. The situation with systemic beta-blockers is less straightforward, but (among other potential ocular effects such as a reduced tear film) there does appear to be a reduction in IOP if administered in certain doses. All of the other factors listed have been associated with a rise in IOP.

15 Which of the following statements regarding an IOP measurement below the normal range within a population is not true?
A It is not of clinical significance.
B It may result from rhegmatogenous retinal detachment.
C It may result from postoperative choroidal detachment.
D It may be associated with a central retinal vein occlusion (CRVO).
E It may be iatrogenic.

The correct answer is A. A reduction in IOP below the expected level may be indicative of a loss of intraocular substance, possibly through a wound or inadequately healed incision, or possibly through a tear or hole in the retina. A drop in IOP in one eye with any tobacco-dust in the anterior vitreous is a very significant finding that warrants immediate medical attention. It is emphasised that the usual association is between CRVO and elevated IOP and that a reduced IOP is only a very rare occurrence as a result of significant retinal damage subsequent to the complications of an ischaemic CRVO.

16 Which of the following factors does not influence the application of the Imbert–Fick principle to the eye?
A Corneal thickness.
B Surface tension of the tear.
C The direction of the force applied perpendicular to the sphere.
D Corneal flexibility.
E Area of applanation.

The correct answer is C. As long as the force is applied perpendicular to the sphere, then the direction of incidence is obviously irrelevant. The other four factors listed are reasons for possible error when trying to equate the human eye with the hypothetical physical sphere proposed by the law.

17 The area of applanation of a Goldmann tonometer probe at which a reading of IOP is made is:
A $3.06mm^2$.
B Between 3 and $4mm^2$.
C $7.35mm^2$.
D $0.5mm^2$.
E $10mm^2$.

The correct answer is C. The diameter of the area of applanation at which the Imbert–Fick law allows a reading of IOP with the Goldmann tonometer is 3.06mm, which gives an area of $7.35mm^2$.

18 Which of the following statements about non-contact tonometers (NCTs) is true?
A They cannot be calibrated.
B They are never as accurate as contact methods.
C They never cause corneal compromise.
D They cannot be used on scarred corneas.
E They may require many readings to be taken to achieve a consistent result.

The correct answer is E. NCTs take an instantaneous reading of IOP, requiring several readings to be taken to prevent the various factors that cause IOP to fluctuate at any one time giving an inaccurate measurement. All NCTs have some calibration mechanism, although adjustment if an inappropriate setting is indicated is usually a matter for the manufacturer. The compatibility of readings between contact and non-contact methods becomes questionable at higher IOP levels, but much research suggests that NCTs operated correctly compare favourably with the Goldmann. There have been reports of corneal changes induced either because of dust in the air chamber of the NCT or in use on very vulnerable corneas. Conversely, the NCT can usually be operated manually even on corneas that do not offer a good reflecting surface, although obviously in this case the accuracy is questionable.

19 Which statement is correct?
A The optic nerve head receives its blood supply from the anterior ciliary arteries.
B The optic nerve head receives its blood supply from the posterior cerebral artery.
C The optic nerve head receives its blood supply from the ophthalmic artery.
D The optic nerve head only receives its blood supply from the posterior ciliary arteries.
E The central retinal artery provides the majority of blood flow to the optic nerve head.

The correct answer is C. Although the posterior ciliary arteries and the central retinal artery do supply the optic nerve, they are both derived from a common source: the ophthalmic artery. The anterior ciliary arteries, again derived from the ophthalmic artery, supply the anterior segment: the ciliary body and iris. Like most end arteries, the ophthalmic artery has a very thick muscular media that, by way of its rich sympathetic innervation and local biochemical factors, allows it to regulate the eye and orbit's blood supply.

20 Which statement is incorrect?
A Pulsatile ocular blood flow (POBF) is the only non-invasive way to measure blood flow in the eye.
B Colour Doppler ultrasound reveals the velocity of retrobulbar arterial blood.
C Digitalised fluorescein angiography can measure retinal blood flow.
D Blue-field entoscopy allows a subjective measure of retinal blood flow.
E Flowmetry uses the Doppler effect to calculate retinal blood flow.

The correct answer is A. Although POBF is the most accessible method of measuring ocular blood flow for optometrists, numerous instruments are now available for its investigation. Each one has certain disadvantages and advantages. Duplex ultrasonography is regarded as the current 'gold-standard' technique. This uses the Doppler shift in reflected ultrasound to calculate blood velocity and, in skilled hands, allows examination of blood velocity in vessels as small as ciliary arteries. Blood travelling towards the ultrasound probe, usually arterial, is coloured (traditionally) red and blood flowing away, usually venous, is coloured blue. Unfortunately, the cost of such colour Doppler imaging techniques limits them to specialised centres.

21 Which statement is correct?
- A   POBF is predominantly a measure of choroidal blood flow.
- B   POBF measures total uveal blood flow.
- C   POBF detects pulsatile retinal blood flow.
- D   POBF is unaffected by gender.
- E   POBF is a measure of pulsatile flow in the posterior ciliary arteries.

The correct answer is A. The choroidal–ciliary vasculature accounts for 95 per cent of the intraocular circulation, the remainder being retinal. Therefore, the IOP variation associated with each heart beat is taken to originate predominantly from the choroidal blood supply. Mean POBF is higher in females than males, because of the higher average heart rate in females and possible hormonal factors.

22 Which statement is incorrect?
- A   Focal ischaemic-type discs commonly have splinter haemorrhages.
- B   Low blood pressure at night may cause ischaemic damage of the nerve head.
- C   Raised IOP is not the sole cause of glaucoma.
- D   Glaucomatous discs have been classified into four distinct types.
- E   Glaucoma is caused by normal-tension blood pressure.

The correct answer is E. Although many variables have been associated with glaucoma, normal blood pressure has not been found to be a risk factor. The true association of blood pressure and glaucoma has yet to be made clear. Some studies have found a greater prevalence of systemic hypertension in glaucoma, while others have not. A number of studies indicate that low ocular perfusion pressure (the difference between ophthalmic artery blood pressure and IOP) correlates with glaucoma: low perfusion would then cause relative, or periods of, optic nerve ischaemia. Furthermore, some patients have been found to have large nocturnal dips in their blood pressure. This has led many ophthalmologists to switch their patients' blood pressure medication regime away from 'just before bed' to another time, to prevent possible overnight hypoperfusion.

23 Which statement is correct?
- A   Systemic medications do not affect POBF.
- B   A diabetic patient with high POBF definitely has proliferative retinopathy.
- C   A patient with a low POBF definitely has normal tension glaucoma.
- D   Other signs of ocular disease should be sought in a patient with a significantly asymmetric POBF.
- E   Optometrists should refer all patients with low POBF.

The correct answer is D. As in other ocular signs, asymmetry is an important clue to pathology. POBF is a relatively new measure and the exact POBF indices that warrant referral still need to be validated. Obviously, from the nature of the measurement, POBF is affected by the rigidity of the eye's vasculature. It is probably better to regard POBF as a measure of the eye's vascular compliance or 'stretchiness' than a measure of absolute flow.

24 Which statement is correct?
- A   POBF can only be measured when used with a slit lamp.
- B   The ocular blood flow (OBF) system only measures POBF and IOP.
- C   The IOP measured by the OBF system is equal to the pulse amplitude.
- D   The OBF system is influenced less by corneal thickness when measuring IOP.
- E   Fluorescein drops are required to measure the IOP with the OBF system.

The correct answer is D. Pneumotonometers, because of the small area of cornea they use to calculate IOP, have been found to be influenced less by corneal thickness. Many studies have found that Goldmann-type tonometers erroneously underestimate a patient's IOP after photorefractive keratectomy (PRK). This results from the reduction in corneal rigidity because of the thinner than average stroma. The reduction in IOP is related to the extent of ablation; that is, the higher the original myopia, the lower the IOP reading after treatment. Typically, applanation tonometers underestimate post-PRK patients' IOPs by about 2–4 mmHg. Incidentally, if an applanation tonometer is used off-axis, on the non-ablated cornea, the problem can be avoided.

25 A 78D slit-lamp indirect fundus lens has:
- A   Lower magnification and field of view compared to a 125D lens.
- B   Higher magnification and field of view compared to a 125D lens.
- C   Lower magnification and greater field of view compared to a 125D lens.
- D   Higher magnification and smaller field of view compared to a 125D lens.
- E   The same magnification and field of view if held at the same distance from the eye as a 125D lens.

The correct answer is D. The higher the power of a positive fundus viewing lens, the lower its magnification and the higher its field of view compared to a lens of the same aperture, but lower power. Thus the 78D lens is excellent for binocular examination of the disc and macula, whereas the 125D lens is better for rapid screening of the retinal periphery.

26 To visualise more of the peripheral fundus using a slit-lamp indirect lens one must:
- A   Pull the lens further away from the eye.
- B   Tilt the lens away from the incident light beam.
- C   Move the lens in the direction one wants to visualise.
- E   Have the patient look towards the area of interest and move the lens in the opposite direction.

The correct answer is E. The view of the fundus through a high-pulse lens is both laterally reversed and upside down (see *Figure 9.2*). However, the patient must look in the appropriate direction to enable the lesion to be seen. Therefore, to examine the superior periphery, the patient must look up; the view of the fundus will then be reversed and upside down. To extend this view out further the lens can be moved.

27 Headset BIO is the most appropriate technique for:
A Screening in children under the age of five years.
B Optic nerve assessment.
C Stereoscopic examination of a fundal lesion.
D A diabetic patient.
E Patients who cannot be dilated.

The correct answer is A. The magnification produced by head-set BIO is too low for detailed optic nerve assessment and dilation is required for adequate examination. The relative degree of stereopsis is quite low and diabetics require careful high-magnification and stereoscopic evaluation of the fundus in general and the optic nerve and macula in particular. However, the wide field of view with long working distance makes this an ideal technique for the young child.

28 The Hruby lens is particularly appropriate for:
A Use when a patient has difficulty maintaining stable fixation.
B Wide-field examination of the posterior pole.
C High-magnification non-inverted stereoscopic examination of the disc and macula through a non-dilated pupil.
D Locating retinal tears in the far periphery.
E High-magnification non-inverted stereoscopic examination of the disc and macula through a fully dilated pupil.

The correct answer is E. The Hruby lens gives a highly magnified small field view of the fundus with excellent stereopsis. The patient's eye must be very stable so a fixation target is essential and it is important to dilate the pupil.

29 The best examination routine on a patient complaining of recent-onset floaters is pupil dilation followed by:
A Headset BIO examination.
B Examination of the anterior vitreous by direct ophthalmoscopy, followed by headset BIO.
C Slit-lamp examination of the anterior vitreous, followed by headset BIO or slit-lamp BIO, followed by mirror contact lens where appropriate.
E Hruby lens examination of the anterior vitreous followed by retinal examination with the central region of a mirror contact lens.

The correct answer is D. It is mandatory to examine the anterior vitreous with the slit-lamp for tobacco dust in all patients with recent-onset floaters, as a positive finding indicates a retinal tear until proved otherwise. Headset or slit-lamp BIO is then the system of choice to screen the retinal periphery for tears. Any suspicious area should then be examined through the peripheral mirror of a contact lens.

30 The various examination techniques in ascending order of stereopsis are:
A Direct ophthalmoscopy, slit-lamp BIO, headset BIO, Hruby lens, fundus contact lens.
B Slit-lamp BIO, headset BIO, Hruby lens, fundus contact lens, direct ophthalmoscopy.
C Direct ophthalmoscopy, slit-lamp BIO, headset BIO, fundus contact lens, Hruby lens.
D Slit-lamp BIO, direct ophthalmoscopy, headset BIO, Hruby lens, fundus contact lens.

E Direct ophthalmoscopy, headset BIO, slit-lamp BIO, Hruby lens, fundus contact lens.

The correct answer is E. Direct ophthalmoscopy provides no stereopsis. Therefore only A, C or E could be correct. The next lowest is headset BIO, so E must be correct.

31 For the majority of conventional, non-mydriatic fundus cameras, the minimum pupil size must be at least:
A 1mm.
B 2mm.
C 3mm.
D 4mm.
E 5mm.

The correct answer is D. With conventional non-mydriatic cameras, a good image is obtained when a minimum pupil size of 4mm is present. Although the Canon CR6 is reputed to produce an image with a pupil size of 3.7mm, with most non-mydriatic cameras pupil sizes less than 4mm will result in a reduction of image quality and resolution by virtue of reflections and shadows. In addition, with smaller pupil sizes the field of view is reduced, and hence it may often be necessary to carry out pupil dilation when using conventional non-mydriatic cameras.

32 Which of the following statements about digital imaging is false?
A Good-quality images are only obtainable when the light levels are high.
B The light level used to grab the image is relatively low.
C Focusing is performed with the aid of an infrared monitor.
D Marked pupil constriction is reduced, which allows rapid, consecutive images to be taken.
E A large field of view of 45° can be obtained with this application.

The correct answer is A. The introduction of digital imaging has had a significant impact on the assessment of the ocular fundus. Since the image is focused using infrared light, pupillary constriction is minimal, and hence not only do these systems allow consecutive images to be captured rapidly, but also they often produce a large field of view, up to 45°. With this form of imaging, good-quality images can be obtained even with relatively low light levels, as image processing via the computer enhances the final picture.

33 In which pathological condition is the scanning laser ophthalmoscope (SLO) most superior to standard imaging for viewing the fundus?
A Blepharitis.
B Conjunctivitis.
C Iritis.
D Cataract.
E Age-related macular degeneration (ARMD).

The correct answer is D. Although it could be argued that the SLO is superior to standard imaging in each of these conditions, research has shown that it is particularly advantageous in patients with cataract. The SLO produces less light scatter than conventional techniques, and thus produces a more useful image in the presence of crystalline lens opacities.

34 The Panoramic 200 SLO utilises two lasers. Images from the red laser mainly relate to the:
 A Level of the photoreceptors.
 B Inner nuclear layer.
 C Inner plexiform layer.
 D Nerve fibre layer.
 E Level of the choroid and retinal pigment epithelium.

The correct answer is E. The two lasers most commonly used in the Panoramic 200 SLO are red (wavelength 633nm) and green (532nm). A third laser channel that is rarely used is the blue, although this can be used for fluorescein angiography. Images from the red laser relate mainly to structures deep in the retina and/or choroid, namely the retinal pigment epithelium and the choroid, while images from the green laser relate to the more superficial structures of the neuroretina.

35 Which of the following statements about the HRT II is true?
 A Its main function is in the analysis of the retinal nerve fibre layer 15° temporal to the macula.
 B Its main function is in the analysis of the optic nerve head.
 C It can be used in the analysis of macular pathologies such as holes.
 D The resolution of this instrument is poor because of the low number of pixels.
 E The HRT II does not allow accurate quantitative analysis of the optic nerve head.

The correct answer is B. The HRT II is a modified version of its sister SLO, the Heidelberg Retinal Tomograph (HRT), which has been used in hospitals and research laboratories for many years. Its sole function is in the analysis of the optic nerve head. The scanning process produces a high-quality image that is 15° by 15°, and thus limits the field of view. The size of each image gives a high-resolution image of 10 microns per pixel. The optic nerve head is analysed in seven areas: global, temporal, temporal superior, temporal inferior, nasal, nasal superior, and nasal inferior.

36 Retinal laser polarimetry can be used to detect early glaucomatous changes in which retinal area or feature?
 A The optic nerve head.
 B The lamina cribrosa.
 C The retinal nerve fibre layer.
 D The small blood vessels at the optic nerve head.
 E The circle of Zinn.

The correct answer is C. A recent advancement in the assessment of the retina is retinal polarimetry. Here a polarised laser beam of 780nm wavelength utilises the bi-refringency of the retinal nerve fibre layer to analyse the thickness of this layer. Utilising these properties, commercially available instruments are used to detect early changes in the thickness of the retinal nerve fibre layer in glaucoma. At present the commercially available instruments are extremely expensive. However, as costs reduce, their use in routine optometric practice will increase.

Multiple-choice answers, Section 3

1 Fibres from the superior peripheral nasal retina pass through the chiasma:
  A Decussating anteriorly.
  B Decussating posteriorly.
  C Laterally and inferiorly.
  D Laterally and superiorly.
  E Decussating centrally.

The correct answer is B. Fibres from the nasal retina decussate in the chiasma, the superior peripheral fibres in the posterior portion and the inferior fibres in the anterior.

2 In the lateral geniculate nucleus (LGN) corresponding retinal points are arranged:
  A In the same layers.
  B In adjacent layers.
  C Always in even layers.
  D Always in odd layers.
  E Randomly.

The correct answer is B. Corresponding retinal points are arranged in adjacent LGN layers.

3 What proportion of cells in the visual cortex have directional sensitivity?
  A About 30 per cent.
  B About 50 per cent.
  C About 70 per cent.
  D About 80 per cent.
  E About 95 per cent.

The correct answer is C. About 70 per cent of cortical cells have directional sensitivity.

4 Which of the following are not components of the Circle of Willis?
  A The internal carotid arteries.
  B The anterior communicating arteries.
  C The anterior cerebral arteries.
  D The middle cerebral arteries.
  E The ophthalmic arteries.

The correct answer is E. The ophthalmic arteries arise directly from the internal carotid arteries and do not form part of the Circle of Willis.

5 If a lesion is affecting one optic tract, which of the following is likely to be an associated finding?
  A A field defect in one eye only.
  B An ipsilateral relative afferent pupil defect (RAPD).
  C Congruous homonymous defects.
  D An acquired colour-vision defect.
  E A contralateral RAPD.

The correct answer is E. An optic tract lesion will be in both eyes, homonymous but not congruous and, although an acquired colour-vision defect might rarely be an incidental finding, it will not be associated with the lesion. As a greater number of fibres decussate, a contralateral RAPD will be found.

6 Which of the following statements is false?
  A Homonymous defects are found in visual cortex abnormalities.
  B Homonymous defects may be found with pupil abnormalities.
  C Homonymous defects will not be found with optic atrophy.
  D Homonymous defects are on the opposite side to the lesion.
  E Homonymous defects can be scotomata.

The correct answer is C. Optic tract lesions will be homonymous and may result in optic atrophy as the lesion is anterior to the nerve fibre synapse in the LGN.

7 Incongruous, heteronymous field defects and optic atrophy describe a lesion:
  A Near the optic tract.
  B Near the visual cortex.
  C Near the chiasma.
  D Near the optic radiations.
  E Near one optic nerve.

The correct answer is C. A heteronymous defect is produced by a lesion around the chiasma. It may be incongruous and there may be optic atrophy.

8 A centrocaecal field defect is found in one eye. Which of the following is unlikely to be an associated finding?
  A RAPD.
  B Optic atrophy.
  C Colour-vision defect.
  D Observable fundus lesion.
  E Reduced visual acuity.

The correct answer is B. A centrocaecal field defect in one eye is a classic defect associated with optic nerve disease. It is unlikely that an associated fundus abnormality will be seen, although optic atrophy may be present.

9 Incongruous, homonymous field defects and a RAPD describe a lesion:
  A Near the optic tract.
  B Near the visual cortex.
  C Near the chiasma.
  D Near the optic radiations.
  E Near one optic nerve.

The correct answer is A. Homonymous field defects must be post-chiasmal. Incongruous defects with an associated RAPD indicate a lesion in the optic tract (see the answer to question 5).

10 Which of the following statements is false?
  A Optic nerve defects may arise as a result of radiation therapy in the region.
  B The majority of optic nerve defects result from demyelinating disease.
  C The chiasma is more likely to be affected by abnormalities than any other part of the visual pathway.

D The vast majority of chiasmal lesions are compressive.

E Isolated optic tract lesions are rare.

The correct answer is B. Optic nerve defects may be caused by meningiomas (of the sheath or the sphenoid bone), arise as a result of previous radiation therapy in the region, or (less commonly) as a result of intrinsic disease such as demyelination.

11 Which of the following is a characteristic associated with temporal lobe abnormalities?

A Agnosia.

B R and L confusion.

C Defects in the lower half of the field.

D Visual neglect.

E Déjà-vu.

The correct answer is E. Déjà-vu is a neurological deficit associated with temporal lobe disease. All the other options are associated with parietal lobe lesions.

12 Which of the following statements is true?

A Many visual cortex lesions are associated with hormonal abnormalities.

B Many visual cortex lesions cause observable optic atrophy.

C Most visual cortex lesions are vascular in origin.

D Most visual cortex lesions result from space-occupying lesions.

E Many visual cortex lesions give rise to colour-vision abnormalities.

The correct answer is C. Most visual cortex lesions are vascular in origin.

13 The earliest perimetrically detectable sign of glaucomatous visual-field loss is relatively steep depressions of sensitivity in small, paracentral areas of the visual field, most commonly:

A Inferotemporally.

B Superonasally.

C Inferonasally.

D Superotemporally.

E Close to the blind spot.

The correct answer is B. The vulnerability of inferotemporal fibres at the disc (where, for example, notching is commonly seen), means that superonasal defects result.

14 Causes of overall depression of the visual field in glaucoma include all of the following except:

A Media changes.

B Beta-blocker therapy.

C Pilocarpine therapy.

D Incorrect spectacle prescription.

E Age.

The correct answer is B. As pupil size is a factor in field depression, pilocarpine is a therapeutic agent likely to affect the visual field. Beta-blockers will not.

15 Compared to high-tension glaucoma (HTG), visual-field defects in normal-tension glaucoma (NTG) tend to be:

A Localised, paracentral, inferior depressions that are closer to fixation with steeper gradients.

B Localised, paracentral superior depressions that are closer to fixation with steeper gradients.

C Localised, paracentral superior depressions that are closer to fixation with shallower gradients.

D Localised, paracentral inferior depressions that are closer to fixation with shallower gradients.

E Localised, paracentral inferior depressions that are away from fixation with shallower gradients.

The correct answer is B. The proximity to fixation and the steepness of gradient of superior scotomata should alert one to the possibility of NTG.

16 In suprathreshold testing, if the intensity of the stimulus is set too high this results in:

A Low test-specificity and high sensitivity.

B Low false-negative response rate and detection of early defects.

C High false-negative response rate and early defects missed.

D High test-specificity and low test-sensitivity.

E High false-positive response rate and early defects missed.

The correct answer is D. The test will miss patients who show early field loss (low sensitivity), while those who fail the test will have a significant scotoma (high specificity).

17 The SITA (Swedish interactive thresholding algorithm) strategy has been developed and achieved by including all the following except:

A Taking more account of prior knowledge of neighbouring test locations.

B Speeding up the rate of stimulus presentation in patients who respond quickly.

C Doing away with the need for false-negative catch trials.

D Analysing the number of responses that fall outside the patient's normal response range.

E Employing frequency-of-seeing curves to shorten the time required to threshold each point.

The correct answer is C. False negatives are still an important factor in SITA strategy.

18 The Heijl–Krakau technique is:

A A technique to establish the threshold increment.

B A new laser-tracking system to monitor fixation.

C A means of estimating the accuracy of fixation using response times.

D A means of estimating the accuracy of fixation by presenting stimuli towards the blind spot.

E A new way to combine false-negative and false-positive responses to monitor fixation losses.

The correct answer is D. Accurate fixation is essential for reliable field assessment, and use of the blind spot provides one method of monitoring this.

19 High false-positive errors:

A   May indicate an observer who is fatiguing.
B   Give rise to decreased sensitivity estimates in threshold tests.
C   Produce 'white out' on the grey scale in 'trigger-happy' patients.
D   Give rise to a high negative mean deviation.
E   Are produced when the patient fails to respond to a previously seen stimulus.

The correct answer is C. Sadly, when a patient is overeager to give results there may well be a 'white-out' result.

20 The threshold of the seventh-highest threshold location or 'general height value' is used to calculate:

A   Total deviation.
B   Short-term fluctuation.
C   All global indices.
D   Glaucoma hemifield test estimates.
E   Pattern deviation.

The correct answer is E. The pattern deviation is achieved by ranking thresholds in order and the seventh highest is adjusted to zero as a gauge against which other results are measured.

21 'Clover leaf' and 'Mickey mouse' fields are associated with a:

A   'Button presser'.
B   Fatiguing patient.
C   Low false-negative rate.
D   Low false-positive rate.
E   High false-positive rate.

The correct answer is B. These artefact defects are classic evidence of fatigue.

22 As field loss increases in severity:

A   Both pattern standard deviation (PSD) and corrected PSD (CPSD) return to lower values.
B   Both PSD and CPSD return to higher values.
C   Both PSD and CPSD remain approximately the same.
D   PSD reduces as CPSD increases.
E   PSD increases as CPSD reduces.

The correct answer is A. These values are greater for smaller localised field loss and, as loss becomes more significant and the overall field is depressed, the PSDs return to lower values.

23 Corrected PSD:

A   Takes into consideration any intra-test variability, as noted by the short-term frequency fluctuation (SF), and is probably the best measure of variation across the field.
B   Will separate out any localised field defects that may be hidden by generalised depression.
C   Is the overall departure of the average deviation of the visual field result from that expected of a normal field of the same age group.
D   Determines change over time by distinguishing random variation from true change.
E   Detects asymmetry between inferior and superior hemifields.

The correct answer is A. CPSD takes into account any intra-test variability and is the best measure of variation across the field.

24 Frequency-doubling perimetry:

A   Is thought to involve the parvocellular (P) pathway.
B   Involves detection of short wavelengths.
C   Involves detection of high-contrast, chromatic stimuli.
D   Is thought to involve the magnocellular (M) pathway.
E   Is dependent on the patient wearing an appropriate refractive correction.

The correct answer is D. Magnocellular pathways are implicated in processing temporal information.

25 The threshold is defined as:

A $\Delta L/L$.
B   L.
C $L/\Delta L$.
D ΔL.
E $L\Delta L$.

The correct answer is A. Sensitivity is defined as the ratio of the background luminance to the minimum light energy needed to evoke a response.

26 Which of the following is false?

A   30dB is a 10,000 times reduction in stimulus luminance relative to the maximum stimulus luminance.
B   0dB represents the maximum stimulus luminance of the perimeter.
C   The decibel scale is a linear scale.
D   A threshold of 36dB on the Henson perimeter is equivalent to a 36dB threshold on the Humphrey field analyser.
E   30dB is equal to 3 log units.

The correct answer is D. 1dB = 0.1 log units.

27 Which of the following is true?

A   50 per cent of the stimuli presented with the Fastpac threshold algorithm are presented from below threshold.
B   The 4-2dB threshold algorithm is 50 per cent faster than the SITA standard.
C   The Fastpac threshold algorithm yields lower variability than the 4-2 dB algorithm.
D   The 4-2dB threshold algorithm crosses the threshold once.
E   The 4-2dB threshold algorithm initially monitors two 'seed' points.

The correct answer is A. This does, however, yield greater variability in measurement.

28 Using a stimulus separation of 6°, an 8.4° diameter scotoma has a probability of detection of:

A   0 per cent.
B   50 per cent.
C   75 per cent.
D   100 per cent.
E   150 per cent.

The correct answer is D.

29 The 10-2 program of the Humphrey field analyser has a stimulus separation of:
A 2°.
B 4°.
C 6°.
D 8°.
E 10°.

The correct answer is A.

30 The pattern deviation plot is calculated from which percentile of the total deviations?
A 95th.
B 85th.
C 75th.
D 50th.
E 5th.

The correct answer is B.

31 Which of the following is a false statement?
A A false-positive rate of 25 per cent classes the visual field as unreliable.
B A high number of false positives decreases the mean defect.
C In SITA, false negatives are calculated using the patient's reaction time.
D False positives and negatives can be used to grade the reliability of the visual-field data.
E Patient reliability is a significant variable in field assessment.

The correct answer is C. SITA assesses false-positive responses using the patient's reaction times.

32 Which of the following statements is true of the mean deviation index:
A It is sensitive to focal loss in the visual field.
B It is increased in the presence of a cataract.
C A high positive value indicates diffuse loss in the visual field.
D A high positive value indicates widespread focal loss in the visual field.
E It is of little consequence, so not employed in modern screeners.

The correct answer is B. Both the mean defect and the mean deviation index may be elevated.

33 Which of the following statements about the normal visual field is false?
A The sensitivity of the visual field decreases with age.
B The hill of vision becomes steeper with increasing age.
C Peripheral stimulus locations exhibit lower variability than central locations.
D If a sensitivity value falls within a given confidence interval, it is deemed to be normal.
E Visual fields are useful indicators of ocular health.

The correct answer is C. Larger receptive fields in the periphery may enhance the reliability of response.

34 In the Glaucoma Hemifield Test, how many sectors is the inferior visual field split into?
A 3
B 5
C 7
D 10
E 18

The correct answer is B.

35 Which of the following statements is false for the Bebié curve analysis?
A A normal visual field would yield a curve that closely follows the 95th percentile line.
B The curve gives information regarding the location of any visual-field loss.
C The curve gives information about focal and diffuse loss in the visual field.
D Focal loss is indicated by a steepening of the curve.
E The curve represents a cumulative distribution of a defect.

The correct answer is B. It does not yield information about the spatial characteristics of visual-field loss.

36 Which of the following is not likely to be the case in a patient who has a hemianopia?
A The PSD will be high.
B The mean defect (MD) will be high.
C The pattern deviation probability plot will show significant probability symbols in either the temporal or nasal visual field respecting the vertical midline.
D The MD will be low.
E Fixation may be a problem.

The correct answer is D. A positive MD represents a loss of sensitivity. One might expect the MD to be high.

37 Which of the following statements about angioscotomata is true?
A They are caused by peripapillary nerve fibres.
B They are only detectable by static perimetry.
C They are more likely near to the blind spot.
D They represent evidence of poor fixation by the patient.
E There are never more than one in any single eye.

The correct answer is C. Blood vessels are larger near the disc.

38 Which of the following statements concerning head position of the patient during field analysis is true?
A It is of no significance.
B A head tilted nasally exaggerates loss because of the nose.
C Head position is a considerable cause of artefactual field loss within the central 24°.
D A head tilt may result in an apparent relocation of the blind spot.
E Facial features cause absolute as opposed to relative scotomata.

The correct answer is D. If the head is not aligned, then the whole field moves with the retina.

39 Which one of the following field disturbances is unlikely to result from migraine?

A Heteronymous hemianopia.
B Macropsia.
C Metamorphopsia.
D Polyopia.
E Scintillating scotoma.

The correct answer is A. Heteronymous lesions arise from chiasmal problems and not migraine, which gives homonymous loss.

40 Which one of the following statements concerning the relationship between the stimulus and the background within a field screener is incorrect?

A Weber's law is only applicable at photopic levels.
B Weber's law represents the relationship between the background intensity and the difference between background intensity and stimulus .
C Miosis will affect the results achieved by instruments that employ lower background luminances.
D Weber's law will not be followed in mesopic conditions.
E Miosis will primarily affect the results from the central field.

The correct answer is E. Miosis is more likely to affect peripheral field assessment.

41 Which of the following is least likely to cause an upper field defect?

A Ptosis.
B Superior retinal detachment.
C Coloboma.
D Eyebrows.
E Glaucoma.

The correct answer is B. Superior detachment would give an inferior field loss.

42 High scores of false negatives are not associated with which of the following?

A Glaucoma.
B Malingering.
C Poor fixation.
D Fatigue.
E Inattentiveness.

The correct answer is A. Reliable patients, even with glaucoma, should not give high false-negative scores.

43 'Trigger-happy' patients on the Humphrey perimeter:

A Have a high false-negative rate.
B Have a high false-positive rate and high fixation-error rate.
C Produce a maple-leaf field.
D Have a high false-negative rate and a high fixation-error rate.
E Have a low fixation-error rate and a high false-negative rate.

The correct answer is B. 'Trigger-happy' patients produce high false-positive and fixation-error rates.

44 Which characteristic pattern in the greyscale plot of the Humphrey perimeter is produced by fatigue?

A Tubular field.
B Maple-leaf field;
C Spiral field.
D Altitudinal defect.
E Paracentral scotoma.

The correct answer is B. The classic fatigue field has a maple-leaf pattern.

45 Ophthalmoscopy may produce after-images that:

A Can be detected with both Amsler and static perimetry.
B Can only be detected with the Amsler grid.
C Can only be detected with static perimetry.
D Affect neither Amsler nor static perimetry.
E Only affect coloured targets.

The correct answer is A. A localised central scotoma may be produced and may be detected by either method.

46 Which one of these statements is false? A tubular field:

A Has the same angular subtense regardless of testing distance.
B Has the same diameter regardless of testing distance.
C Is a characteristic of functional field loss.
D Is a concentrically reduced field.
E May be found in the second eye tested with a spiral field in the first eye tested.

The correct answer is A. The normal field has the same angular subtense regardless of the testing distance, whereas the tubular field maintains its diameter.

47 Which of the following statements is true? In aphakic patients:

A An intraocular lens (IOL) contracts the visual field.
B A contact lens gives a smaller field than a spectacle lens.
C A spectacle correction magnifies the image size by approximately 30 per cent.
D The blind spot is enlarged with a spectacle correction.
E Peripheral sensitivity increases with a spectacle correction.

The correct answer is C. The image is about 30 per cent larger, but the field contracts, and the blind spot is smaller with a spectacle correction. Peripheral sensitivity is reduced. Neither IOLs nor contact lenses contract the field significantly, so the field is larger than with a spectacle correction.

48 Which of the following statements is true?

A Defocus has no effect on visual fields.
B Refractive errors over 1.00D should be corrected.
C Defocus results in an artificially high threshold setting.
D Defocus causes increased false positives.
E Defocus has less effect with smaller targets used.

The correct answer is B. Refractive errors over 1.00D should be corrected. Defocus may cause the threshold to be set too low, and may increase false negatives, and the effect is worse with smaller targets.

49 What is the approximate percentage of patients who have no false-positive responses to catch trial presentations?

A   30 per cent.
B   40 per cent.
C   50 per cent.
D   60 per cent.
E   70 per cent.

The correct answer is E. These data come from a research project using threshold perimetry. Similar results have been obtained with suprathreshold perimetry.

50 The variability in a visual-field test is not dependent on:

A   The test location's threshold.
B   The test strategy.
C   Fixation errors.
D   The age of the patient.
E   The size of the test stimulus.

The correct answer is D. There is no relationship between variability and age. Research excluded patients with dementia. Threshold variability actually increases as the sensitivity reduces. Variability is dependent upon the test strategy. The threshold of the full test strategy is less variable than the threshold of the fast test strategy. The more fixation errors the patients make, the more variable the results will be. This is not, however, the major cause of variability in the visual field. Variability in threshold measures reduces as the size of the stimulus increases. Larger stimuli are not used for perimetry as it has not been established whether the decrease in variability is accompanied by a reduction in sensitivity.

51 Which of the following is not a measure of patient reliability?

A   False-positive response errors.
B   False-negative response errors.
C   Fixation losses.
D   The global index mean deviation or mean defect.
E   Patient responses that fall outside the normal response window.

The correct answer is D. The global index mean deviation is a measure of the extent of visual-field loss. It is derived from threshold tests and is not a measure of reliability. False-positive response errors are used as a measure of patient reliability. The higher the percentage of false-positive responses to catch trials, the less reliable is the patient. False negatives are again used as a measure of patient reliability. The number of false-negative responses is, however, dependent upon the extent of visual-field loss, being greater in large defects. Fixation losses are higher in less reliable patients. False-positive responses occur with a wider range of response times than true-positive responses. By looking at the distribution of response times, it is possible to obtain an estimate of the patient's reliability.

52 Which is the best technique for monitoring fixation?

A   Direct observation by the perimetrist.
B   A built-in eye movement recorder.
C   A built-in eye movement recorder with feedback that excludes results collected while fixation was inaccurate.

D   Blind spot sampling, the Heijl–Krakau technique.
E   Direct observation backed up by objective measurement.

The correct answer is E. The combination of direct observation with an objective measurement, such as the Heijl–Krakau technique, is currently the best option. Direct observation by the perimetrist is a good technique, but does not give a numerical value. The eye-movement recorders used in perimeters cannot differentiate between a rotation of the eye and a translation of the eye. The latter can result from patients simply realigning themselves and need not include a loss of fixation. Built-in eye-movement recorders are also of relatively low resolution and cannot detect small, but significant, fixation errors. Direct observation backed up by objective measurement only samples fixation and does not monitor it. The size of the blind spot means that it is unlikely to detect small, but significant, fixation errors. Mislocation of the blind spot at the onset of the examination can result in a large number of apparent fixation errors in a patient whose fixation is very good.

53 A false-positive catch trial response is:

A   When the patient presses the response key to a non-existent stimulus.
B   When the patient fails to respond to a previously seen stimulus.
C   When the patient presses the response key too late.
D   When the patient presses the response key too early.
E   When the patient presses the response key twice.

The correct answer is A. A false-positive response is when the patient presses the response key, signalling that they saw the stimulus, when no stimulus was presented. A false-negative response error is when the patient fails to respond to a previously seen stimulus. It occurs more often when variability is high, that is, when the sensitivity is low. When the patient presses the response key too late this, again, is a false-negative response error in that their response would not have been logged, even though they pressed the key. With elderly patients, it is important that they are given plenty of time to press the response key. When the patient presses the response key too early this is a false-positive response if the stimulus was not presented. If a stimulus was presented, it is recorded as a true positive response. Pressing the response key twice normally has no effect upon the data.

54 The Heijl–Krakau technique:

A   Uses response times to estimate patient reliability.
B   Is a new technique for establishing the suprathreshold increment for suprathreshold perimetry.
C   Is a means of estimating the accuracy of fixation that involves presentations directed towards the blind spot.
D   Is a new way of integrating false-positive and false-negative responses to catch trials.
E   Is an automatic fixation monitor that uses an eye-movement recorder.

The correct answer is C. The Heijl–Krakau technique gives an estimate of fixation accuracy. At the onset of the test, the position of the blind spot is established by presenting a series of stimuli in the most likely blind spot locations. The location at which the stimulus is not seen is taken as the blind spot location. Throughout the test, stimuli are occasionally presented at the blind spot location. If they are seen then it is assumed that the eye was not fixating accurately.

Index

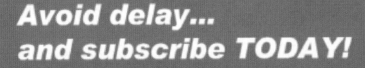